T0361465

Modern Chinese Medicine Food Cures

MODERN CHINESE MEDICINE FOOD CURES

A Personalized Approach to Nutrition

Dr. Melissa Carr

SINGING DRAGON
LONDON AND PHILADELPHIA

Singing Dragon London and Philadelphia

First published in Great Britain in 2025 by Singing Dragon,
an imprint of Jessica Kingsley Publishers
Part of John Murray Press

4

A CIP catalogue record for this title is available from the
British Library and the Library of Congress

ISBN 978 1 80501 319 8
eISBN 978 1 80501 320 4

Printed and bound in the United States by Integrated Books International

Jessica Kingsley Publishers' policy is to use papers that are natural, renewable
and recyclable products and made from wood grown in sustainable
forests. The logging and manufacturing processes are expected to conform
to the environmental regulations of the country of origin.

Singing Dragon
Carmelite House
50 Victoria Embankment
London EC4Y 0DZ

www.singingdragon.com

John Murray Press
Part of Hodder & Stoughton Limited
An Hachette UK Company

The authorised representative in the EEA is Hachette Ireland,
8 Castlecourt Centre, Dublin 15, D15 XTP3, Ireland (email: info@hbgi.ie)

Contents

Recipes

Acknowledgments

Writing a book was a much bigger task than I ever thought it would be. I'm fortunate to have family that supported me while I worked on this during any "free" moments. Thanks to my loving husband, Sean Wilkinson, for going on those annual two-person writers' retreats we created so we could each work on our own books, and for listening to me read out bits of my book, whether you were interested or not. Thanks, Mom and Dad, for letting us staycation at your house for one of our annual week-long "writers' retreats."

Thank you to my colleagues and friends who read through my book or parts of it and gave me helpful feedback! That's you, Dr. Yvonne Farrell (Dr. TCM), Dr. Maryam Mahanian (Dr.TCM), Dr. Jennifer Mackenzie (ND), Sonja Huber (CST), Dr. Kyla Drever (Dr.TCM), Clayton Willoughby (R.Ac.), Dr. Eyal Lebel (Dr.TCM), and Tania Mercuri (CNP, NNCP). Thank you, Chef Luisa Rios, for helping me with recipe ideas and possibly a future book using more of the recipe work we did!

Acknowledgments to my Nana who passed at 103 years old the day before I received notice that this book was accepted for publication. She had a huge love of food, and I think I inherited that.

Preface

Why This Book?

An apple a day keeps the doctor away. But if you're allergic to apples, then eating one would put you in a real pickle. While one person might go bananas over a specific superfood, that might be forbidden fruit for another. It's no piece of cake to find your ideal diet. There are so many books and people out there trying to tell you that their diet is the greatest thing since sliced bread, and that if you just listen to them, your life will be a bowl of cherries. But I'm not spilling the beans when I remind you that you and I are different and it's hard to compare apples to oranges, so perhaps you should take that one-diet-fits-all approach with a grain of salt. In a nutshell, this book is written to help you understand the basics of nutrition, learn the foundations of Traditional Chinese Medicine's[1] approach to health and to food, and provide steps so you can make healthier food choices, so I'll drop the half-baked, cheesy food expressions before I make you nuts.

For many of you, Traditional Chinese Medicine might seem too foreign or too dated to be applicable to your life. How would the philosophers, doctors, and healers from thousands of years ago know anything about addressing the ills of today? TCM is a complete medical system and is well described as a "living tradition." This means it continues to maintain its connection to its history, origins, and foundational principles while it is allowed to grow, expand, and evolve with adjustments made to our clinical practice as new knowledge, lifestyle and environmental changes, innovative technology and resources, and other factors come into play. What I most love about TCM is that it is a modern practice because it has gone through centuries of ongoing questioning and criticizing, trial and error, and a going back and forth between theory and practice—and this continues onward today.

---

[1] Note that, throughout this book, I use the term "Traditional Chinese Medicine" or "TCM" as that's the terminology we commonly use in Canadian schools, but it may also be referred to as "Chinese Medicine," "East Asian Medicine," "Zhong Yi," or other terms.

With TCM's several-thousand-year history of analysing, interpreting, and treating health based on our personal and individual symptoms, medical history, age, sex, emotional and mental state, and even character traits, it employs many treatment methods to improve health status, but food is one of the most foundational. TCM assessed the health value of foods long before Hippocrates' famous quote, "Let food be thy medicine and medicine be thy food."

Food is also my favorite subject matter. Years ago, when I taught English in Japan, my students often asked me why food always ended up being the central conversational topic. For example, I might mention and explain a food idiom like the ones above, and then veer off into conversational practice about their favorite meal. Now, my patients are used to seeing me enter the treatment room still chewing my snack as I ask them about what restaurant they like. Some things never change.

I'm not the only one who loves talking about food—it's a hot topic for many of us. Nutrition and recipe books are abundant, but recommendations are often contradictory—vegan, paleo, low-carb, low-fat, gluten-free, allergen-free, raw, juicing, food combining, intermittent fasting, and so forth. So how do we know what foods are right for us as individuals? And how can we enjoy foods that are tasty and easy to make, while still being healthy?

Every day, I see patients who can benefit from eating the right foods. But they are confused. People have told them that one diet or another is *the* ideal diet, but so many pieces of advice about nutrition are contradictory. They've seen healthcare providers who've only given them their "don't eat" food list. They have cravings for foods that they know aren't healthy, and healthy foods have a reputation (though untrue) for tasting horrible. My patients often feel overwhelmed about choosing, buying, and making foods that are healthy for them—they feel they simply don't have enough time, energy, or money.

If you've felt frustrated about knowing what you should eat, I understand. I've felt that too!

It's also important to remember that food is more than its nutritional value, and it should be enjoyed. It's deeply integrated into many of our cultural and societal rituals, celebrations, and gatherings. Preparing and sharing food can strengthen our relational ties, and most people have at least a few food-related stories to tell. Depending on our upbringing, some foods make an appearance at nearly every meal, while others are reserved for special occasions. The smells and tastes of certain foods can trigger nostalgia and emotions (both good and bad), and secret family recipes can be passed along as valued treasures.

Food is complex, but what we eat doesn't have to be complicated for us to get both nutritional value and enjoyment.

My Take on Food

When I was a kid, my house was the place to go to for all the chips, cookies, and pop you could manage. As long as we could also eat our veggies, we could also have all the treats. I could eat it all because I was known as the kid with the hollow legs. I once had a friend's mom stop me from eating after I had devoured my fourth grilled cheese sandwich and row of Oreo cookies because she was afraid that I was going to make myself sick. As a preteen, going out to celebrate a birthday, I once polished off my 8 oz steak, baked potato, Caesar salad, and dinner roll (or two), and still finished my aunt's filet mignon and my sister's lobster before having my black forest cake for dessert. In university, I came in second in an impromptu pizza-eating contest with (mostly male) friends.

As a kid, I was very active, figure skating four to five days a week, playing on the school volleyball team, and going to weekly dance lessons, so it makes sense that my metabolism was fast. But my food choices, particularly my sweet-tooth food choices, were already impacting how I was feeling.

When I started studying TCM, I was just a week into classes when I went into the student clinic to get a treatment. I figured that I had better see what acupuncture felt like, as I had never had it, and here I was studying it for my future profession! The clinic students asked me what I'd like to have treated. I said, "Nothing really, I'm healthy. I just want to see what it feels like." They asked me how I felt at that moment. I said, "Fine." They continued questioning, and I eventually told them that I had a headache, but that it was no big deal. When they found out that I had headaches nearly daily, they told me that was not okay. I had figured that it was just normal for me. At least I didn't get the debilitating migraines that many of my mom's family got. They decided to treat my headaches anyway. Thankfully! I was given herbs, acupuncture, and dietary changes. My daily muffin and sweetened "fruit" drinks were the first foods to go. I hadn't realized how much sugar were in those. I now rarely get headaches. But I am reminded to watch my sugar intake when I overdo it because that will trigger a headache, and now that I know the bliss of a clear head, I don't want to go down that road again.

It was since then that I've recognized that I can't just eat anything and everything that's put in front of me. At least not in the quantities that I used to eat them. But I'm also generally opposed to restrictive diets (though I'll cover a few for specific reasons in this book). I think that most people have a pretty good idea about what foods are generally not healthy, so I'd rather focus on the what-you-can-eat list. And that list will vary from person to person and perhaps change over time for one person depending on their age, health condition, or even the season.

Tips for Using This Book

This book is designed as a reference for TCM practitioners, other healthcare providers, and those just interested in learning more about making healthy food choices for themselves and ones they care for.

I know many may flip past the introduction, past the basics about TCM, and past the foundations of nutrition, delving instead into what seems like the meat (or chickpea stew or big salad) of the book. You might choose to start by checking out the foods by symptom or disease or trying to figure out which element you are. If you have already studied TCM or grew up with its principles, absolutely, skip the TCM intro chapter. If you've studied nutrition, flip past the fundamentals of nutrition chapter. However, I encourage you to read it through from the start if all this is relatively new to you.

Imagine trying to read a Spanish novel without learning some Spanish first. It'd be tough, perhaps impossible, and you'd likely give up soon enough. The starting chapters in this book are designed to help you understand the reasons for the food recommendations, and to help you figure out for yourself what foods are most likely to benefit you.

- If you want to learn more about TCM and its approach to food, start with Chapter 1: *Basics of TCM* and Chapter 2: *How to Classify Foods Using TCM.*
- For general information about nutrition—calories, macronutrients, and micronutrients—read Chapter 3: *Foundations of Nutrition.*
- If you have a specific health issue you want to address, go to Chapter 4: *Nutrition Tips for Common Symptoms and Illnesses.*
- If you just want to dive right in with food choices right for you, go to Chapter 5: *Five Elements Quiz—What Am I?* to find out what TCM pattern you fit under so that you can make your best food choices. You can then head to Chapter 6: *Foods by Element* to the TCM element category (or categories) that best suit you.
- Chapter 7: *Modern Food* covers some of the pluses and minuses of the growing, processing, preserving, and marketing of our food.
- Take a read through Chapter 8: *Food Allergies, Sensitivities, and Intolerances* to learn about some of the challenges and ways to work around or through reactions to foods.
- Don't get too excited about Chapter 9: *Common Diets and Cleanses* because...well, you'll see.
- But do check out Chapter 10: *Basic Healthy Eating Tips* for some simple things you can do to get the most out of your food, including actual enjoyment of healthy meals!

Consider keeping a food diary for one to two weeks (included at the back of this book) to sort out if some foods feel particularly good or not, and to get a clearer sense of what you're actually eating.

When I was a nutrition instructor, my students would sometimes ask me what they needed to know for the test. While I would have loved for them to hang off my every word (as if!), I would tell them to pay attention to the things I repeated because those were more important bits of information. In this book, there is a lot of repetition for key elements because repetition is one of the ways we learn best.

CHAPTER 1

Basics of TCM

Welcome to the World of TCM

To understand how TCM approaches nutrition, it's essential to know at least the basics, so here's your crash course. TCM has been around for 2000–5000 years, depending on which source you use and how you identify the beginnings of this medicine. History was never my forte, but for a comparison of how old that is, the wheel was invented about 5500 years ago, the alphabet was conceived about 3700 years ago, iron began to be widely used to make tools and weapons about 3000 years ago, and paper was created less than 2000 years ago. It was with the creation of paper that TCM could be more regularly documented.

TCM's beginnings were largely rooted in Daoist (also spelled Taoist) philosophies. The study of nature was key to understanding how our bodies work. TCM is a holistic medicine that considers the whole person, including the body, mind, and spirit as interrelated and inseparable. It also recognizes that our external environment plays an essential role in how our own health manifests.

The wording used in TCM can sound both familiar and foreign, such as when a TCM practitioner diagnoses you as having "Heart Fire," but your main symptom is insomnia, not heartburn. Or perhaps you were told you have "Wind in the Channels," not because you have gas but because you have a tremor. You may also be told you have something long-winded like "Liver Qi stagnation attacking the Spleen causing Spleen Qi deficiency and Dampness." But your liver enzymes were tested recently and are fine, no medical doctor has ever even mentioned your spleen, and you are not sweaty.

If all this is starting to sound confusing or difficult to you, you're not alone. When I was a TCM student, I spent a chunk of my first weeks in school confused and wondering if I had made a mistake. I just couldn't reconcile what I already knew about health with what I was being taught in TCM school. I had to allow myself to approach the lessons with a beginner's mind, opening it up to new concepts, language, and philosophies without judgment. Only after the completion of my TCM foundations courses could I then think in my new "TCM language" and start to re-incorporate the health concepts and information I had previously learned in university, finding ways to combine the best of both worlds.

My plan for you is to speed up that process considerably because if you're studying to be a TCM practitioner, you have other teachers. If you don't want to become a TCM professional, but simply want to apply the basics so you can make healthy food choices for you and your family, the nitty-gritty is enough to get you started.

The concepts can get complex, but they don't need to be confusing. English is said to be one of the most difficult languages to learn, but if you grew up with English as a first language, Japanese or Swahili or Portuguese can seem much harder to learn from scratch. But once you become proficient in that new tongue, you won't have to translate everything in your head, as you'll simply think in that language. The same can be said of learning about "TCM language" as I introduce some new concepts.

A common way of managing the fact that many of the TCM terms are recognizable words, but that they have different meanings than our everyday current definitions and use, is to capitalize the TCM terms. Thus, we write Liver, Wood, Blood, Phlegm, Cold, and so forth, when we mean the TCM version of these words.

Yin Yang

This is one of the most foundational aspects of TCM. Yin and Yang represent opposing but mutually supporting energies—a part of everything we are and everything around us. The Chinese character of the word Yin symbolizes the shady side of a mountain, while the character for Yang shows the sunny side of the mountain. Neither is better than the other. Both are equally important. Additionally, nothing is pure Yin or Yang. There is a seed of Yin within all Yang and vice versa. This whole idea is simply embodied in the well-recognized Tai Ji symbol (see Figure 1).

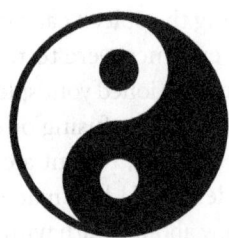

Figure 1: Tai Ji Symbol

There should be a balance between Yin and Yang, though that doesn't necessarily mean an equal 50:50 split all the time. Nighttime tends to have more Yin energy, while daytime tends to have more Yang (see Table 1 for more examples). Note the words "tends to," as that's not the case for every location and every day. Look to nature and you will see that in the northern hemisphere (opposite in the southern hemisphere) there's more Yang energy in the summer as the temperatures climb, people want to get more active, and flowers and plants are actively blooming and growing. In winter, more Yin energy means that there's a greater tendency toward hibernation and recuperation as the weather turns cold and seeds store up the plants' energies. We are a part of nature, so we too are affected by nature's to and fro. Yang cannot exist without Yin, and Yin is absent without Yang.

Table 1: Yin and Yang

Yin	Yang
Moon	Sun
Night	Day
Cool/Cold	Warm/Hot
Storing/Conserving	Moving/Activating
Dark	Light
Winter	Summer
Feminine	Masculine
Matter	Energy
Below	Above
Back	Front
Water	Fire
...and so forth	

Do you have a tendency toward an excess or deficiency of either of these energies? For example, do you often find yourself overheated and hyperactive (mentally or physically), and have a hard time winding down for sleep? You may need to support more Yin in your life—maybe meditation, getting to bed earlier, eating more cooling foods with fewer stimulants. Conversely, if you're often cold, feel depressed, and have low energy, you could perhaps use a bit of a Yang kick. Warming foods and time in the sun may help.

It's the relationship between Yin and Yang that is important. You can have an excess or deficiency in either—or both. For example, if you feel hot, that could be because you have an excess of Yang or a deficiency of Yin. Which of those relational imbalances it is will affect the treatment steps you should take. In this case, if you have an excess of Yang creating Heat, you'd be best to decrease your Yang heating foods. If you have a deficiency of Yin creating Heat, you should increase your Yin cooling foods (see Figure 2).

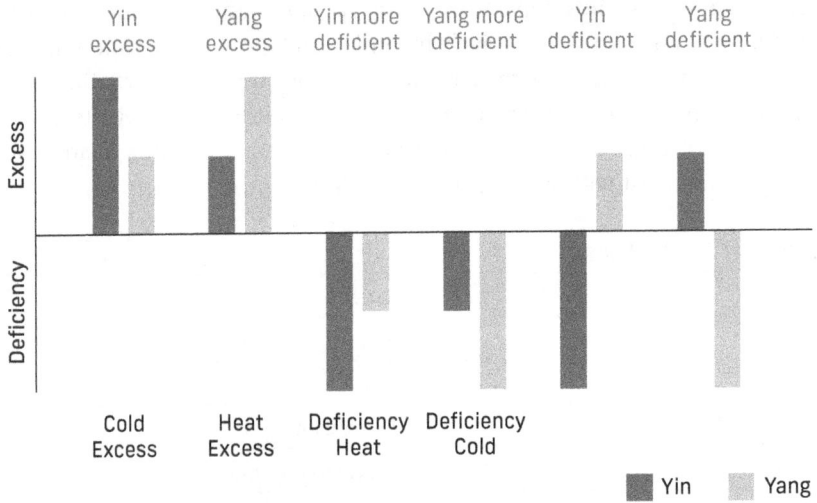

Figure 2: Relative Yin and Yang for Hot and Cold

Eight Guiding Principles

TCM took the Yin Yang principle of Daoism and included it in the eight guiding principles that consist of four opposite imbalances that can occur in the body. They are:

- Cold/Hot: If there is too much relative Cold in the body, the tendency is toward poor circulation, feeling cold, slow metabolism, and pale complexion. Too much relative Heat creates fevers, feeling hot, fast metabolism, flushed complexion, irritation, and inflammation.
- Deficiency/Excess: Deficiencies are marked by not enough of something, like not enough Blood, energy (Qi), or fluids. Excess conditions are too much of something, such as Blood, energy (Qi), fluids, or pathogens (virus, bacteria, fungus, etc.). Chronic conditions tend to be marked by deficiencies, while acute conditions tend to be the result of excesses, but this is not always the case.
- Internal/External: Internal conditions are ones that affect the interior of the body—the organs, bones, deep blood vessels and nerves, the spinal cord, and the brain. External conditions tend to be acute

conditions, ones that are caused by pathogens, with symptoms that affect the skin, peripheral blood vessels and nerves, and muscles.

- Yin/Yang: We can have deficiency or excess of either Yin or Yang.

A TCM practitioner considers all eight of these principles when assessing a patient. Thus, someone with a cold resulting in a fever, sore throat, and cough would be diagnosed as having a Hot, Excess, External, and Yang Excess process happening. Someone with chronic fatigue syndrome, poor circulation, and slow metabolism would be assessed as Cold, Deficiency, Internal, and Yang Deficiency or perhaps both Yin and Yang Deficiency.

And because we're much more complex than this, there's more…

Five Elements

Because TCM was developed through many years of observation of people and nature, there are five elements from nature that are used to help us define patterns of imbalances within our bodies. These elements are Water, Wood, Fire, Earth, and Metal (see Figure 3). Each of these elements supports the production of one element and helps keep in check another element. This is represented in Figure 4.

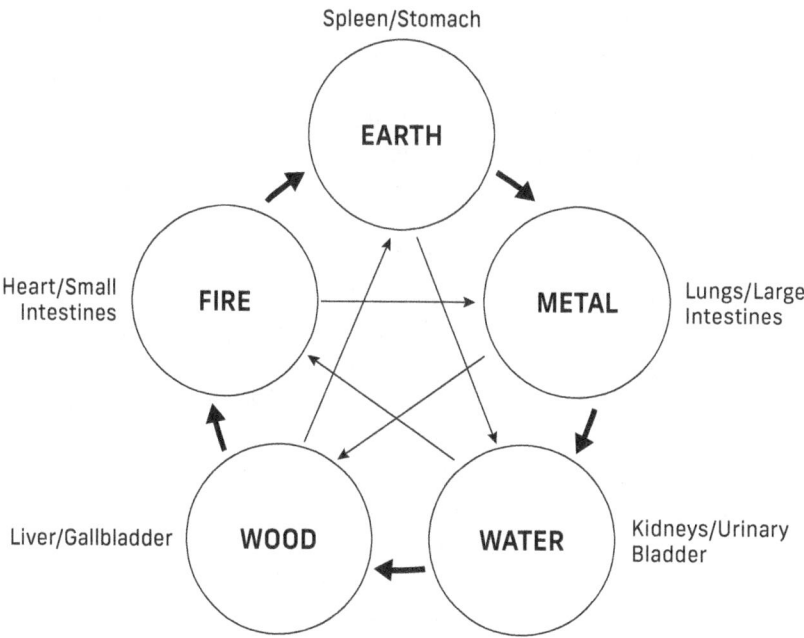

Figure 3: Five Elements

Production Cycle: Each element produces the next

Earth produces Metal (metals are found in the earth)
Metal produces Water (water condenses on metal)
Water produces Wood (wood grows from water)
Wood produces Fire (fire burns from wood)
Fire produces Earth (earth is made from the ashes of fire)

Control Cycle: Each element keeps the next in check

⎯⎯⎯⎯⎯⎯⎯⎯→

Earth controls Water (earth dams water)
Water controls Fire (water puts out fire)
Fire controls Metal (fire melts metal)
Metal controls Wood (metal chops wood)
Wood controls Earth (wood blocks earth, like a fallen tree on a dirt path)

Figure 4: Five Elements Production and Control Cycles

One of the tricky things to explain about the organs assigned to each of these five elements is that they don't necessarily directly relate to the actual physical organs within your body. They are names assigned to help understand patterns of symptoms and imbalances. So, when a TCM practitioner states that you have Heart Fire, it doesn't mean you have heartburn or that your physical heart is overheated. But you are likely struggling with insomnia, anxiety, or possibly canker sores or urinary tract infections. Nor does having Spleen energy (Qi) deficiency mean that your physical spleen is not getting enough energy. But you may be tired, foggy-headed, bloated, and/or bruising easily.

When I started studying TCM, the five-elements principles simultaneously provided some of my most "aha!" moments of understanding at the same time as they produced a lot of "huh?" thoughts. I found that the easiest way for me to get around my confusion was to start off with putting aside what I already know about physiology (my background is a degree in kinesiology, and I studied hard to know all I could about how our organs and bodies as a whole work, so that was hard to do). For instance, I know that the spleen is not involved in digestion. However, the TCM Spleen is central to digestion. This is because the pancreas is not discussed in TCM, but it is instead assigned to be a part of the TCM Spleen system (the ancient creators of this system probably didn't have the tools to be able to specify the functions to the correct organ, in this case). Thus, the pancreas secretes digestive enzymes and the hormones insulin and glucagon that balance blood sugar, but the functions are assigned to the Spleen.

Note that when the organ name is capitalized, it is referring to the TCM organ system; otherwise, it is kept all in lower case.

I find it fascinating that a lot of people with asthma and allergies also often have eczema and issues with constipation, diarrhea, or other bowel irregularities. TCM has long seen a link in issues with the lungs, skin, and large intestines. They categorized them all under the element of Metal.

Because of the importance of the five-elements system to TCM, I've chosen that as the focus for classifying foods. To see which element(s) you might be best to address to improve your health, check out Chapter 5: Five Elements Quiz—What Am I?

Qi

A whole book can be written about this very small word, Qi (pronounced *chi*). The Chinese character for Qi is composed of two symbols that combined signify the steam rising from rice as it cooks. Qi is most often defined as "energy," but it is more complex than this. It has also been translated as "vital energy," "life force," "breath," and "oxygen." China is not the only country to come up with the idea of Qi. Indian culture calls it *Prana*, ancient Greeks called it *pneuma*, Hawaiians call it *mana*, Japanese call it *Ki*, Tibetan Buddhists call it *lüng* (*rlung*), and Hebrews call it *ruach*.[1]

Everything has Qi. We now understand that everything is composed of molecules that are in continuous movement. Everything has either kinetic (moving) energy or potential (storing) energy. Gee, those ancient scholars were smart; that's Yang (kinetic) and Yin (potential) described in physics terms that we use now.

As living beings, we receive energy from various sources, including the energy we are born with (genetic or ancestral), energy from the air we breathe, and energy from the food and drink we consume. This latter Qi, the one we get from our food, called Gu Qi (no, not Gucci®, the famous fashion line) or Food Qi, is more than just calories. It's more than vitamins and minerals. It's the energy of the sunshine that feeds the plants we eat. It's the earth it grows in. It's the complex combination of things that make

---

1   Note that there is not always agreement on spelling and capitalization of words like Qi, Ki, Prana, pneuma, mana, rlung, and ruach, so I've tried to choose what I've found to be most common. For example, "ruach" may more generally mean "God's breath," while "Ruach" may mean "God." And "Prana" refers to cosmic energy as a whole and "prana" means its manifestations.

an apple different from a pear, a spinach leaf different from a chili pepper, a home-cooked meal different from a frozen microwave dinner.

Blood

Of course, you know what blood is. It's the red stuff that flows out of you when you are cut. It's what carries oxygen and nutrients to your cells. It's what medical professionals take from you to test the function of many of your body's organs and tissues. In TCM, it's that and more.

Blood and Qi are strongly interrelated. Blood is the "mother" of Qi, nourishing the organs that form Qi. Qi moves Blood, giving it life and carrying it to where it's needed. Thus, you may often hear Qi and Blood mentioned together, such as "Qi and Blood stagnation" or "Qi and Blood deficiency." They are different components, but they strongly affect each other.

There is a lot more to know about Blood, but for the basics of understanding, if a TCM practitioner tells you that you are Blood deficient, you may or may not be anemic. Your Blood deficiency might be causing dry skin, dry eyes, blurred vision, dizziness, insomnia, palpitations, poor memory, fatigue, weakness, and paleness.

Blood stagnation or stasis, similarly, doesn't necessarily mean blood clots. Blood stagnation commonly causes pain, particularly pain that is fixed, stabbing, or sharp, and worse at night, and there may be a purplish tinge to the nails, complexion, lips, or tongue.

Jing (Essence)

The English translation most often used is "Essence." This is probably one of the hardest TCM terms to pin down. Many online products claim to be able to "boost your Jing," meaning increased virility for men, in particular, but there are two main problems with this. For one, while a deficiency in Jing may result in impotency or infertility, it is not only—or even mainly—related to sexual prowess. Second, it is very difficult to take something that will magically restore depleted Jing. It is possible to build up more Jing with certain foods and herbs, exercises, and practices, but it is not easy. The main thing you can do is slow its depletion.

There are a few types of Jing. There is the Jing you are born with, called Prenatal Jing. This is somewhat like your genetics. It is the energy passed from your parents to you, and it determines your constitution, strength, and vitality. For this type of Jing, basically you get what you got. Some people can get away with unhealthy lifestyles because they started with strong Prenatal Jing, while others must work hard to stay healthy because their Prenatal Jing starting point was weaker. Another type of Jing starts to build after you are born, so, suitably, it is called Postnatal Jing. It is derived from eating, drinking, and breathing, and the Qi we get from those activities can be stored as Jing. Finally, we have Kidney Jing. The Kidneys, shaped somewhat like seeds, are most closely associated with reproductive materials—eggs and sperm. Kidney Jing is determined by what we are born with and can be partially replenished by Postnatal Jing. It is the foundation for our ability to grow, develop, and reproduce.

So, what are your take-home pieces of information about Jing?

- Prenatal Jing was passed on to you from your parents.
- Moderation and balance are key to slowing the loss of Jing.
- Eating and living healthy can help build Qi, some of which can replenish some of your Postnatal Jing.
- Having enough Jing is one of the keys to a long and healthy life.

Jin Ye (Body Fluids)

Basically, these are your bodily fluids. There are "pure" forms of these fluids that lubricate, moisten, and nourish organs and tissues in the form of saliva, tears, synovial fluids, cerebrospinal fluids, mucosal linings, and part of the blood. And there are "impure" forms that are eliminated from the body in the urine, feces, and vomit.

With that introduction, welcome to the World of TCM!

CHAPTER 2

How to Classify Foods Using TCM

Your Foods Give You Hints About How They Affect Your Body

One of the coolest things about TCM is that you don't have to memorize everything to have a basic and workable understanding. TCM was developed in large part through observations—look, listen, feel, smell, and taste. As a result, you can get a sense of some of the properties of any food, even one you've never seen or eaten before.

The Appearance of a Food: Carrots Are Good for Your Eyes

We've all heard that carrots are good for our eyes. They—along with many other foods—are rich in beta-carotene, a precursor for vitamin A which helps with eye health, preventing and slowing the progression of eye diseases. But if you didn't know anything about vitamins and their benefits, might you have a clue about one of their health benefits? Sure! Cut a carrot crosswise and look at the flat side. You'll see that it looks very much like an eye, even showing a darker central area just like the pupil and radiating lines in what would be the iris (see Figure 5).

How about an avocado? It looks like a womb. It amazes me that even the pit/seed in the middle represents where a fetus would grow and eventually become a full-grown adult, just as the pit would grow a new avocado plant! Avocados can help balance hormones (Panahi *et al.*, 2011) and they are a good source of folate, a key nutrient to prevent birth defects like spina bifida.

Check out a grapefruit (or orange, lemon, lime, or other citrus fruit). When you cut it open, you'll see that the compartments look like mammary glands found in breasts. Citrus fruit contain limonoids, a substance that helps inhibit the development of cancer cells in breasts (Guthri *et al.*, 2000).

The comparison that I think is the most fascinating is the walnut and the brain. Walnuts look like a brain—even split in two, like our two hemispheres (see Figure 6). What's more, it's encased in a hard shell to protect it, just like our brain is encased in a hard skull. Well, guess what? Walnuts contain essential fatty acids (EFAs) that are needed for a healthy brain.

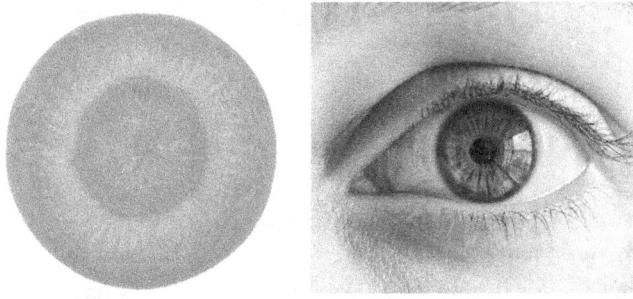

Figure 5a and 5b: Carrot and Eye

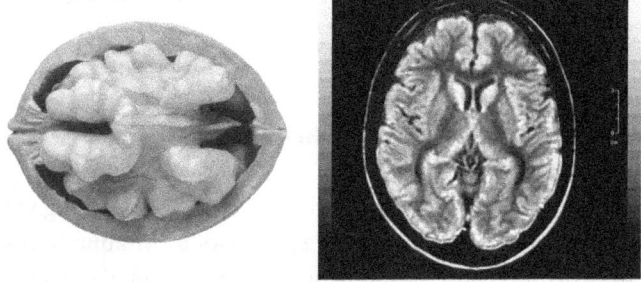

Figure 6a and 6b: Walnut and Brain

Those are just a few examples, but I'm sure you can think of others.

Warming and Cooling Foods: Roots Are Warming, Leaves Are Cooling

Because TCM is such an integrated part of my life, I've long thought that calling a food warming or cooling is obviously clear. However, in a recent conversation with a medical student interested in nutrition, I mentioned how a raw food diet may not be suitable for some because it can be too cooling. She asked me what I meant by that—how does a food warm or cool the body?

Is a cooling food one that is served cold, while a heating food one that is served hot? Partly, but not really. The physical temperature of a food can have some impact on its overall effect. But it's more than that.

Remember that TCM is based on observations. How do you feel when you have a hot pepper? If you're like me, you'll scream "hot, hot, hot!" and go looking for something to cool the mouth. You'll feel the heat, even if it's served cold out of the fridge. If you're feeling a chill, you might also crave a nice chai tea. The spices in it—cinnamon, cardamom, cloves, ginger, and black peppercorn—are all warming. Wine is also warming. The sensation of warmth and rosy cheeks that some of us get (some of us more than others!) tells us that.

What about a hot summer day? What do you crave? Maybe watermelon. That's cooling. Cucumbers? Salads? Also cooling. But what about green tea when you drink it hot? Or tofu when it's served cooked and hot? Although their initial sensation might feel warming, their overall impact will be cooling.

Not sure if you feel more cooling or warming effects from a food? There are other things that can indicate whether it is hot, warming, neutral, cooling, or cold. One of the things that impacts the temperature of a food is how it's prepared. From raw being the coolest to most cooked being the warmest, there may be some disagreement about the exact positioning, but Figure 7 shows the premise.

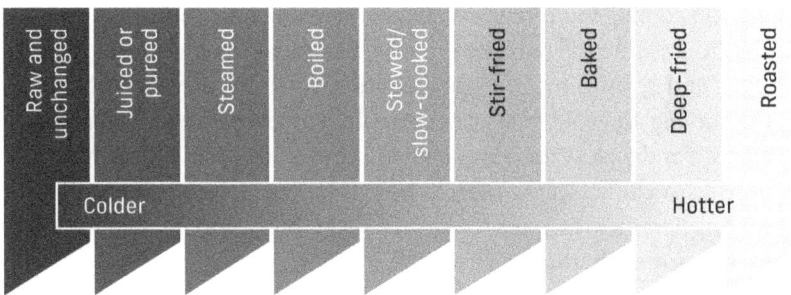

Figure 7: Temperature of Food by Preparation

- Cooked foods are warmer than raw foods, and some forms of cooking are warmer than others. Even fine cutting, pureeing, blended, and juicing can slightly warm a food's property.
- The temperature of the food when consumed will affect its temperature effect on you.
- Plant foods that grow underground tend to be warmer than those grown above. Roots and rhizomes are usually warmer than leaves and fruit. If a plant grows in sunshine and air, it tends to be more Yang; if a plant grows in darkness and earth, it tends to be more Yin.

- Plants that grow faster are often cooler than those that take longer to grow. It takes only about 60 days for a cucumber to grow, while it takes 75 to 100 frost-free days to grow a pumpkin.
- Foods that are red, orange, or yellow are commonly warmer than foods that are green, blue, and purple. Red apples, grapes, and peppers have warmer properties than green ones.
- Mother Nature wisely supplies the right foods to balance our bodies in the context of where we are living. When winter weather turns colder, locally available foods tend to be those grown underground, with warmer resulting properties. As spring and summer bring warmer weather, more plants grow above ground, giving us an abundance of leaves, fruits, and flowers we can eat—foods that cool us off during hotter months. This is one of the reasons why emphasizing locally and seasonally available foods is healthier for you.
- Chewing our food well warms it up because it gets broken down and releases its energy and nutrients.
- Some foods are determined warming or cooling by their observed effects on the body.

Note that balance is found by appropriately combining *both* warming and cooling foods that are suitable to your constitution, current condition, and external environment. Unless you have extreme heat signs and symptoms, it is not advised for you to select only from the cooling and cold foods categories (not an excuse to binge on ice cream!) and vice versa. Simply be mindful to select more from the heating or cooling categories. Even TCM herbal formulas add some cooling herbs to a formula designed to heat things up; they just select more warming herbs.

Let's go into a bit more detail about the temperature of foods, according to TCM.

Hot and Warm Foods
Remember from the Yin Yang section in Chapter 1 that Yang energies are warming. Obviously, hot foods are going to have more of a heating impact than warming foods. Their effects on the body are:

- dispelling cold
- increasing circulation

- stimulating activity of the organs and body.

Heating foods are particularly suitable for those with cold symptoms. Cold in your body has the same impact as cold on the environment. Cold slows movement, contracts, and becomes solid like ice. See Table 2 for a list of hot foods and Table 3 for a list of warm foods.

Some of the common symptoms that may be treated by warming foods include:

- feeling cold or chilled (hands, feet, whole body)
- poor circulation
- paleness
- loose stools (though some cases of acute diarrhea are caused by heat)
- bloating, slow digestion
- low energy
- symptoms aggravated by cold (such as cold weather aggravating arthritis)
- tendency toward water retention.

Hot Foods
Table 2: Hot Foods List

Vegetables	Fruit	Grains, legumes, nuts, and seeds	Meats, seafood, and dairy	Spices, herbs, and miscellaneous
• cayenne • chili • hot peppers	• durian (very warm)	• soybean oil (very warm)	• lamb	• black and white pepper • cinnamon bark • dried ginger • horseradish • mustard • spirits (alcohol)

Note that, like almost all health (and science) topics, there is always debate. Some of the foods I have listed here have been placed in the warm category by one source and in the neutral category by another. This is nature, always on a scale, so the definition of warm to neutral or neutral to cool is subjective.

Warm Foods
Table 3: Warm Foods List

Vegetables	Fruit	Grains, legumes, nuts, and seeds	Meats, seafood, and dairy	Spices, herbs, and miscellaneous
• bell peppers • chive • fennel • leek • mustard greens • onion • oyster mushroom • parsnip • pumpkin • scallions/ spring onions • squash	• blackberry • cherry • date • guava • kumquat • longan • lychee/litchi • nectarine • peach • pineapple • pomegranate • raspberry • umeboshi plum	• oat • quinoa • sweet rice • black bean • chestnut • coconut • pinenut • pistachio • pumpkin seed • sunflower seed • walnut	• anchovy • beef • butter • chicken • eels • goat milk • ham • lobster • mussel • shrimp/ prawn • turkey • venison	• anise • caraway seed • cilantro/ coriander • clove • coffee • cumin • fennel seed • fresh ginger • garlic • ginseng • nutmeg • rosemary • sweet basil • thyme • vinegar • wine

Neutral Temperature Foods

These are foods that are neither significantly warm nor cool, so are nourishing for both hot and cold constitutions (see Table 4 for a list of neutral foods).

Neutral Foods
Table 4: Neutral Foods List

Vegetables	Fruit	Grains, legumes, nuts, and seeds	Meats, seafood, and dairy	Spices, herbs, and miscellaneous
• beetroot	• apple	• rice bran	• abalone	• honey
• Brussels sprout	• apricot	• rye	• carp	• licorice
• cabbage	• fig	• white rice	• chicken egg	• saffron
• carrot	• grape	• almond	• cow's milk	• sage
• cauliflower	• kohlrabi	• black sesame seed	• duck	
• corn	• lotus fruit, seed, and root	• broad bean	• oyster	
• corn silk	• olive	• cashew	• pork	
• green bean	• papaya	• adzuki bean		
• potato	• plum	• kidney bean		
• shiitake mushroom	• raisin	• lentil		
• sweet potato		• pea		
• turnip		• peanut		
• yam		• soybean		
		• soy milk		

Cooling and Cold Foods

Cooling foods are Yin in nature, and they can vary in degree of coolness from mildly cool to cold. Their effects are:

- clearing heat
- dispelling toxins
- calming and sedating hyperactivity of the organs.

Cooling foods help treat those with too much heat in their body. Warmth is important in the body, but too much heat causes inflammation, irritation, and disruption of organ function. See Table 5 for a list of cooling foods and Table 6 for a list of cold foods.

Some heat symptoms that can be treated with cooling foods include:

- feeling hot
- excessive perspiration, spontaneous sweating, night sweats
- thirst

- symptoms of dryness
- constipation or diarrhea with strong smelling stools or blood
- strong appetite
- bad breath
- nosebleeds
- acne
- rashes and other skin eruptions
- high blood pressure
- anxiety
- irritability
- vivid dream and/or insomnia
- mouth ulcers, cold sores
- heartburn.

Cooling Foods

Table 5: Cooling Foods List

Vegetables	Fruit	Grains, legumes, nuts, and seeds	Meats, seafood, and dairy	Spices, herbs, and miscellaneous
• alfalfa sprouts • bok choy • broccoli • button mushroom • celery • cucumber • daikon • eggplant/ aubergine • lettuce • radish • spinach • summer squash • Swiss chard • tomato • watercress • zucchini/ courgette	• cantaloupe • green apple • kiwifruit • lemon • lime • loquat • orange • pear • strawberry • tangerine	• amaranth • barley • buckwheat • millet • wheat bran • whole wheat • lima bean • mung bean • tofu	• cheese • chicken egg white • yogurt	• green tea • marjoram • peppermint

Cold Foods
Table 6: Cold Foods List

Vegetables	Fruit	Grains, legumes, nuts, and seeds	Meats, seafood, and dairy	Spices, herbs, and miscellaneous
• bamboo shoot • bitter gourd • romaine lettuce • water chestnut	• banana • grapefruit • persimmon • star fruit • watermelon		• clam • crab • octopus	• salt • seaweed (dulse, kelp, nori, etc.)

Flavor: You've Got Taste

No, I don't mean your style in clothes or design (though perhaps you *do* have good taste!), but your sense of tasting flavors. Flavor is what most people love about food. It's also why many find eating healthily difficult. The challenge is that we're designed to crave two flavors in particular—sweet and salty.

These flavors were once difficult to come across in large quantities, and they were much less intense than the whammo punch of sweet and salty that we have today. Other, generally less popular, flavors we consider in TCM are bitter, sour, pungent/spicy, and bland. Many foods, of course, offer up more than one flavor at a time, sometimes combining flavors, like oranges that are both sweet and sour.

Sweet: The Search for More Changed the World

Sugarcane was first domesticated about 10,000 years ago on the island of New Guinea, where people would chew the stem. It was used for medicinal benefit, religious ceremonies, and even starred in myths about the creation of man.

Sugar Mamma

One mythical story about the creation of man related to sugarcane is that the first man made love to a stalk of sugarcane and created humans—what a sweet (but strange) love story. Another myth tells about two fishermen, the first two people on earth, who found a piece of sugarcane in their net. At first, they thought it was useless and tossed it out. But after catching it for three days in a row, they decided to plant it in the ground. From that plant the first woman appeared.

By day, she would cook for the men and, at night, would disappear back into the cane. Sugarcane is still used in traditional ceremonies in New Guinea with priests sipping sugar water from coconut shells. That sugar water has now been replaced by Coke.

After spreading through the Polynesian islands, sugar finally reached the Asian mainland, and by 500 AD India was processing it into a powder that was used for medicine. In fact, it was once used to treat some of the symptoms that our excess consumption of sugar now causes: headaches, stomach issues, and impotence. Of course, sugar's popularity didn't stop there. Once it reached Persia, the head honchos there started to serve it in delicious sweets to their guests. Everywhere the Arabs conquered, they brought sugar. When I visited Turkey, the stacks upon stacks of amazing, sweet desserts lined up in the windows of many stores made my mouth water.

The first sugar to reach Europe was so rare that it was considered a spice and only consumed by nobility. It was sometimes called "white gold," such was its value. The call for more sugar was so strong—what would you do to keep eating your favorite sweet?—that it was, in part, cause for the "age of exploration," with Europeans looking for tropical lands where they could grow more sugarcane. The growing, harvesting, and processing of sugar was very difficult and labor-intensive work, so the rapidly increasing demand for more sugar tragically began the slave trade. Despite the thousands of people suffering and dying, and despite acres of land being destroyed, our appetite for this addictive substance continued to grow. In 1700, the average Englishman ate four pounds of sugar per year. By 1800, he was up to 18 pounds per year, and just 70 years after that, he was consuming 47 pounds yearly (Arthur, 2023). In 2004, Canadians ate about 22 *times* that amount annually! That equates to about 26 teaspoons daily, or 21.4 percent of our total daily calorie intake (Langlois and Garriguet, 2011). The good news (maybe) is that, in 2015, our numbers came down slightly with 18.8 percent of our total daily caloric intake (Canadian Sugar Institute, n.d.). Still, this is way, way, way too much.

It is now thought that too much sugar intake is one of the reasons we are seeing a record number of chronic illnesses like diabetes, cardiovascular diseases, strokes, inflammatory disorders, and obesity.

The point of my sharing some of the history of sugar—beyond its fascinating story—is twofold. First, that it's no wonder that we have such a hard time cutting back. In fact, biologically, our brains are wired with reward triggers when we eat sugar. Eating sugar causes a release of opioids and dopamine—brain chemicals that make us feel good—similar to drugs such as heroin (Avena, Rada, and Hoebel, 2008). And second, that eating small quantities of foods that are naturally sweet has traditionally been medicinal, and it can once again be healthy.

Sweet Flavor in TCM

By TCM standards, sweet flavor relates to the Earth element (see Chapter 6: Foods by Element to learn more about the Earth element), and in particular to the body's ability to process and digest. Sweet foods are Yang in nature.

Sweet foods can help:

- build up a weakened body
- gain weight, strengthen digestion
- slow down and neutralize the toxic effects of other foods
- calm the nervous system.

Sweet Foods

Table 7: Sweet Foods List

Vegetables	Fruit	Grains, legumes, nuts, and seeds	Meats, seafood, and dairy	Spices, herbs, and miscellaneous
• bamboo shoot • beet • cabbage • carrot • celery • corn • cucumber • eggplant/ aubergine • kohlrabi • lettuce • mushroom • potato • pumpkin • radish • spinach • squash • string bean • sweet potato • taro • tomato	• apple • apricot • banana • cherry • coconut • date • fig • grape • grapefruit • guava • longan • lychee/ litchi • mango • orange • papaya • peach • pear • persimmon • pineapple • plum • raspberry • star fruit • strawberry	• amaranth • barley • buckwheat • flax • kamut • millet • oats • rice • rye • spelt • wheat • adzuki bean • black bean • chickpea • kidney bean • lentil • navy bean • soybean • tofu • all nuts • all seeds	• beef • chicken • clam • egg • fish • lamb • milk • oyster • pork • shrimp/ prawn • yogurt	• cinnamon • coffee • ginseng • licorice • saffron • sesame oil • sugar • wine

Sweet foods are not just cookies, candies, cakes, and pop. Those are among the modern-day foods that have contributed to many of our current chronic diseases. Naturally sweet foods include fruits. They also include roots, rhizomes, and tubers like carrots, beets/beetroot, yams, potatoes, and fennel. Many grains, such as rice, millet, and wheat, are also mildly sweet. These foods are all rich sources of complex carbohydrates. Sources of protein, like meats, legumes, nuts, and seeds, also have some level of sweetness to them.

As you can see from Table 7, many foods are categorized as sweet, so you have lots to choose from.

Salty: It Resulted in the Creation of our Cities

If you're not seduced by sweet stuff, chances are you're swayed by salty snacks. Salt is another part of food that is necessary to our lives, was once hard to come by, and is now available in abundance.

Deeper Meanings to Salt

A Cochiti Native American myth tells of an elderly, impoverished woman named Old Salt Woman, traveling with her grandson, asking for food. She is denied assistance by several households, but when she is given food, she offers in return part of her flesh—salt.

The Bible also mentions salt over 30 times, including when Lot's wife Adit is turned into a pillar of salt for not following instructions to avoid looking back, and in the phrase "salt of the earth." Salt is often used to represent purity and salvation (another alteration of the word "salt").

Salt even makes its way into superstition and symbolism. In the painting *The Last Supper* by Leonardo da Vinci, Judas is shown with an overturned salt cellar in front of him. For the superstitious among us, we now throw a pinch of spilled salt over our left shoulder to temporarily blind evil spirits that appear there. Salt is used to repel evil spirits in Buddhist traditions and purify an area—such as a sumo wrestling ring—in Shintoism. In India, salt is a symbol of good luck in reference to Mahatma Gandhi's liberation of India.

Salt comes from oceans, either living ones or dried-up ones. The growth of our civilization depended upon salt. We followed and ate animals that would lick salt from rocks. Those animal paths became roads, and we created settlements along those roads. As we started to grow and eat more grains, we needed more salt to supplement our diet. Salt's scarcity and usefulness made it a valuable commodity.

Long used to flavor foods and to preserve them, salt was literally worth its weight in gold at times, traded ounce for ounce with gold in the sub-Sahara in the sixth century. We've learned in our history lessons about the spice routes, travels between Asia and the Mediterranean. But did you know that one of the most valuable spices was salt? In fact, our word "salary" comes from the word "salt," as it was once used to pay Roman soldiers, who were evaluated based on their "worth in salt."

Salt has played a prominent role in history, driving exploration, trade, governance, technology, and innovation. Wars have even been waged, won, and lost because of salt. For example, it's been recorded that Napoleon's troops died during their retreat from Moscow because a lack of salt meant their wounds would not heal.

Once again, we've taken a valuable food and overdone it. According to a 2023 report from the World Health Organization (WHO), adults the world over are consuming a mean average of 4310 mg of sodium daily (equivalent to almost 11 g of salt)—more than twice what is recommended (WHO, 2023). The problem isn't usually what you pour out of your saltshaker. It's often how many processed and packaged foods and drinks you are consuming that elevates your sodium consumption.

And the result of too much sodium is dangerous as our bodies hold on to water in order to dilute its excess, increasing the amount of fluid around cells and the volume of blood in the bloodstream. This increased blood volume means the heart must work harder. It also means more pressure on the blood vessels which, over time, can make them stiffer. Less flexible blood vessels and more blood volume leads to higher blood pressure, increasing the risk for heart attacks, heart failure, and strokes.

Even without increasing blood pressure, high sodium can still cause damage to the tissues of the heart, major blood vessels, and the kidneys. It has also been linked to osteoporosis, stomach cancer, and asthma.

This problem of excess sodium is aggravated by our relative under-consumption of potassium. We need way more potassium than sodium, but the average American, according to a 2018 study on sodium and potassium intake, gets only about 2000 mg of potassium daily, less than half of what's recommended (Whelton, 2018). Where sodium excess increases blood pressure, potassium relaxes blood vessels and helps with the excretion of sodium, thus lowering blood pressure. Those with the highest ratio of dietary sodium to potassium are twice as likely to die from a heart attack than people with the lowest ratio, and 50 percent more likely to die from any cause (Yang, 2011).

Conversely, other studies have found that too little sodium is also associated with higher risk for heart disease (O'Donnell *et al.*, 2011) and a potentially faster onset of insulin resistance (Garg *et al.*, 2011). Sodium replacement is also important for those participating in endurance sports.

While salt is important to our health, too much or too little salt causes problems. Balance can be achieved by eating more fresh vegetables and fruit, naturally rich in potassium and low in sodium, and eating less processed foods. Luckily, salty flavor is found naturally in some foods, and it can be enjoyed in a healthy manner.

Salty Flavor in TCM

According to TCM, salty flavor is connected to the Water element (see Chapter 6: Foods by Element to learn more about the Water element). Salty foods are Yin in nature.

Salty foods can help:

- dissipate accumulations and soften lumps
- nourish blood and moisten dryness
- lubricate the intestines to purge bowels.

Salty Foods

Salty foods aren't just potato chips, crackers, and pretzels. They include foods that are prepared using salt, like pickles, some grains and meats, and foods from the ocean (see Table 8).

Table 8: Salty Foods List

Vegetables	Fruit	Grains, legumes, nuts, and seeds	Meats, seafood, and dairy	Spices, herbs, and miscellaneous
• bladder-wrack • dulse • kelp • kombu • all seaweed • pickled vegetables		• amaranth • barley • millet • miso	• abalone • clam • crab • duck • ham • mussel • oyster • pork • sea cucumber • shrimp/prawn	• salt • soy sauce

Bitter: It's Tricky, as It Can Signal Either Friend or Foe

"It left a bitter taste in his mouth." This is not a complimentary expression. Bitter is most often associated with something negative. In the word "bittersweet," bitter is the negative part and sweet is the positive part. Bitter is not a flavor that most of us crave, because we've evolved to be wary of it. After all, poisonous things tend to taste bitter. The thing is, many medicinal and healing ingredients are also bitter, so it's important to at least develop a tolerance for (if not a liking of) this contradictory flavor.

Genetics and Taste

Whether you like vegetables or not may depend partially on your genetics. Research has found that we have 25 different bitter-tasting genes, so our genetics may affect how we perceive the taste of foods. In fact, those who are more sensitive to tasting bitterness eat about 25 percent fewer vegetables. And because each bitter food acts through different receptors, we can notice the bitterness in one food but not another. For example, you can be a high responder to the bitter flavor in grapefruit but not in coffee. This may cause you to dislike grapefruit but like coffee. In addition, since bitter and sweet oppose each other in the brain, you will experience less sweetness if you notice more bitterness. But don't let that give you an excuse to avoid eating your veggies. As with all things genetic, you can influence your genetic expression by making lifestyle changes. In this case, gradually increase your exposure to eating bitter-tasting vegetables so that your taste buds can become accustomed, and you can actually start to enjoy them.

What's more, appreciation for taste starts very early—surprisingly, even as early as in the womb. In one study, pregnant women and breastfeeding mothers drank carrot juice for three weeks. When the babies were eventually switched to solid foods, the babies of the carrot-juice-drinking mothers liked carrots more than those babies who did not have this early exposure (Mennella, Jagnow, and Beauchamp, 2001). Other studies have demonstrated that babies who normally disliked bitter and sour flavors began to enjoy them when they were exposed to them by being given a variety of vegetables. When it comes to adult picky eaters, one might say, "Don't be such a baby." But in this case, maybe you should be like a baby and learn to like those flavors over time.

While bitter foods haven't made many friends for their flavor, they have been recognized for centuries for their medicinal benefits. In fact, most of our powerful medicinal herbs land squarely in the bitter flavor category. This is why we've been taught to take "a spoonful of sugar to help the medicine go down." (It's okay if you just broke into Mary Poppins' song when you read that phrase.) Sweet flavor—which we tend to love—counters bitter flavor.

Orange Juice and Toothpaste

I recall getting ready for school when I was a kid and brushing my teeth before my mom reminded me to finish drinking my orange juice. Yuck. If you've ever done this, you know that awful flavor, but did you know why it tastes like that?

Many commercial toothpastes contain a chemical called sodium lauryl sulfate (SLS). It's used as a foaming agent in toothpastes, shampoos, and detergents. As a side gig, SLS suppresses receptors in your taste buds that pick up on the flavor of sweet while also breaking apart phospholipids (fatty molecules) on your tongue that would reduce your ability to taste bitter. So you get more bitter, less sweet out of anything you drink or eat afterward.

Besides simply not eating after you brush your teeth, you can also choose toothpaste that doesn't contain SLS, as it's not needed, unless you love the Cujo foaming-mouth look. Fewer unnecessary chemicals in and on your body is better for you anyway.

While I do sometimes tell my patients it's okay to add a bit of honey to their Chinese herbal formulas if they have a hard time getting them down, most find that the "can't stand it" reaction they initially get to their herbal medicinal drinks is replaced by a "not my favorite flavor, but I don't hate it" response after a week or so of regular consumption. Believe it or not, some even come to love the taste of their Chinese herbs, especially as their bodies reap the health benefits.

Bitter Flavor in TCM

TCM classifies bitter flavor with the Fire element (see Chapter 6: Foods by Element to learn more about the Fire element). Bitter foods are Yin in nature.

Bitter foods can help:

- improve digestion and thus support nutrient absorption
- detoxify the body and support the liver

- reduce symptoms of Dampness, such as high cholesterol, candida yeast overgrowth, skin eruptions, mucus excess, tumors and cysts, edema, and obesity
- cool Excess Heat (and fever) in the body
- reduce inflammation (not a coincidence that, in TCM, inflammation is usually associated with Heat)
- reduce sweet cravings and support weight loss by stimulating metabolism
- induce bowel movement
- fight infections
- calm emotions and help focus the mind.

Bitter Foods
Table 9: Bitter Foods List

Vegetables	Fruit	Grains, legumes, nuts, and seeds	Meats, seafood, and dairy	Spices, herbs, and miscellaneous
• alfalfa • artichoke • arugula/rocket • asparagus • broccoli • Brussels sprouts • burdock root (gobo) • cabbage • cauliflower • celery • chard • cilantro/ coriander • dandelion leaf • endive/chicory • kale • kohlrabi • lettuce • mushroom • parsley • radish • rhubarb • romaine lettuce • scallions/spring onions • turnip • watercress	• bitter melon • bitter orange • citrus peel • grapefruit • papaya	• amaranth • barley • hops • quinoa • rye • sesame		• alcohol • aloe • basil • beer • chamomile • chicory • coffee • dill • dark chocolate • echinacea • fenugreek seed • goldenseal • horseradish • milk thistle • nettle • tonic water • turmeric • valerian • vinegar • white pepper • wine

Many bitter foods are thankfully mixed with other flavors, while many of the more strongly flavored bitter foods are recognized as medicinal herbs, though they are sometimes used as food as well. See Table 9 for a list of bitter foods.

Sour: Is it the Comeback Kid?

In researching about the flavor sour, I was surprised to see that a search brought up several website links that discussed either "bitter" or "bitter/ sour." I've always thought of those two flavors as mutually distinct. Bitter is bitter; sour is sour. But, apparently, particularly in English-speaking countries, these two are often confused, most likely because of a lack of exposure and a misunderstanding of definition.

If you are one of the many who interchange these two words, you'll want to pay particular attention to the differences in taste for the bitter foods listed above versus the sour foods listed below. TCM has long recognized their different health benefits, and now chemistry shows that the compounds that give them their flavor are indeed different.

Sourness is the ability to taste acidity, and in studies, a diluted HCl (hydrochloric acid) solution is often used. When I was in high school, in fact, we used to be given a bit of acid and base to dilute so we could taste the differences—sour vs. slippery. I'm not sure if this classroom experiment is still being offered, particularly as I recall one student not diluting her solutions enough and burning her tongue!

Fermentation Feature

Once a commonly employed method to prepare and preserve foods, except for the making of alcohol, cheese, and bread, much of the process of fermentation lost its popularity for many years, as refrigerating, freezing, and canning became widely available. However, fermentation has regained its "cool kid" status as people are searching for it in their grocery stores, and even going back to their grandmothers' recipes for fermented foods. In North America, the most commonly chosen fermented foods include yogurt, cheese, alcohol, bread, sauerkraut, and pickles.

Some other fermented foods have a more particular following. These are foods with a love it/hate it reputation, and typically those who love it grew up on it. Some of my Japanese relatives love natto, a fermented soy product that has a texture that is, quite frankly, disturbingly similar to mucus, and smells like nothing I would willingly consume. My great uncle used to make tsukemono, Japanese pickles that we appropriately named "stinky pickles." While I was studying in China, I stayed in a city that I was told is famous for its fermented tofu. When my classmates and I were invited to a fancy dinner, our hosts kept trying to turn the revolving tray in the center of our table so that the most revered dish would be closest to us, their honored guests. We kept trying to graciously turn it back to them, wanting to be careful not to offend, but that tofu dish's overpowering stench was making us nauseous. While I lived in Japan, a friend from New Zealand was convinced he was going to make me a fan of Marmite, a thick and sticky spread made from yeast extract, similar to Vegemite that Australians often love. Its smell repelled me, and I refused. But he snuck a bit of it into the sandwiches he made me, adding a bit more with each visit, until he eventually showed me what I had been unknowingly eating. I had to admit that it didn't taste bad, as I had become accustomed to it.

Fermented foods are both sour and salty. When prepared traditionally, they may start with salt or some starting lacto-fermentation or "mother" starter, but modern commercially sold products are now often cheated with a faster route of using vinegar instead. In addition, some of these foods are also pasteurized for a longer shelf life, which leaves them devoid of some of the health benefits of the good bacteria and flavor.

Raw fermented foods have many health benefits, including supporting healthy digestion, improving the balance of good bacteria, and providing a well-absorbed source of nutrients. Keep in mind, however, that some fermented foods are high in sodium, and also that eating too many pickled foods has been associated with higher levels of stomach cancer. Too much of a good thing makes it no longer a good thing.

Which raw fermented foods did your ancestors eat? How can you fit them into your diet?

Sour Flavor in TCM

TCM classifies sour flavor with the Wood element (see Chapter 6: Foods by Element to learn more about the Wood element). Sour foods are Yin in nature. Just as sucking on a lemon can make you pucker your lips, sour has an astringent effect. It pulls things in and is used to treat abnormal leakages in the body.

Sour foods can help:

- treat urinary incontinence, bedwetting, diarrhea, excessive sweating, nocturnal emission, excessive menstrual bleeding, and hemorrhage
- lift sagging tissues to treat prolapsed organs, hemorrhoids, and flaccid skin
- help gather a scattered mind
- support liver function
- assist in the breaking down of dietary fats and proteins; sour helps digest greasy, rich foods
- cleanse, detoxify, and stimulate the appetite.

Sour Foods

While you will likely expect foods like lemons and limes to fit in this category, you might be surprised to see other foods in Table 10 that seem more dominant in the sweet (e.g., grape, mango) or salty (e.g., soy sauce), but they do also have a sour element to them.

Table 10: Sour Foods List

Vegetables	Fruit	Grains, legumes, nuts, and seeds	Meats, seafood, and dairy	Spices, herbs, and miscellaneous
• fermented vegetables like kimchi, pickles, poi, and sauerkraut • leek • rhubarb	• blackberry • grape • hawthorn berry • huckleberry • kumquat • lemon • lime • mango • olive • raspberry • sour apple (crab apple) • sour plum • tangerine • tomato (technically a fruit)	• sourdough bread • adzuki bean • fermented soy bean products like miso, natto, soy sauce, and tempeh	• cheese • kefir • yogurt	• kombucha • rosehip • tamarind • vinegar

Pungent: Fire in Your Mouth or in Your Nose

Of all the flavors, this is probably the one to bring about the most heated discussions (pun intended). "My mouth is on fire!" says one person at a dinner table. Another, eating the very same dish, laughs and replies, "What? It's not spicy at all." This is a discussion I often have. I'm the first person portrayed in this brief example. It has been joked that I think tomatoes are spicy. And I've noted that I think that a lot of restaurants try to cheat flavor by adding hot spices.

In fact, one of the historical reasons for the rapid growth of the popularity of hot spices around the world is that it can hide the "off" taste that foods have when they start to become rancid. Luckily, it also helps to kill off some of the microbes as well, so it's not just hiding a wolf in sheep's clothing.

In TCM, the category of pungent doesn't refer only to the hot spices. It also includes acrid and aromatic flavors. This means that foods like garlic, onions, and turnips also fit this classification.

Fire in the Mouth: Chemesthesis

The hot burning sensation of spicy food is not really a taste sensation, as the feeling of heat is not signaled by the taste buds. It is, instead, another kind of nerve signaling called chemesthesis that makes you feel fire in your mouth. Chemesthesis is a chemical-induced reaction that activates receptors to signal your trigeminal nerves to communicate heat, cold, and pain in your eyes, nose, mouth, and throat. So it tells you that your tongue feels a burn or warmth with chili pepper, ginger, or cinnamon; your nose stings with horseradish, wasabi, and mustard; your eyes water when cutting onions; your tongue tingles with coolness from peppermint and spearmint; and your nose and mouth are tickled by carbonated drinks.

Because chemesthesis can also signal pain, extremes of hot and cold can be perceived as pain. To me, chilies taste like my-mouth-is-on-fire-my-eyes-are-watering-my-stomach-hurts-why-would-anyone-willingly-eat-this pain. Many animals don't like hot spices, and they won't eat them if they can perceive the heat. Interestingly, birds can eat spicy foods because they can't feel the burn from hot peppers and chilies. A professor of psychology at the University of Pennsylvania, Dr. Paul Rozin, tried to condition rats to like chilies to see if it's a simple matter of exposure and adaptation. One group of rats were fed food with chilies from birth. The other group of rats had chilies added gradually into their diet. Both groups continued to prefer non-spicy food. Even after he added a compound that makes rats feel sick when eating the non-spicy food, they still preferred that over the chili-laced option (Rozin, Gruss, and Berk, 1979). In other words, they preferred eating the food that made them vomit to eating the food that burned their mouths. So why do some of us love to add a spicy kick to our foods?

Maybe we've learned to tolerate the sensation because of some of the health benefits, like its anti-microbial and blood-circulation-boosting effects. However, the level of spiciness that some people like is way beyond health benefits. Competitions are held to see who can eat the hottest peppers (see Table 11 for a list of the spiciest peppers—the Scoville Heat Chart). Hot sauces are proudly given names that indicate pain, like "Bomb Laden Mad Blast Habanero Hot Sauce," "Crazy Jerry's Brain Damage Mind Blowin' Hot Sauce," and much ruder variations of "Brenda's Bootie Burner Hot Sauce." This has been called "benign masochism" by Dr. Rozin. When Dr. Rozin gave groups of people food flavored with differing amounts of chili pepper and asked them to rate the taste, the variance between "just right" and "ouch" was minimal, with the preferred hotness level just below each individual's rating of unbearable pain. In many areas of the human brain, neurons that respond to pleasure and pain are closely placed (Rozin and Schiller, 1980). It's a kind of thrill seeking that, though it can cause discomfort, generally won't (at least immediately) kill you. Personally, I prefer roller-coaster rides, bungee jumping, or some other non-mouth-burning thrill.

Table 11: Scoville Heat Chart

	Scoville Heat Units (SHU)
pure capsaicin	15,000,000
pepper spray	2,000,000–5,300,000
Caroline red reaper	1,400,000–2,200,000
Trinidad scorpion	1,200,000–2,009,231
ghost pepper/bhut jolokia	800,000–1,041,427
chocolate habanero	425,000–577,000
red savina habanero	200,000–350,000

fatali	125,000–325,000
Scotch bonnet	100,000–250,000
habanero	100,000–250,000
Thai pepper	50,000–100,000
cayenne pepper	30,000–50,000
Tabasco	30,000–50,000
seranno pepper	10,000–23,000
jalapeño pepper	3500–8000
poblano	1000–1500
Anaheim pepper	500–2500
chile verde	500–1500
pepperoncini	100–500
bell pepper	0

Pungent Flavor in TCM

TCM classifies pungent flavor with the Metal element (see Chapter 6: Foods by Element to learn more about the Metal element). Pungent foods are Yang in nature.

Pungent foods can help:

- clear the lungs of mucus
- stimulate blood circulation
- support the heart
- help clear obstructions
- improve sluggish liver.

Pungent Foods

Pungent foods are significantly different based on their temperature, so in Table 12, warming pungent foods are identified with "(W)," cooling pungent foods are labeled with "(C)," and neutral pungent foods with "(N)."

Table 12: Pungent Foods List

Vegetables	Fruit	Grains, legumes, nuts, and seeds	Meats, seafood, and dairy	Spices, herbs, and miscellaneous
• anise (W) • fennel (W) • garlic (W) • kohlrabi (N) • leek (W) • mustard greens (W) • all onions (W) • radish (C) • scallions/ spring onions (W) • taro (N) • turnip (C)	• kumquat (W) • all hot peppers (W)	• rice bran (N)		• basil (W) • black pepper (W) • caraway seed (W) • cilantro/ coriander (W) • cinnamon (W) • clove (W) • dill (W) • ginger (W) • horseradish (W) • marjoram (C) • mustard seed (W) • nutmeg (W) • peppermint (C) • rosemary (W) • saffron (N) • spearmint (C) • thyme (W) • white pepper (W) • wine (W)

Direction of a Food: In and Out, Up and Down

Usually when we think of directions, we are thinking of a map, of turning left or right, or maybe looking up to the sky or down to the earth. We don't normally consider that the foods we eat have a preference for action toward a direction—upward (above the waist), downward (below the waist), inward (internal regions of the body), and outward (skin and body surface)—or to particular organ systems within our bodies. TCM considers this.

Outward Foods

Outward-moving foods bring the action of the body from internal toward the skin. They can:

- induce perspiration and reduce fever
- treat a cold or flu (especially if caught early).

Foods with an outward movement are often Hot, Warm, Pungent, or Sweet. They are helpful to eat in the summer (see Figure 8 for a list).

black pepper	hot peppers
cinnamon bark	onions
garlic	parsley
ginger	peppermint
horseradish	radish

Figure 8: Outward-Moving Foods

Inward Foods

Foods that move inward move the energies inward to the internal organs. They can also slow loss of fluids. They can:

- ease abdominal swelling
- treat excessive perspiration, frequent urination, seminal emission, and premature ejaculation.

Inward foods are Cold foods that are Bitter or Salty, with benefits related to the winter months (see Figure 9).

bitter gourd	kelp
clam	lettuce
crab	salt
hops	seaweed

Figure 9: Inward-Moving Foods

Upward Foods

Foods that move upward in our body bring an action of lifting. They can:

- relieve diarrhea
- support a lift of prolapsed organs
- help hernias
- treat problems in the upper part of the body.

Leaves and flowers tend to be upward-moving foods, although there are exceptions. Warming, Hot, Pungent, Sweet, and Bitter foods tend to move upward. These are particularly helpful foods to have in the spring, just as flowers and grasses are coming to surface from the ground (see Figure 10 for a list of upward-moving foods).

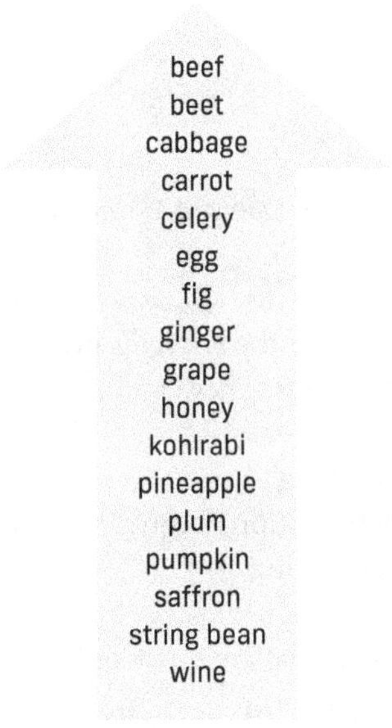

beef
beet
cabbage
carrot
celery
egg
fig
ginger
grape
honey
kohlrabi
pineapple
plum
pumpkin
saffron
string bean
wine

Figure 10: Upward-Moving Foods

Downward Foods

Foods that move downward in our body are grounding and reverse upward movement. They can:

- stop vomiting and relieve nausea
- treat hiccups
- reduce coughing and asthma
- address constipation.

Roots, seeds, and fruits tend to have a downward action, although there are some exceptions. Downward foods can be Cold, Cool, or Warm and Sweet or Sour. They are good in autumn, as leaves fall (makes this one easy to remember, doesn't it?) to the ground (see Figure 11).

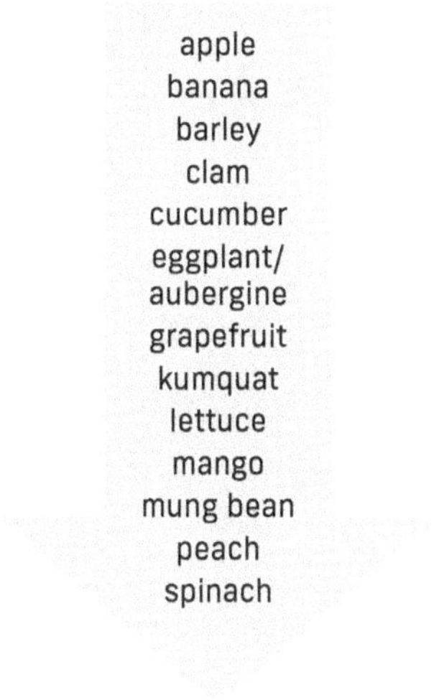

apple
banana
barley
clam
cucumber
eggplant/
aubergine
grapefruit
kumquat
lettuce
mango
mung bean
peach
spinach

Figure 11: Downward-Moving Foods

CHAPTER 3

Foundations of Nutrition

The Anatomy of Nutrition: Simply Complicated

Food should be one of the simpler things in our lives, don't you think? We need food for its calories, vitamins, minerals, and other essential compounds, and nature supplies what we need, though most of us no longer need to chase after and kill our food or travel great distances on foot to forage for it. For those of us lucky enough to have access, we have a bounty of options in one large, brightly lit space—organized by category and conveniently labeled. And, we even have people offering to tell us what to eat, when to eat what, and how to prepare and serve it.

And that's the problem. So many choices. So many opposing opinions.

Before you can understand nutrition, it's important to get to know some of the foundations. Just as a Traditional Chinese Medicine provider should have a strong understanding of human anatomy and biology, in addition to knowing the acupuncture meridians and points, so too should we grasp the "anatomy" of nutrition prior to delving in TCM food cures.

Note: In my listing of foods that are good sources of each nutrient, it is just a listing, not an indicator that you should eat that particular food, especially if you know you have challenges with that food item. For example, dairy is an excellent source of calcium, but it is not suitable for everyone. Additionally, there are many considerations you may want to make, like if it's organic, from grass-fed cows, from other ruminant sources like sheep or goat, the amount of fat in it, and its pasteurization.

So, let's get down to the basics. Let's pull it all apart first before putting it all back together. What is food?

The Building Blocks
Macronutrients

Macronutrients are those nutrients—carbohydrates, proteins, and fats—that provide calories (energy) that we need. "Macro" means big, signifying here that we need these nutrients in large quantities, though, for many, our problem now more often stems from getting too much.

What's a Calorie?

Everyone knows what a calorie is, right? It's the thing that you count and limit when dieting, right? It's the thing you try to pile on when you're the skinny kid trying to bulk up, right?

Well, yes. And not entirely.

A calorie is actually the amount of energy that is needed to increase the temperature of one gram of water by one degree Celsius at a pressure of one atmosphere (say what?!). The world calorie comes from the Latin word "calor," which means heat.

But that's no longer how we define it. That definition is now more commonly called a joule.

What we now more commonly call a calorie is actually a "Calorie" with a capital C. It is 1000 of those original small "c" calories. Each food calorie is technically a kilocalorie (kcal).

However, if you had skipped this sidebar altogether, you'd still be right in continuing to call a calorie (with a small c) the energy that food gives you. In the common world, outside of labs, we've essentially given up the word's original meaning and we mean food calories whenever we refer to "calorie."

Carbohydrates

We often call them carbs. We've nicknamed them, shortening their name, as if doing so makes them our buddies, our friend we reach for when we're feeling down or lonely. It's a complicated relationship. We love carbs. We hate carbs. We blame carbs. We need carbs.

Carbs can invoke feelings for many, but they are just one of the most abundant sources of energy for our bodies, providing 4 Calories per gram.

Carbohydrates are generally broken down into simple carbohydrates (one or two sugars strung together) and complex carbohydrates (three or more sugars strung together). A carb family tree (see Figure 12) can give you a better overall picture, but just like any family tree, it can start to get complicated, and much of the for-general-public nutritional information available is over-simplified, and thus not quite accurate. I've tried to strike a balance between accurate and not overly confusing. Trust me, that's not easy!

Origin Story

Are you a word geek like me? Then perhaps you'd like to know where the word "carbohydrate" came from.

Carbohydrates are biological molecules made up of carbon, hydrogen, and oxygen. Because there are usually twice as many hydrogen atoms as oxygen atoms, just like water (H_2O), they have been named "hydrates of carbon"—or carbohydrates.

Cool, right?

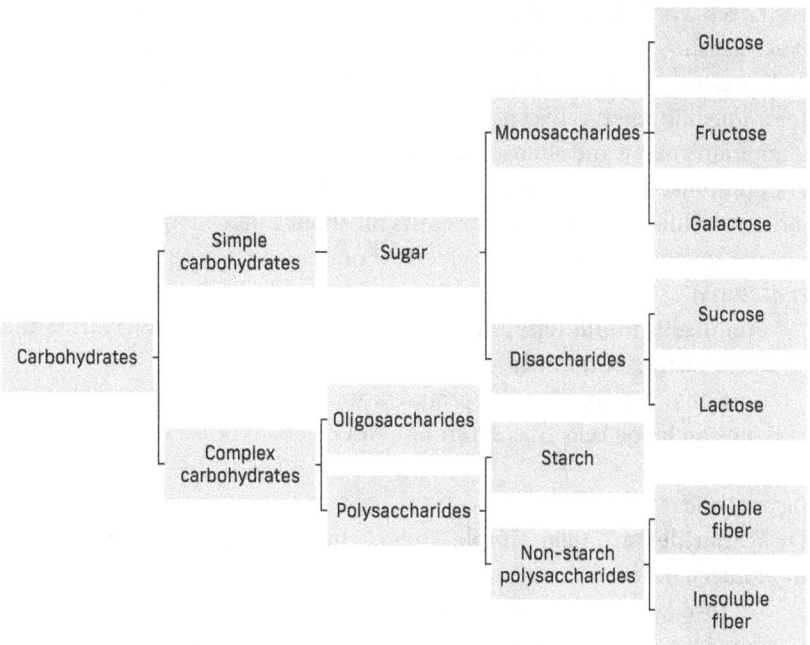

Figure 12: Carbohydrate Family Lineage

Simple Carbohydrates
Sugar

Sugars are found in every living organism, as they are vital sources of energy and form part of the backbone of DNA molecules. So, if you tell someone they're sweet, you're kind of being literal! Simple sugars are either monosaccharides or disaccharides.

Although carbs have become part of the line of usual suspects when people look for the culprit guilty of causing weight gain and a slew of health issues and symptoms, sugar has become villainized as the most evil of the carb family. All families have their "good" and their "bad," their helpful and their destructive members. Keep in mind that some healthy foods naturally contain sugar, including fruits and vegetables. Other foods with "refined sugars" provide calories but not vitamins, minerals, or other beneficial nutrients, so they are called empty calories. You'll likely recognize them by their brightly colored packages that are designed to entice, though they sometimes hide under the cloak of healthy food.

Monosaccharides

Monosaccharides are the simplest forms of sugar.

Glucose is the most common monosaccharide, and its name comes from the Greek word *glukus*, meaning "sweet." Unfortunately, if you eat too much *glukus*, it shows on your *tukus* (Yiddish word for buttocks). The "-ose" suffix indicates sugar. Once absorbed into the bloodstream, glucose can be used for immediate energy. Except for prolonged periods of starvation, glucose is your brain's major and almost only source of energy. Your brain doesn't store energy (unlike the *tukus*), so to function well, it needs a continuous source of glucose. While the brain only accounts for about 2 percent of the total body weight, it consumes about 20 percent of our glucose energy (Mergenthaler *et al.*, 2013).

Fructose is found naturally in fruits, vegetables, and honey. It is the sweetest-tasting of the sugars.

Galactose is found in milk products and sugar beets and is part of the antigens on blood cells that determine ABO blood types.

Disaccharides

Disaccharides are also simple sugars, but they are made from two monosaccharides.

Sucrose, whose name comes from the Latin word *sucrum* for "sugar," is the most recognized disaccharide, and it is commonly known as table sugar. Sucrose is made up of the monosaccharides glucose and fructose, and can be quickly broken down into these components for rapid absorption into the bloodstream. Sucrose is found in large quantities in sugar beets and sugarcane. It is also often found in high quantities in hyper little kids. My little (he's an adult now and bigger than me, but I still think of him as little) cousin used to say that he'd go "crazy off the wall"—his wording for hyperactive—if he ate red dye or too much sugar.

Lactose is a disaccharide consisting of the monosaccharides galactose and glucose. It is found in mammalian milk and is broken down by the enzyme lactase. You can blame lactose if you've had to give up ice cream and milk-shakes because you produce insufficient lactase and are lactose intolerant.

Maltose is a disaccharide made up of two molecules of glucose. Germinating grain, such as barley, contains maltose, also known as malt sugar, and it is important for the brewing of beer (and thus also beer bellies and some bar brawls).

Complex Carbohydrates

Complex carbohydrates contain three or more sugar molecules that are strung together in long, complex chains. Considered the "good guys" in the carbohydrate family, they are found in whole plant foods alongside lots of vitamins and minerals. Fruits, vegetables, legumes, and grains are good sources of complex carbs.

Oligosaccharides

Oligosaccharides have not received as much attention as their carbohydrate family members: sugars, starches, and fiber. Oligosaccharides contain 3 to 10 (though some sources state 3 to 9) sugar molecules. "Oligo" comes from the Greek word for "few." Oligosaccharides are divided into two even longer name divisions, fructo-oligosaccharides (FOS) and galacto-oligosaccharides (GOS). Thank goodness for acronyms! Found in plant foods like legumes, asparagus, onions, chicory root, and barley, many oligosaccharides are not well absorbed in the small intestine.

Although about 90 percent of oligosaccharides avoid digestion in the small intestine, once they reach the large intestine, they have a different role to play. They become prebiotics. You've likely heard of probiotics (beneficial bacteria in the body), but maybe you've not heard as much about prebiotics, the food of probiotics. Prebiotics from oligosaccharides (also from resistant starches and fermentable fiber) support the growth of probiotics.

Because oligosaccharides are poorly digested, they may cause digestive distress for some, and those people may benefit from following the FODMAP diet (see Chapter 8: Food Allergies, Sensitivities, and Intolerances).

Polysaccharides
Starches

Starch is the energy storage form for most green plants. They store much of the starch in their roots, fruits, or grains, so starch is found in the highest amounts in root and tuber vegetables like potatoes and yams, whole grains like wheat and rice, and also in corn. These foods have become staple foods in many areas of the world—rice in Asia, maize (corn) in Central America, and taro in the Pacific Islands, for example—because they are generally widely available in the region, grow well, and store easily.

Starch must be broken down in the body into glucose before it can be used for energy. Whatever is not used right away is stored in the form of glycogen in the liver or muscles. Once those stores are full, glucose is then stored as body fat.

Starchy foods have formed the basis of some healthy diets, offering readily available sources of calories, and also providing vitamins and minerals. It's important, however, to consider individual needs when choosing how many or how much of these foods to include in your diet. That's the whole point of this book, after all!

Non-Starch Polysaccharides

Non-starch polysaccharide is not an easy term to remember, or to market as part of a nutritious diet. More commonly termed *dietary fiber*, it includes cellulose, hemicellulose, and pectins (though it gets complicated here with the terminology often expanding and changing).

If sugar is considered the "bad boy" in the carbohydrate family, then fiber is treated like the "golden child." You probably know fiber as the thing that you know you should eat more of, but that doesn't seem that appetizing. It's generally not something that your taste buds will crave because it has no taste. Plus, though you have to make the effort to eat it, it leaves your body mostly undigested.

So, what's the point?

Fiber helps support digestive health, regulate blood sugar fluctuations, lower elevated cholesterol, help eliminate toxic waste products from the body, prevent colon cancer, and more.

Dietary fibers are most commonly divided into soluble and insoluble fibers. It's not a perfect division (what in the world is?), but here are some of the benefits and types of food that provide each of these categories. Most whole plant foods contain a mix of both soluble and insoluble fibers.

Soluble fiber attracts water, so it turns to a gel when it enters your body, thus slowing your digestive process. Note that if you are supplementing with psyllium husk or any other soluble fiber product, make sure to consume it with a lot of water. Because it creates a gel, insufficient water will make it act more like a plug, causing constipation—uh-oh!

- Although fiber is commonly thought of as something that "makes you go," because it slows the speed of digestion, it also helps manage diarrhea and loose stools.
- It helps regulate blood sugar levels.

- It lowers total cholesterol and low-density lipoprotein (LDL) cholesterol.
- It reduces the risk of getting intestinal ulcers.
- It may increase the number of healthy bacteria in the colon.
- It provides a feeling of satiation (feel full) without added caloric count.

To get more soluble fiber in your diet, include:

- oats/oat bran
- psyllium husk
- other grains like barley, bran, brown rice, and rye
- black beans, navy beans, kidney beans, and other beans
- tofu, edamame
- vegetables like asparagus, beets/beetroot, collard greens, broccoli, Brussels sprouts, eggplant/aubergine, green beans, peas, sweet potato, turnip
- fruits like apples, apricots, avocado, figs, pears, plums, prunes
- almonds, chia seeds, flax seeds, hazelnuts, sunflower seeds.

Insoluble fiber does not bind itself to water and turn to gel, like the soluble fiber, but it does absorb water while moving through the digestive system, making for an easier passage. Insoluble fiber is found in many whole foods, but the highest amounts are often found in the parts of the foods that are tougher to chew, like cabbage, onions, bell peppers, and the skin of apples, cucumbers, and grapes.

- It promotes regular bowel movements.
- Because it absorbs water, it adds bulk to the stool to relieve constipation.
- Speeding intestinal transit time helps it move toxic waste through the colon more quickly.
- It assists in blood sugar regulation.
- By optimizing intestinal pH, it helps prevent colon cancer.
- It may increase the number of healthy bacteria in the colon.
- It provides a feeling of satiation (feel full) without added caloric count.

To get more insoluble fiber in your diet, include:

- wheat bran
- most whole grains, including barley, millet, rye

- most legumes, including kidney beans, lentils, navy beans, and pinto beans
- most vegetables, including broccoli, carrots, kale, okra, peas, potatoes, spinach, sweet potatoes, squash, and turnip
- dried fruits, including dates and prunes
- berries, peels of apples, apricots, pears, and plums
- almonds, flax seeds, hazelnuts, sunflower seeds, and walnuts.

Fats

"Low fat," "No fat," "Fat-free."

These were labels that once proudly adorned package after package lining our grocery store shelves. Fingers of blame were pointed squarely at fats for our escalating problems with obesity and many of its associated health issues, particularly cardiovascular diseases. So, on our doctors' advice, we cut back on dietary fat.

"Fat-free" became our mantra, and we anticipated dropping the pounds and seeing obesity become a thing of our past. But it didn't happen. Obesity rates climbed.

Look at Figure 13. Starting in 1977, the American government started telling people to eat less fat. Throughout the 1980s, the number of low-fat and fat-free products was on a steep incline. We thought that "low-fat" equaled healthy. The problem is that as we started getting access to more low-fat foods, the companies making those foods increased the products' simple carbohydrate quantity. That is what later brought on the "low-carb" craze. So what are our guidelines regarding dietary fat?

We still don't know the definitive answer. Scientists and nutritionists can't seem to come to agreement. In fact, with the publication of just one guest editorial article in 2011 on "The importance of reducing SFA [saturated fatty acids] to limit CHD [coronary heart disease]" in the *British Journal of Nutrition* (Pedersen *et al.*, 2011a), many well-referenced back-and-forth retorts and defense responses have ensued (Hoenselaar, 2011, 2012; Pedersen *et al.*, 2011b; Ravnskov *et al.*, 2012).

Fat provides the biggest caloric hit per gram, at 9 Cal/g. But it also creates a feeling of satiation—it helps you feel full for longer, as it does not provide the same quick blood sugar as most carbohydrates. Fats are also needed for the absorption of the fat-soluble vitamins A, D, E, and K.

Some might say that fats can be classified as "the Good, the Bad, and the Ugly."

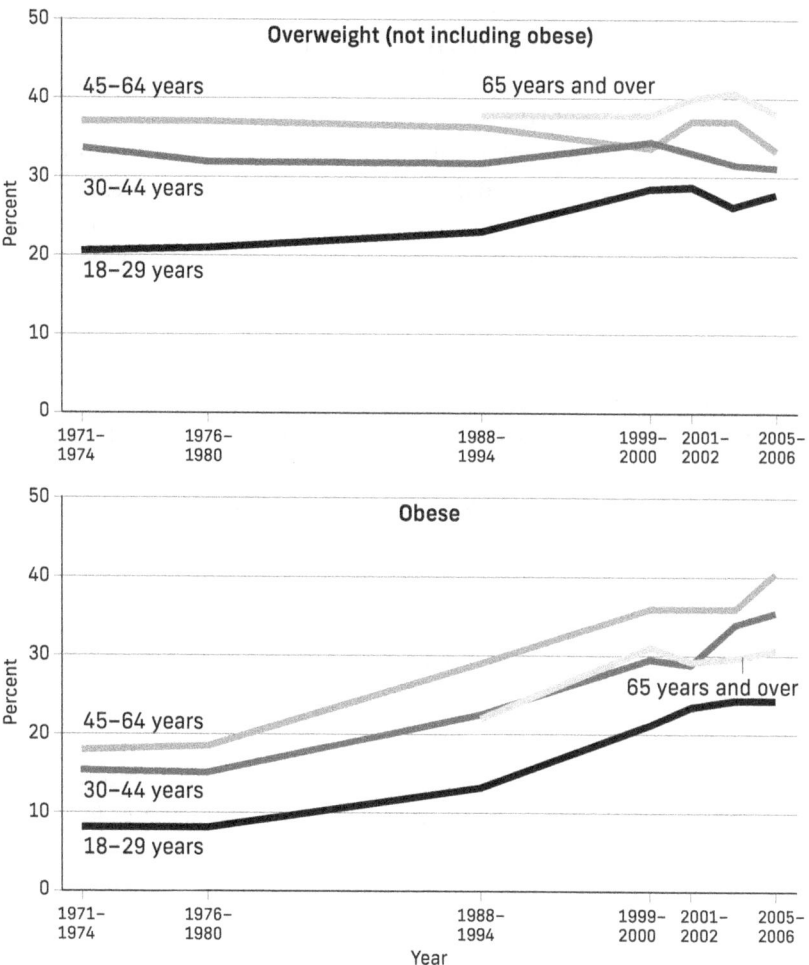

Figure 13: Percentage Overweight or Obese Over Years

SOURCE: NATIONAL CENTER FOR HEALTH STATISTICS (2009)

Unsaturated Fats—the Good

The saturation of fats doesn't refer to how deeply the grease from your burger settles in when you accidentally dribble it on your shirt. Saturation refers to the type of chemical bonds. Remember basic chemistry? Me neither (but shhhh, don't tell my dad as he has a PhD in chemistry and spent a lot of time helping me with my science homework when I was a kid).

If you want to, you can read the more detailed science part in the box below, but if you'd rather skip that, what you really need to know is that the basic building blocks of fats are fatty acids. How many carbon atoms in a chain of fatty acids, the type of bonds between the carbons, and how many hydrogen atoms there are all determine the type of fat.

Unsaturated fats are sometimes called the "good fats." (Isn't it funny how we always like to classify things as "good" or "bad"?)

One thing to keep in mind with unsaturated fats is that they are light sensitive, so keep them stored in glass containers that are shaded or store them in a dark place. Cool temperatures are better too, as they are heat sensitive as well. The more unsaturated the fat, the less stable, so some (essential fatty acids, for example) need to be kept refrigerated.

Chemistry of Fat

Fat is composed of carbon, oxygen, and hydrogen (Figure 14). Each of those atoms has sites for binding to another atom. Carbon has four binding sites, oxygen has two, and hydrogen has one.

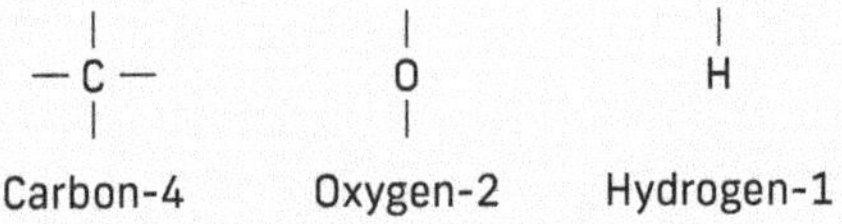

$$-\overset{|}{\underset{|}{C}}-\qquad \overset{|}{\underset{|}{O}}\qquad \overset{|}{H}$$

Carbon-4   Oxygen-2   Hydrogen-1

Figure 14: Carbon, Oxygen, Hydrogen

When only one atom binds at a binding site, this is called a saturated bond. When two binding sites are taken by one atom, it is called an unsaturated bond (see Figure 15).

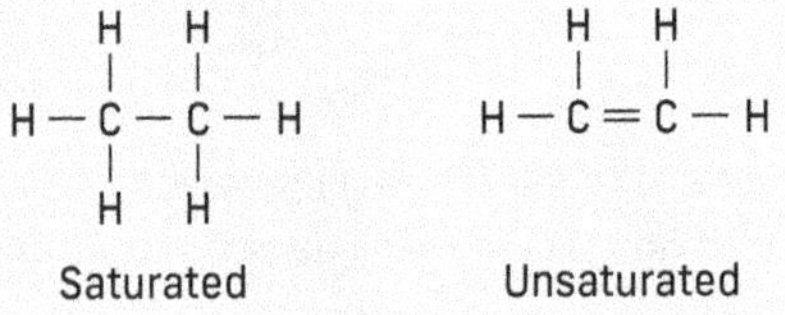

$$H-\overset{\overset{\displaystyle H}{|}}{\underset{\underset{\displaystyle H}{|}}{C}}-\overset{\overset{\displaystyle H}{|}}{\underset{\underset{\displaystyle H}{|}}{C}}-H \qquad H-\overset{\overset{\displaystyle H}{|}}{C}=\overset{\overset{\displaystyle H}{|}}{C}-H$$

Saturated   Unsaturated

Figure 15: Saturated and Unsaturated Bonds

Although the image here is drawn in a straight line, where there is an unsaturated bond, the molecule tends to bend. Because the chains bend, they can't pack in as closely, so unsaturated fats are liquid at room temperature.

Fats are made up of fatty acids, which are a string of carbon atoms, holding "hands" (bonds) in a chain, hydrogen atoms on each carbon, and an acid group (called carboxyl) on one end (Figure 16).

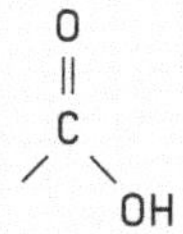

Figure 16: Carboxyl Group

Where there is one unsaturated bond in the fatty acid chain, it is called a monounsaturated fat. Where there is more than one unsaturated bond, it is called a polyunsaturated fat (see Figure 17).

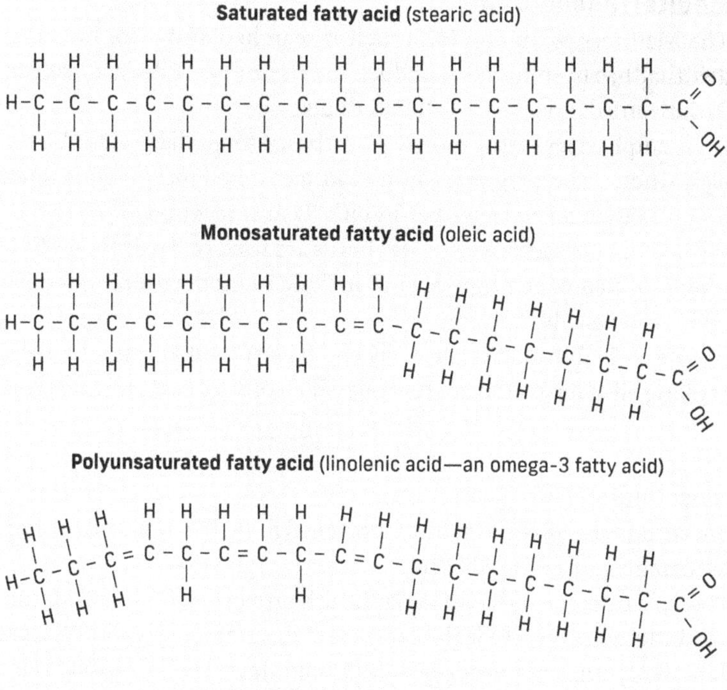

Saturated fatty acid (stearic acid)

Monosaturated fatty acid (oleic acid)

Polyunsaturated fatty acid (linolenic acid—an omega-3 fatty acid)

Figure 17: Fatty Acids

Monounsaturated Fats

Monounsaturated fats have just one unsaturated bond. The only thing we seem to like as much as labeling things as "good" or "bad" is making acronyms. Monounsaturated fats are sometimes referred to as MUFAs.

Monounsaturated fats have been shown to lower the risk of heart disease and stroke, improve blood cholesterol levels, reduce the risk of breast cancer, help stabilize blood sugar and insulin levels, and support healthy weight loss.

Examples of foods that are high in monounsaturated fats include:

- olive oil
- sesame oil
- canola oil
- peanut oil
- safflower oil
- avocados
- many nuts and seeds.

Mediterranean Diet

The Mediterranean diet is a much-researched and recommended diet that has been found to reduce the risk of heart disease, cancer, Parkinson's disease, and Alzheimer's disease.

It emphasizes eating mostly plant-based foods like fruits, vegetables, whole grains, legumes, nuts, and seeds. Red meat is consumed no more than a few times per month. Fish is recommended two to three times per week. Spices and herbs are used to flavor foods, limiting salt. Red wine is optional to include in moderation. And olive oil is used heavily.

Although olive oil is a healthy and flavorful oil, it is not the best cooking oil. Keep reading to find out which oils are best for which use.

Polyunsaturated Fats

Polyunsaturated fats, conveniently shortened to PUFAs, are fats that include more than one unsaturated bond.

Polyunsaturated fats have similar health properties as monounsaturated fats, and additionally include the category of essential fatty acids (EFAs). EFAs are fats that your body needs but can't manufacture. That's why they are essential to our diet. The most talked about EFAs are omega-3 and omega-6 fatty acids.

Examples of foods that are high in polyunsaturated fats include:

- corn oil
- fatty fish (e.g., salmon, tuna, cod, halibut, sardines, herring, mackerel)
- flax seeds, flaxseed oil
- safflower oil
- soybean oil
- sunflower seeds

- walnuts.

Saturated Fats—the Bad(?)

Saturated fat is solid at room temperature because all the bonds between the carbons are single bonds, which allows the fatty acid chain to be straight and lets the chains sit closely together. Saturated fats have long been considered the "bad fats." You'll find these fats in:

- animal fat (you can easily see it in meats like beef, lamb, and pork)
- poultry skin
- lard
- cream, butter, cheese, milk
- many baked goods
- fried foods
- palm oil
- palm kernel oil
- coconut oil
- avocado.

Saturated fats have been blamed for raising cholesterol and contributing to heart disease. Even the vegetable source saturated fats have been frowned upon.

However, coconut oil, though highly caloric, actually increases your metabolism, helping you to burn fat faster. It has also been researched for its ability to decrease excessive abdominal fat (Assunção et al., 2009) and lower blood cholesterol (Nevin and Rajamohan, 2004), counter to our notion about the evils of all foods high in saturated fats.

While we were in the midst of a "fat war," with health professionals recommending everything low-fat, awareness started to arise in the scientific world that there seemed to be a problem with the idea that saturated fats were at fault. How was it that the French somehow manage to eat a lot of saturated fats and dietary cholesterol, while still showing low rates of coronary artery disease? They called this the "French Paradox" (Ferrières, 2004). It's been theorized that the love of red wine in France may have abated the heart health issues. However, it is interesting to note that they also eat a whole load of fresh vegetables, fruit, and whole grains, and that's likely also part of the picture.

Trans Fatty Acids—the Ugly

These are definitely the ugly. Although some meat and dairy products naturally contain small amounts of trans fats, most trans fats are man-made. Because unsaturated fats are less stable and more likely to spoil, scientists (in what seemed at the time like a good idea) processed the fats to make them more stable. They chemically forced hydrogen into omega-6 polyunsaturated oils in a process known as hydrogenation (more accurately named "partial hydrogenation"). This makes those supposedly healthy fats less likely to spoil, but unfortunately also creates some significant health issues.

The body has a hard time trying to metabolize trans fats, causing them to contribute to heart disease; they may also increase the risk of diabetes (Willett and Mozaffarian, 2007) and of cancer (Slattery *et al.*, 2001).

It goes almost without saying that we should avoid hydrogenated (or partially hydrogenated) oils so that we can limit our intake of these ugly trans fats. Commonly hydrogenated fats and sources of these fats include:

- store-bought baked goods: cakes, cookies, crackers, and pie crusts often contain shortening, which is normally made using hydrogenated vegetable oil
- fried food: deep-fried foods like fried chicken, french fries, and donuts
- margarine and creamer: you're better to use real butter and real cream
- refrigerator dough: I used to love popping open the Pillsbury dough containers (remember how you'd whack the side on a table or counter and then twist it open and it would "pop"?), but these are sadly really unhealthy with their "partially hydrogenated soybean and/or cottonseed oil," not to mention the high-fructose corn syrup, artificial flavor, and other chemical ingredients
- so many convenience foods: chips, microwave popcorn, frozen meals, instant mashed potatoes, etc.

Check your labels, as not all these foods use partially hydrogenated oils. Better yet, limit your processed foods all round!

How Do I Store My Oils?

As with almost all food products (honey is an odd exception), oils can go rancid. Depending on the type of oil, some will spoil faster than others, so it's important to know how to properly store them, and how to identify oils that have gone bad (not to the dark side—as you'll see, oils generally stay "good" longer in the dark).

Rancid oil smells different—sharp, bitter, or unpleasant. I think it tastes like Playdough, but others might say it tastes like crayons or putty. Keep in mind that the "best before" date may not tell the whole story. If you have an open half-used bottle of olive oil that has been sitting for a while, smell it to see if it's still okay. The air in the bottle is called "headspace," and oxidation from that air causes free radicals (usually "free" is a positive word, but not in this context) that can cause us health damage if consumed regularly. You won't likely get sick from just a few doses, but the taste will also be altered, potentially ruining the flavor of your food.

Heat, oxygen, and light are all enemies of oil. The more saturated the oil, the more stable it is. This is why coconut oil makes a good cooking oil and is often jarred in clear containers, while olive oil makes a better salad oil and comes in dark glass bottles. The most sensitive oils are the essential oils and polyunsaturated fats. They often have to be stored in the fridge.

I know it's convenient to have your cooking oils stored on or around your stove, but if they are exposed to heat, they will deteriorate more quickly.

Check your oil containers to find out how they should be stored, but here are some general rules.

Keep in the Fridge

Polyunsaturated oils are best kept in the fridge once opened. Some of these oils may become more solid and cloudy while being stored in the fridge. If they do, remove them from your fridge and leave at room temperature for an hour or two before use.

- flaxseed oil
- grapeseed oil (can be stored at room temperature—assuming your room is less than 21°C (70°F)—for up to three months or in the fridge for up to six months)
- hazelnut oil (same as grapeseed oil)
- hemp oil
- safflower oil
- sunflower oil
- truffle oil
- walnut oil (same as grapeseed oil)

Keep in a Cool, Dark Place

Some of these oils can also be kept in the fridge to keep them lasting longer, though because of their higher quantity of saturated bonds, they are more likely to become solid.

- avocado oil
- coconut oil (very stable, this oil is often solid or semi-solid at room temperature)
- macadamia nut oil (though high in polyunsaturated fats, it is also naturally high in antioxidants that help keep it stable)
- olive oil
- peanut oil

Proteins

Proteins are the building blocks of the tissues of your body. In fact, you contain at least 10,000 different proteins—they make up your muscles, skin, hair, blood, enzymes, DNA, and more.

Proteins are broken down into 21 standard **amino acids**. Nine of those amino acids are essential—we need to eat them—as our bodies can't make them. We found this out because scientists fed rats only corn protein for some time, and all the rats got sick. When they added milk protein, the rats recovered, but without that, they died (awful, I know). The corn was lacking some amino acids that the milk provided.

Nonessential amino acids are ones that our bodies can produce, even if we don't get them from our food. Conditional amino acids are not usually essential unless we are ill or stressed.

Amino Acids

Essential amino acids:

- histidine, isoleucine, leucine, lysine, methionine, phenylalanine, threonine, tryptophan, and valine

Nonessential amino acids:

- alanine, asparagine, aspartic acid, and glutamic acid

Conditional amino acids:

- arginine, cysteine, glutamine, glycine, ornithine, proline, serine, and tyrosine

For a long time, people worried whether they would get enough of all the amino acids if they didn't eat animal-source foods. But while non-meat sources of food may not each contain all the amino acids, combining foods can easily help us meet our needs. This is called eating "complementary proteins." For example, grains are low in the amino acid lysine (called a "limiting amino acid"), while the limiting amino acid in some legumes is methionine. So eating grains and beans together ensures the full range of essential amino acids. You can also make up a complete protein by combining legumes with nuts or seeds or by choosing the vegan-friendly complete protein foods quinoa, buckwheat, or soy.

Myth Busting: Vegetarians and Vegans Can't Get Enough Protein

For a long time, vegetarians and vegans have been warned that they are not getting enough protein. The Harvard educational website page on protein states, "Vegetarians need to be aware of this. People who don't eat meat, fish, poultry, eggs, or dairy products need to eat a variety of protein-containing foods each day in order to get all the amino acids needed to make new protein."

In 1971, Frances Moore Lappé wrote a book called *Diet for a Small Planet*. As a sociologist, she was trying to end world hunger by using vegetable protein instead of animal protein, as the former involves less waste. She wrote about the theory of protein complementing, which she has since modified in light of new awareness about amino acid storage.

It was once believed that athletes would not be able to get enough protein from a vegetarian or vegan diet. More and more high-level and professional athletes are now doing just that. Of course, they are not eating only bread, pasta, and bananas.

The good news is that it's really not that hard to get enough protein from a vegetarian, or even vegan, diet. Your body can store amino acids for later use. So, while it's important to eat a range of foods, you don't have to stress over which amino acids are the limiting ones in each food.

When amino acids are strung together into long chains (like beads on a necklace), then looped, spiraled, and zigzagged to form three-dimensional shapes, they become proteins. Those shaped strands can be combined with other strands to make even bigger proteins.

Like carbohydrates, proteins contain 4 Calories per gram.

Micronutrients

"Micro" may be thought of as less important than something labeled "macro," but though they are only needed in small amounts in relation to macronutrients, micronutrients are vitally important. Vitamins and minerals are micronutrients, and without them we wouldn't function.

When I first started the chapter on nutrition basics, I thought it would be a relatively short discussion. However, as you'll soon see, it's a big topic! I decided to include some foundational information about the vitamins and minerals in food, even though TCM never considered these individual components, because we want to be able to identify possible deficiencies or excesses. If someone is eating a complete and whole diet, is relatively healthy, and leads a balanced life, it may not be important to pay attention to these individual nutrients. However, there are many who eat a limited diet, whose digestive systems are impaired, who have poor health, who have deficiencies because of lifestyle choices (e.g., smoking, alcohol, drugs, extreme physical activities), who take medications, who are pregnant, or who are very young or elderly, leading to a need to make food and supplement choices to meet nutrient requirements.

Vitamins

Vitamins are organic compounds that you need to get from an outside source (usually food) because your body cannot make it in sufficient quantities. There are 13 vitamins, nine of which are water-soluble and four that are fat-soluble.

Water-Soluble Vitamins

These are vitamins that dissolve in water and are excreted easily from your body. Because your body doesn't store them readily, they need to be consumed regularly. Vitamin C and all the B vitamins fit this category.

Vitamin C: Ascorbic Acid

Detailed information about vitamin C and its benefits can and already has taken up a whole book, but we'll leave that to Linus Pauling's followers to get into details. In case you don't know, Linus Pauling was a double Nobel Prize winner (for chemistry and for peace) who, among many other things, studied the health benefits of taking vitamin C in high quantities.

The main functions of vitamin C are:

- produces collagen, a protein essential for making skin, blood vessels, tendons, ligaments, cartilage, bones, teeth, corneas, and more
- heals wounds
- forms scar tissue
- helps absorb iron
- protects against free radicals, as it is a powerful antioxidant that can help prevent cellular damage
- makes some neurotransmitters—chemicals that communicate with your brain and nervous system to relay messages of thoughts, feelings, and commands—including serotonin.

Vitamin C deficiency most recognizably causes the disease called **scurvy** (see box), but can also lead to a lot of health issues, including (to name a few):

- poor wound healing
- easy bruising
- poor immune function
- irritability
- anorexia
- alopecia
- non-alcoholic fatty liver disease.

Odd Bits of Trivia About Vitamin C
Sickly Sailors

Vitamin C is probably the most recognized vitamin, with most people being able to identify at least a few vitamin-C-rich foods. But prior to its discovery in the 1930s, people didn't know why sailors away at sea for long periods of time would suffer from swollen and bleeding gums, loose teeth, poor wound healing, and hemorrhaging under the skin—a disease known as scurvy.

Because they didn't have access to fresh fruit and vegetables, scurvy was a major cause of disability and death on long voyages. Danish sailors knew to bring lemons and limes with them, but British mariners didn't do so until the mid-1700s when they started to bring lime juice on board—thus the derogatory (so don't use it) name, Limey, sometimes used for British.

In university, I was able to observe the start of scurvy firsthand in one of my friends. Living in a co-ed dorm, a group of us shared a kitchen which was often full of unwashed dishes, pots, and pans. Since one friend didn't want to have to spend much time either shopping for food or making meals, he stuck with the university's four food groups: KD (short for Kraft Dinner to Canadians—I know Kraft has made more than macaroni and cheese, but this is their most famous food by far), ramen noodles, hot dogs, and ketchup. Oh, and beer. So five food groups. This is all I saw him ever eat for months. When he started to complain that his gums were bleeding when he brushed them, I asked him if he had had any fruit or vegetables of late. He had not. Crazy but true. After a few days of including an orange or two, his gums stopped bleeding.

Evolutionary Evidence

As humans, we need to consume vitamin C to survive. So too do our primate cousins, our evolutionary ancestors. At some point in history, one of the genes that helped our ancient relatives to make vitamin C mutated (Drouin, Godin, and Page, 2011). We still have that gene, but our bodies can't turn the gene on to make it active. Thus, we have to eat vitamin C, while our pet dogs, cats, elephants (not sure my strata will approve that one!), and other pet and non-pet mammals won't get scurvy. They can make their own vitamin C.

Interestingly, two other mammals—bats and guinea pigs—also can't make vitamin C, but it's a different mutation that caused that.

Oops! Too Much!

Although high doses of vitamin C (1000–10,000 mg) can be well tolerated, you'll likely discover you've had too much when you reach what's called "bowel tolerance." Yup, that is what you probably think it is. Get too much and you'll end up with diarrhea, as your body eliminates excesses.

Of course, it's impossible to list all foods containing vitamin C, and most know that citrus fruits are a good source, but here are some that are high in this important nutrient:

- citrus fruits (oranges, lemons, limes, grapefruit)
- papaya
- kiwifruit

- strawberries, raspberries
- pineapple
- cantaloupe
- green leafy vegetables
- parsley
- broccoli
- squash
- green beans
- tomatoes
- bell peppers.

For those taking high doses or with sensitive stomachs, a buffered vitamin C, called Ester-C, may be a better option when supplementing. The Ester form uses an alkaline mineral like calcium to increase the pH of the acidic ascorbic acid.

B Vitamins

There are eight B vitamins, with six of those being numbered. Although they are important as a group—all key in energy production—each has individual functions.

Vitamin B1: Thiamin

The main functions of B1 are:

- helps the body metabolize carbohydrates, branched chain amino acids, and fatty acids into energy, providing fuel for the body
- takes part in the synthesis of DNA and RNA
- assists in muscle contraction and the conduction of nerve signals
- plays a key role in the structure and integrity of brain cells.

Thiamin deficiency was first identified in countries that began to eat a lot of polished rice (rice that removed the outer covering that contains vitamin B1). Those people developed a disease called **beriberi** (four types of beriberi—wet, dry, gastrointestinal, and infantile) with symptoms of weight loss, edema, impaired sensations, weakness and pain in the limbs, increased heart rate, heart failure, problems breathing, digestive issues, and emotional disturbances.

Another disease associated with thiamin deficiency is **Wernicke's disease** or **Wernicke's encephalopathy**, a neurological disorder that causes abnormal involuntary eye movements, problems with voluntary coordination of muscle movements, imbalance, and confusion.

Korsakoff syndrome is a chronic disease that may follow an episode of Wernicke's disease. Most commonly caused by alcohol misuse, it can also occur with AIDS, chronic infections, poor nutrition, malabsorption, and other health issues. Symptoms include memory loss, difficulty understanding information and putting words into context, confabulation, and hallucination.

When both these two latter diseases occur together, the syndrome is called **Wernicke-Korsakoff syndrome**. Left untreated, mortality is high, but early treatment before irreversible damage has occurred can bring better outcomes.

Best sources of B1 include:

- lentils and other legumes
- asparagus
- onions
- green peas
- kale, spinach, cabbage, broccoli, Brussels sprouts
- carrots
- tomatoes, eggplant/aubergine
- mushrooms
- nuts and seeds
- whole grains
- beef liver and pork.

Vitamin B2: Riboflavin
The main functions of B2 are:

- is a basic building block for normal growth and development
- helps release energy from carbohydrates
- takes part in red blood cell production
- assists in recycling the body's antioxidant glutathione.

We All Live in a Flavus Submarine...

Riboflavin is unique among the vitamins in that you can actually see if you've eaten a lot of it in your diet or supplement form because your urine will turn bright yellow. I always try to let my patients know this if they are new to supplementing because they may otherwise think that something has gone terribly wrong when they note the dramatic change in their urine. The "flavin" in riboflavin comes from the Latin word for yellow, *flavus*.

Signs of riboflavin deficiency include:

- anemia
- swelling of mucous membranes
- mouth or lip sores
- skin disorders
- sore throat
- preeclampsia in pregnant women
- poor metabolism of vitamin B6, folate, niacin, and iron.

Vitamin B2 has also been used therapeutically to help prevent migraines. Best sources of B2 include:

- soybeans
- green leafy vegetables
- asparagus
- broccoli, Brussels sprouts, cauliflower
- peppers
- root vegetables
- squash
- beef, turkey
- salmon, sardines
- eggs
- milk
- nuts
- mushrooms
- fortified grains.

Vitamin B3: Niacin

Vitamin B3 comes in several forms, including niacin (also called nicotinic acid) and niacinamide (also called nicotinamide). Niacin is the precursor to niacinamide, and the two vitamins are incorporated into two vital coenzymes, nicotinamide adenine dinucleotide (NAD) and nicotinamide adenine dinucleotide phosphate (NADP)—say that three times fast! In short, they are needed for producing energy.

The main functions of B3 are:

- helps convert dietary carbohydrates, fats, and proteins into energy
- helps protect the body's cells from free radical damage via NAD and NADP.

Are You Blushing?

One of the most recognized vitamin side effects is the niacin flush. Because niacin dilates blood vessels, it creates a sensation of heat and causes the skin to blush. A slight niacin flush that lasts for about 15 minutes is an external sign that you've taken enough of it. Too much flush lasting too long can indicate you took too much.

Most people find that their tolerance for the flushing effect builds over time, so it's easier to start with lower doses and increase them gradually.

Another way to avoid the flush is to take niacin in a "flush-free" format, which is niacin in combination with inositol, a vitamin-like nutrient. Niacinamide also doesn't cause flushing, but it may not have all the same health benefits as niacin.

Deficiency of vitamin B3 in its severe form causes a disease called **pellagra**. Pellegra was first recorded in the 1700s after the widespread cultivation of corn in Europe, and it was again documented in the southern United States in the early 1900s. It was particularly the poor who suffered this deficiency disease because corn became a major staple of their diets. Corn actually does contain vitamin B3, but it is in a bound form not available to the digestive systems of humans. However, in Mexico, where corn is also a dietary staple, corn tortillas are traditionally prepared by soaking the corn in a lime solution before cooking it, releasing the bound niacin.

The symptoms of pellagra are called the three Ds—dermatitis, diarrhea, and dementia—though not all three symptoms are needed for diagnosis. If left untreated, a fourth D can occur. Death. The word pellagra comes from the Italian words *pelle agra*, meaning raw skin and referring to the scaly, darkly pigmented rash that develops when exposed to sunlight. Digestive symptoms include a bright red tongue from inflammation, constipation, vomiting, abdominal pain, and then diarrhea, which further aggravates the nutritional deficiencies. Although dementia is one of the Ds, headaches, depression, disorientation, memory loss, and fatigue are more common.

Niacin specifically, and not niacinamide, is used for treating high cholesterol and for improving blood circulation. Niacinamide is sometimes used for treatment of diabetes, both type 1 and 2. Vitamin B3 has also been studied for its potential benefits in treating schizophrenia, Alzheimer's disease, depression, attention deficit hyperactivity disorder (ADHD), alcohol dependence, osteoarthritis, cancer, and acne, among other symptoms and diseases.

Best sources of B3 include:

- tuna, salmon, sardines
- chicken, turkey, beef
- asparagus
- tomatoes, bell peppers
- sweet potato
- peanuts, sunflower seeds
- lentils
- brown rice, barley
- mushrooms.

Vitamin B5: Pantothenic Acid

The main functions of B5 are:

- plays a role in the breakdown of carbohydrates, fats, and protein for energy
- is needed for the manufacture of red blood cells
- is involved in the production of sex- and stress-related hormones
- helps maintain a healthy digestive tract
- supports the body's use of other B vitamins, especially B2
- participates in the synthesis of cholesterol.

Because pantothenic acid is plentiful in our foods, deficiency is rare. In fact, the word *pantothen* is a Greek word meaning "from all sides" or "from everywhere." However, food processing can destroy this vitamin, as it can the other B vitamins as well, so don't expect to get sufficient vitamin B5 from most fast food or junk food!

There is some evidence that vitamin B5 may help lower LDL (bad cholesterol) and triglycerides and raise HDL (good cholesterol) in those with high cholesterol. Vitamin B5 has also been called the "anti-stress" vitamin because of its involvement with manufacturing stress-related hormones, but there is no evidence that taking it reduces stress. Too bad because taking a B5 pill would be a lot easier than making lifestyle changes!

Best sources of B5 include:

- brewer's yeast
- cauliflower, broccoli, kale
- mushrooms
- avocados
- tomato
- potato, sweet potato
- legumes

- egg yolks
- beef, turkey, duck, chicken, organ meats
- whole grains (though milling can remove a lot).

Vitamin B6: Pyridoxine

Vitamin B6 comes in six forms: pyridoxine, pyridoxal, pyridoxamine, pyridoxal 5′-phosphate (PLP), pyridoxamine 5′-phosphate (PMP), and pyridoxine 5′-phosphate (PNP).

The main functions of B6 are:

- helps with protein, carbohydrate, and fat breakdown for energy
- is needed for red blood cell formation
- assists in synthesis of important brain neurotransmitters, including GABA, dopamine, and serotonin
- is involved in the formation of the myelin sheath, a layer that covers nerve cells and is needed for nerve signal transmission
- maintains normal levels of homocysteine, an amino acid found in the blood that may be involved with cardiovascular disease and Alzheimer's disease (along with B12 and folic acid)
- supports a healthy immune system.

Common signs of vitamin B6 deficiency include:

- cracking at the corners of the mouth
- dermatitis
- swollen tongue
- microcytic anemia
- depression and confusion
- convulsive seizures in newborns.

Deficiencies most often occur in alcoholics, smokers, and those who are obese or who have hyperthyroidism, kidney disease, Crohn's, ulcerative colitis, or celiac disease. It is also more common in pregnant women, especially with preeclampsia or eclampsia. Over time, some medications—including some antiepileptic drugs, theophylline (a medication for lung disease), and cycloserine (a broad-spectrum antibiotic)—can lead to deficiency (National Institutes of Health, 2017a).

There is some evidence to suggest that supplementing vitamin B6 could help reduce premenstrual syndrome (PMS), carpal tunnel syndrome, nausea and vomiting during pregnancy, memory loss, diabetes, ADHD, acne, atherosclerosis, and asthma attacks.

Excessive supplementation with vitamin B6 can become toxic over time, resulting in nerve damage, numbness and tingling in the extremities, oversensitivity to sunlight, abdominal pain, and changes in liver function tests. It may also interfere with the Parkinson's disease treatment levodopa.

Best sources of B6 include:

- brewer's yeast
- cereal grains
- legumes
- carrots, peas, potatoes, spinach
- milk, cheese
- fish, eggs, liver
- sunflower seeds.

Vitamin B12: Cobalamin

Vitamin B12 comes in a few forms, but because all contain the mineral cobalt, they are collectively called "cobalamins." The active forms of this vitamin are methylcobalamin and 5-deoxyadenosylcobalamin. Other forms you'll find are cyanocobalamin and hydroxycobalamin, both of which need to convert into one of the first two forms to become biologically active.

The main functions of B12 are:

- helps make DNA
- forms healthy red blood cells
- keeps nerves working properly
- maintains normal levels of homocysteine, an amino acid found in the blood that may be involved with cardiovascular disease and Alzheimer's disease (along with B6 and folic acid).

To absorb vitamin B12 from food, hydrochloric acid (HCl) in the stomach must first separate B12 from the protein to which it is attached. Then, vitamin B12 combines with a protein in the stomach called intrinsic factor. If there is either insufficient HCl or intrinsic factor, then vitamin B12 absorption is impaired. In addition, vitamin B12 is found almost exclusively in animal-source foods. As a result, vitamin B12 deficiency is not uncommon, particularly in:

- vegans and others who eat no or little animal-source foods
- older adults, as HCl and intrinsic factor production decreases with age
- those with pernicious anemia, a type of anemia that causes a decrease in intrinsic factor production

- people taking medications to reduce stomach acid—proton pump inhibitors (PPI) and H2-receptor antagonists
- those taking the medications chloramphenicol (an antibiotic) or metformin (commonly used for diabetes)
- those who have a digestive disorder like celiac disease, Crohn's, or ulcerative colitis, or who have had gastrointestinal surgery.

Vitamin B12 deficiency can result in **megaloblastic anemia** as well as:

- fatigue
- weakness
- numbness and tingling in hands and feet
- constipation
- loss of appetite
- weight loss
- poor memory
- confusion
- depression
- problems with balance
- soreness in the mouth
- infant failure to thrive.

If someone is supplementing high doses of folic acid, this can also cause a vitamin B12 deficiency.

Vitamin B12 supplementation is commonly found in B complex or multivitamin supplements, but in low quantities. It can be found on its own in tablets or capsules that are swallowed, in sublingual form (tablets that are dissolved in the mouth), or in injection form. This type of shot in the arm (or buttocks) really can give you renewed energy or enthusiasm, as the expression goes, if you are deficient.

Best sources of B12 include:

- beef liver, clams
- meat, poultry, fish, eggs, milk, dairy products
- fortified breakfast cereals and other fortified foods
- nutritional yeast.

It is controversial whether we can utilize edible sea algae or chlorella as a B12 source, as these forms generally do not appear to be biologically active in our bodies.

Folate

Folate includes the naturally occurring folate found in foods, as well as the synthetic folic acid added in supplements and fortified foods.

The main functions of folate are:

- plays a key role in cell division
- is needed for the synthesis of amino acids and DNA
- helps form red blood cells
- is required for normal fetal development of the spine, brain, and skull, particularly within the first four weeks of pregnancy
- maintains normal levels of homocysteine, an amino acid found in the blood that may be involved with cardiovascular disease and Alzheimer's disease (along with B6 and B12).

Folate is now fortified in many foods because of its importance to proper fetal development, particularly when a woman may not yet know that she is pregnant. Because pregnancy results in an increased use of folate by the body for fetal growth, supplementation is recommended for women who are trying to get pregnant or who are pregnant to prevent neural tube defects like spina bifida and reduce the incidence of preterm delivery, slow fetal growth, and low infant birth weight.

Folate deficiency can cause megaloblastic anemia, resulting in:

- fatigue
- weakness
- problems with concentration
- headaches
- shortness of breath
- heart palpitations.

Deficiency can also cause canker sores and changes in skin, hair, and fingernail pigmentation.

Other causes of folate deficiency include chronic alcoholism and malabsorption health issues like Crohn's, ulcerative colitis, and celiac disease. Some medications can also interfere with folate absorption. These include methotrexate (a drug used for cancer and autoimmune disorders) and sulfasalazine (used mostly for treating ulcerative colitis). Some antiepileptic medications can reduce serum folate levels. Additionally, folic acid supplementation can interfere with antiepileptic medications. That last issue obviously makes things a bit tricky, so someone in that situation would have to consult with their medical professional.

Best sources of folate include:

- dark green vegetables
- legumes
- fortified grain products
- corn
- oranges.

Biotin

Have you ever heard of vitamin H, B7, or coenzyme R? No? Well, you're not alone. I hadn't heard it called that either, though I know plenty about biotin. Conveniently, they are one and the same, so here's an introduction to the often-forgotten B vitamin.

The main functions of biotin are:

- helps convert carbohydrates, fats, and protein into energy
- builds healthy fat in the skin
- is needed for healthy hair, eyes, liver, and nervous system
- plays an important role in normal fetal development.

Deficiency is not common but can cause:

- cracking at the corners of the mouth
- swollen red tongue
- dry eyes
- hair loss
- dermatitis
- seizures
- fatigue
- insomnia
- depression.

Some causes of biotin deficiency include long-term use of intravenous (IV) feeding devoid of biotin, anti-seizure medication, a rare hereditary disease called biotinidase deficiency, and digestive issues like Crohn's, ulcerative colitis, and celiac disease. Prolonged consumption of raw egg whites can also cause biotin deficiency because it contains a substance that binds to biotin in the large intestines, preventing it from being absorbed. I have observed biotin deficiency from this last situation, as it used to be quite popular for body builders to drink six or more raw eggs daily. There are better ways to supplement protein, if needed, so skip that disgusting mucus-like drink.

Best sources of biotin include:

- brewer's yeast
- cooked eggs, especially the yolk
- root vegetables
- legumes
- sardines
- nuts
- mushrooms.

Fat-Soluble Vitamins

Fat-soluble vitamins, logically, dissolve in fat. As a result, low-fat diets are sadly lacking in the vitamins A, D, E, and K. The good news is that the body is better able to store these vitamins, especially vitamins A and E, in the body's tissues. It is more likely, on the other hand, to have an excess of these vitamins if too much is consumed or supplemented. And in the nutrition and health world, those numbers of safe, ideal, and excessive have changed.

Vitamin A

Vitamin A is not a single nutrient but a group of related nutrients that are divided basically into two groups:

1. Preformed vitamin A are retinoids that are found in animal-source foods. The retinoids include retinol, retinal, retinoic acid, and retinyl esters—sounds like chemistry class.
2. Provitamin A carotenoids (carotenes and xanthophylls) are found in plant-source foods. Carotenes include alpha, beta, gamma, delta, epsilon, or zeta-carotene—sounds like a fraternity or sorority. You'll most likely recognize beta-carotene but may not have known about its Greek siblings. Xanthophylls include astaxanthin, beta-cryptoxanthin, canthaxanthin, fucoxanthin, neoxanthin, violaxanthin, zeaxanthin, lutein, and lycopene. About 500 carotenoids have been identified, so this is nowhere near a complete listing! You may have heard of lutein (found in supplements for eye support) and lycopene (naturally found in tomatoes and commonly included in supplements for prostate and heart health). Some of these provitamins can be converted in the body into the retinoid form of vitamin A.

The main functions of vitamin A are:

- Supports healthy vision. The name sort of gives it away. Retinoid.

Retina (layer at the back of the eye that has light-sensitive cells to carry signals to the brain). Carotenoids have also been found to help with vision. Lutein, beta-carotene, and zeaxanthin have been shown to help repair tissue in the eye that is damaged by age-related macular degeneration.

- Supports a healthy immune system. It's required to synthesize immune cells to increase immune reaction, but also helps with the immune and inflammatory "braking" system that stops the immune system from becoming overactive (e.g., allergies, autoimmune disorders).
- Is essential for normal cell growth and development.
- Maintains epithelial and mucosal tissues.
- Helps normal bone development and maintenance.
- Supports healthy reproductive systems of both men and women. Is required for proper production of sperm.
- Helps prevent cellular damage through its role as antioxidant.
- Deficiency can be serious, as a weakened immune system can allow for infections like pneumonia and measles to become deadly. It can also result in blindness, with one of the earliest signs of deficiency being night blindness. Vitamin A deficiency is most common in:
  - periods of high nutritional needs like pregnancy, lactation, infancy, and childhood, particularly in developing countries
  - those with chronic diarrhea; unfortunately, vitamin A deficiency also leads to diarrhea
  - people with cystic fibrosis
  - alcoholics: it's best to consume foods rich in vitamin A, as supplementation should be monitored when the liver is not functioning well.

Best sources of vitamin A include:

For retinoids:

- organ meats like liver
- butter, cheese, dairy
- eggs
- fish.

For carotenoids:

- sweet potato, yam

- pumpkin, squash
- carrot
- Swiss chard, collard, kale, spinach
- apricot
- cantaloupe
- mango.

Vitamin D

For years, we were warned off excessive intake of vitamin D from supplemental sources. As a fat-soluble vitamin, vitamin D can be stored in the body. However, we have become increasingly aware that many of us are deficient in this nutrient, and so recommended supplemental dosages and upper intake limits have increased. Some say that those upper limits are still too conservative. And now, there's even a Vitamin D Society that's declared November as Vitamin D month, and large health organizations like the Canadian Cancer Society, the Arthritis Society, and the World Health Organization have identified that vitamin D deficiency is relatively common, particularly in the Northern hemisphere.

The main functions of vitamin D are:

- promotes calcium absorption
- supports healthy bone growth and remodeling
- modulates cell growth
- plays a role in immune function and inflammation.

When I first studied nutrition in university (more than a few years ago), almost all I learned about vitamin D was that deficiency would cause **rickets** in children and **osteomalacia** in adults. Rickets and osteomalacia are usually caused by prolonged vitamin D deficiency in children and adults, respectively, and result in a softening and weakening of bones. Now there is a lot of research investigating vitamin D's role in preventing diabetes, colorectal cancer, breast cancer, cardiovascular disease, multiple sclerosis, and more.

Vitamin D deficiency can result in:

- weaker bones
- bone deformities and pain
- hypocalcemic seizures
- dental abnormalities
- muscle weakness and spasms
- possibly higher risk for some types of cancer
- increased mortality with cancer

- possibly higher risk for heart disease
- possibly higher risk for multiple sclerosis
- increased risk for type 2 diabetes
- poorer immune system response.

Vitamin D deficiency is further augmented in those aged 50 and older, as the body's ability to convert vitamin D from sun exposure declines with age. It is also recommended for pregnant women, babies and infants, those not eating the foods listed below, and those who have limited sun exposure to supplement.

The challenge is that there are limited natural food sources of vitamin D. Best food sources of vitamin D include:

- egg yolks
- fatty fish like salmon, tuna, sardines, mackerel, and herring
- beef liver
- mushrooms: can contain some vitamin D
- fortified foods: cow's milk, goat's milk, milk alternative beverages, orange juice, yogurt, cheese, infant formula, and margarine may have vitamin D added.

Our main source of vitamin D is from the sun—the reason why vitamin D is nicknamed "the sunshine vitamin." Guess what? We were never meant to spend most of our lives indoors, working by artificial light. Humans evolved close to the equator tens of thousands of years ago, living outdoors in the sunlight, with no clothing to cover our skin. We would naturally get somewhere around 90 percent of our vitamin D through our skin. The problem is that we now have to balance sun exposure for vitamin D with risk of skin cancer and sunburn. Plus, in northern areas of the world, the UVB levels from sunlight are too weak for four to six months of the year.

Vitamin E

Vitamin E is another of those vitamins that is not just one but a family of eight vitamins. There is the "mama" alpha-tocopherol (yes, I chose the alpha to be the mom), "papa" beta-tocopherol, and their two kids, gamma-tocopherol and delta-tocopherol. And then there is a repeat of alpha, beta, gamma, and delta within the tocotrienols. Alpha-tocopherol is thought to be the most active vitamin E in our bodies, but all appear to be important. In supplement form, vitamin E is usually alpha-tocopherol alone, but labels noting "mixed vitamin E" would generally indicate all eight forms.

It's worth mentioning that, in supplement form, you can find both natural and synthetic forms of vitamin E. Most commonly, you'll see d-alpha-tocopherol as one of the natural forms. If you see an added "l" in the name, as in dl-alpha-tocopherol, that's an indication that you have a synthetic form of vitamin E, a form which is made using refined oils and is much more poorly absorbed, not staying long in the tissues.

The main functions of vitamin E are:

- It is a powerful antioxidant, protecting the body from the damaging effects of free radicals caused by aging, cigarette smoke, air pollution, UV radiation from the sun, and more. In this role, vitamin E may help prevent cancer, eye disease such as age-related macular degeneration, and cognitive impairment.
- Protects LDL cholesterol, helping to prevent atherosclerosis and cardiovascular disease.

Vitamin E deficiency is not common, but for those who are malnourished, those who cannot absorb dietary fat properly, or for premature or very low-birthweight babies, deficiency can result in neurologic symptoms, muscle weakness, damage to the retina of the eyes, greasy stools, chronic diarrhea, and inability to secrete bile.

Low vitamin E status (not true deficiency) may be more common, with a possible connection to an increased risk of miscarriage. Cigarette smokers also appear to have lower levels of vitamin E than non-smokers.

Vitamin E deficiency may cause:

- peripheral neuropathy
- ataxia
- skeletal myopathy
- retinopathy
- impaired immune response.

There may be, however, an increased risk of bleeding when vitamin E is supplemented by those on blood-thinning medications or with vitamin K deficiency. Additionally, those on statins (cholesterol-lowering drugs) are recommended not to take more than 800 IU of vitamin E, as it may impair the benefits of the medication.

Best food sources of vitamin E include:

- green leafy vegetables
- nuts and seeds like sunflower seeds and almonds
- olives

- avocado
- broccoli
- bell peppers
- shrimp/prawn, sardines.

Vitamin K

You might think the next vitamin in line after A, B, C, D, and E would be F, but you'd be wrong. That would seem to make sense, but first identified for its role in blood clotting, vitamin K was so named after the German word *koagulation* (English: coagulation, meaning "clotting").

Vitamin K comes in three forms. K1 (phylloquinone) is found in plants, as it is involved in the process of photosynthesis. K2 (menaquinone) can be synthesized in our intestines by good gut bacteria and is also found in fermented foods and in animal livers. K3 (menadione) is a synthetic form of vitamin K.

The main functions of vitamin K are:

- is required for blood clotting
- assists in proper bone formation, structure, and strength
- helps prevent calcification in arteries, thereby aiding in preventing cardiovascular disease (particularly vitamin K2 along with vitamin D).

Vitamin K deficiency is most common in neonates because vitamin K does not cross the placental barrier, breast milk is low in this nutrient, and there is minimal colonic bacterial synthesis in newborns. Although vitamin K deficiency in healthy adults is not common, it can occur in those with liver disease, gallbladder or biliary disease, inflammatory bowel disease and other malabsorption issues, cystic fibrosis, polycythemia vera, nephrotic syndrome, and leukemia. It can also occur in alcoholics, those with serious burns, and those on blood thinners (like warfarin or high doses of aspirin), cholesterol-lowering drugs, long-term broad-spectrum antibiotics, high doses of vitamin A or E, or long-term hemodialysis.

As you might figure out, one of the most common signs of a vitamin K deficiency is excessive bleeding with poor clot formation. Osteoporosis is another possible sign of vitamin K deficiency.

Those on blood-thinning medications and hemodialysis may be restricted in vitamin K quantities recommended for consumption.

Natural vitamin K is otherwise safe, with no known toxicity. The synthetic vitamin K3 is not recommended, as it may interfere with an important antioxidant in the body called glutathione.

Best sources of vitamin K include:

- dark leafy greens like kale, spinach, mustard greens, collard greens, and Swiss chard
- broccoli
- Brussels sprouts
- kiwifruit
- blueberries
- prunes
- animal liver
- fermented soybeans, natto (this is one of the best, but for many its smell and texture may be hard to get past), miso, and tempeh
- sauerkraut.

Minerals

Minerals are elements found in food, soil, and water, and are necessary for our health. There are at least 20 that we currently know of, and they are subdivided into the categories of macrominerals and trace minerals.

Macrominerals

Although they are not more important than the trace minerals, our bodies do need them in larger quantities. There are currently seven recognized macrominerals.

Calcium

Calcium is the most abundant mineral in the body, with our bodies storing most of it (99%) in our bones and teeth. The other 1 percent is tightly regulated in the blood and fluid surrounding our body's cells. If calcium levels in this fluid change, the body quickly acts to get rid of the calcium, store excesses, or pull calcium out of bone storage.

The main functions of calcium are:

- forms bones and teeth as the major structural element
- mediates the constriction (vasoconstriction) or relaxation (vasodilation) of blood vessels
- plays a role in muscle contraction
- aids in the transmission of nerve signals
- is involved in the secretion of hormones, including insulin.

Of course, the major worry with calcium deficiency is a weakening of bones and teeth. Osteomalacia (softening of the bones), osteopenia (reduced bone density less severe than osteoporosis), and osteoporosis (loss of bone density that elevates risk of fractures) are all worrying outcomes of calcium deficiency. While nutritional calcium insufficiency is not the only cause of these bone diseases, it is one of the aspects essential to consider.

Osteoporosis is not a minor inconvenience to be taken lightly. An increased risk of bone fracture means that an osteoporotic person can break a bone even with something as simple as coughing. Broken bones caused by osteoporosis are more common than heart attacks, strokes, and breast cancer combined for women over the age of 50. Additionally, almost 1 in 3 people who sustain a hip fracture because of osteoporosis will re-fracture within one year, and 28 percent of women and 37 percent of men die within a year of that fracture (Schnell *et al.*, 2010).

Insufficient calcium intake, through diet, may also be linked to a higher incidence of kidney stones. It might seem contradictory, as most kidney stones are made of calcium oxalate or calcium phosphate. However, large, long-term studies have indicated this to be the case (Curhan *et al.*, 1993, 2004; Taylor, 2004; Taylor and Curhan, 2013).

Calcium in sufficient doses of 1000–2000 mg daily has also been associated with lower risk of developing high blood pressure, preeclampsia, and eclampsia during pregnancy; stroke; colon cancer; and premenstrual syndrome (Oregon State University, 2014) (premenstrual syndrome is also known as PMS—Provide Me Sweets, Pass My Shotgun, Psychotic Mood Shift, Pardon My Sobbing, Pimples May Surface, Puffy Mid-Section, and Pass My Sweatpants).

Things that can increase the likelihood of calcium deficiency include vitamin D deficiency, low blood magnesium levels, excessive sodium intake (lay off having too much salt), drinking soft drinks, smoking, alcoholism, and chronic kidney failure. Abnormal parathyroid function will also affect calcium blood levels.

Best sources of calcium include:

- dairy, including milk, cheese, yogurt (of course, everyone knows this)
- dark leafy greens like collard greens and kale (note that while spinach and chard are also rich in calcium, they also contain oxalic acid, which can make the calcium less readily absorbable by the body)
- sardines, anchovies, mackerel—because when you eat the whole of these small fish, you are also eating their bones
- legumes, including navy beans, black beans, and baked beans
- tofu
- almonds
- calcium-fortified milk alternative beverages and orange juice.

If you are taking calcium supplements, keep in mind a few things. Calcium carbonate is often the least expensive, but in this case, you are getting what you pay for. The over-the-counter antacid TUMS uses calcium carbonate, so some people take it, thinking they are doing their bones a favor. The problem is that calcium needs stomach acid for absorbing the calcium from it, and calcium carbonate decreases stomach acid. Kind of a catch-22, right? The problem is worse for older individuals, as we tend to produce less stomach acid as we age. So, an elderly woman takes calcium carbonate to try to decrease her risk of a hip fracture, but further impairs her digestive process, weakening her absorption of calcium and other nutrients, and not getting the bone health benefits.

Better calcium supplement forms include calcium citrate, calcium gluconate, calcium lactate, and the tongue-twister microcrystalline hydroxyapatite calcium (also called MCHC calcium—much easier to remember and say!).

Is Calcium All I Need to Build My Bones?

In short, no.

In fact, though your bones are a major storage place for calcium, and though sufficient calcium is essential for healthy bones, some research has pointed to potential dangers in having too much dietary/ supplemental calcium. A study of 926 men from the Physicians' Health Study found that men eating three or more servings of dairy daily had a 141 percent increased risk of death from prostate cancer compared with those men who ate less than one dairy food per day (Yang *et al.*, 2015). A meta-analysis study found that high intake of dairy products, but not supplemental or non-dairy calcium, may also increase prostate cancer risk (Aune *et al.*, 2015). For women, large studies have found intake of dairy to be associated with a greater risk of endometrial cancer (in postmenopausal women not receiving hormone therapy) (Ganmaa *et al.*, 2012) and of breast cancer (Fraser *et al.*, 2020). There is thought that the connection between dairy and these hormone-related cancers may be due to changes in the milk's hormone composition because of modern milk industry methods. For example, some countries, like the United States, allow for the growth hormone recombinant somatotropin (rBST), a genetically engineered growth hormone, to be fed to dairy cows. Canada, the European Union, the United Kingdom, Australia, and New Zealand do not allow it. Note that they may allow imported milk from the US, however, because they deem it safe for consumption (BCPP, 2019).

Other nutrients that are key to bone health include vitamin D, magnesium, vitamin K, boron, potassium, silica, zinc, manganese, copper, and chromium.

If you want strong bones, just do it. Weight-bearing exercise, that is. We usually think of the word "stress" in a negative light. But stress through some strain on the bone is what's needed to make bones denser and stronger. Weight-bearing exercise works our bones against gravity, and includes activities like walking, running, climbing stairs, dancing, weightlifting, and push-ups. Keep in mind that only the bones that are stressed will get stronger, so if walking is your main activity, you'll also need to include some upper-body exercise as well.

You might also limit how many cups of coffee and other caffeine sources you have. Caffeine tends to cause you to lose calcium through urination, and four cups of coffee or more daily has been shown to increase the risk of bone fractures.

Ideally, you'll say goodbye to pop (maybe you call it soda, cola, or soft drink—no matter, you're best to break up your relationship with it and call it "your ex"). In addition to being a source of unneeded extra sugar or artificial sweeteners that are damaging to your health, it may also weaken your bones. The oft-quoted Framington Osteoporosis Study found lower bone density at some of their tested bone sites in older women who consumed soft drinks daily versus those who had it less than once a month (Tucker *et al.*, 2006).

Again, in the category of no health benefits, stop smoking. Smoking has been associated with lower bone density in adolescents, leading to poorer future bone health.

Don't wait until you are elderly to take care of your bones! Although we sometimes don't think about a health issue until it becomes an actual problem, prevention is always our best option. And bone health is no exception. We build bone density early in our lives, having achieved 90 percent of our peak bone mass by the time we are 18 years old (girls) or 20 years old (boys). We top out for bone mass by about age 30.

Magnesium

I don't have nearly enough room in this section (or this book) to cover all the things that magnesium does for our bodies. There are over 300 enzyme systems that use magnesium as a cofactor. Clearly, this is an important mineral!

The main functions of magnesium are:

- plays a key role in bone metabolism, with 50 to 60 percent of magnesium stored in bone
- is essential in cellular energy production
- is needed for the synthesis of DNA, RNA, proteins, and glutathione
- affects the conduction of nerve impulses and muscle contraction, including the very important normal heart rhythm
- helps with the transport of ions like calcium and potassium into and out of cells
- maintains nervous system balance, with deficiency of magnesium being related to depression
- supports blood sugar control
- helps manage inflammation and wound healing.

Magnesium deficiency has been linked to an increased risk of cardiovascular disease, hypertension, osteoporosis, and type 2 diabetes. Other signs of deficiency include:

- loss of appetite
- nausea and vomiting
- weakness
- numbness and tingling
- muscle cramping
- restless leg syndrome
- seizures
- abnormal heart rhythms
- irritability
- confusion
- insomnia.

The incidence of magnesium deficiency seems contradictory: although magnesium is found in a lot of foods, unfortunately, a vast number of people still don't get enough magnesium for optimal wellness. In addition, trying to figure out an individual's magnesium status is difficult because most of it is inside the cells or bone.

Magnesium deficiency is more common for those with digestive disorders like Crohn's, malabsorption disorders, chronic diarrhea, celiac disease, and pancreatitis; those with diabetes mellitus, hyperthyroidism, or kidney impairment; and the elderly. It is also more likely in those on long-term diuretics; those who drink too much alcohol, caffeine, or pop; those who eat too much salt; those with heavy periods or who sweat excessively; and for those in times of prolonged stress. Additionally, long-term use of proton pump inhibitor (PPI) drugs used to treat heartburn, acid reflux, and stomach ulcers can cause magnesium deficiency.

Best sources of magnesium include:

- spinach, Swiss chard, beet greens, turnip greens, kale, cabbage
- squash, broccoli
- pumpkin seeds, sesame seeds, sunflower seeds
- cashews, almonds
- soybeans, tofu, tempeh
- black beans, navy beans, pinto beans, kidney beans
- quinoa, buckwheat, brown rice, barley, millet, oats, rye, wheat.

Phosphorus

Although it's the second most abundant mineral in the body, this important mineral is often forgotten about. Another mineral that is stored mostly in the bones and teeth, but is also in every cell in the body, it makes up about 1 percent of our total body weight.

The main functions of phosphorus are:

- plays a vital role in basic cell functions—growth, maintenance, and repair
- is needed to make DNA and RNA—genetic maps and building blocks
- helps the body make ATP, a molecule the body uses to store energy
- assists in acid-base balance
- works with B vitamins for healthy kidney function, normal heartbeat, muscle contractions, and nerve signaling.

Phosphorus deficiency is very rare because it is found in many foods, and your kidneys reabsorb phosphorus if for some reason you don't eat enough of it. Signs of phosphorus deficiency include:

- loss of appetite
- anemia
- bone pain
- loss of bone density
- muscle weakness
- fatigue
- irregular breathing
- numbness and tingling of the extremities
- higher susceptibility to infection.

Deficiency of phosphorus is possible in anorexics or those who are near starvation; those with malabsorption issues like Crohn's, ulcerative colitis, and celiac disease; alcoholics; diabetics; and those taking diuretics and some antacids.

More common is phosphorus excess because this abundant mineral is found in high quantities in a lot of processed foods, as it is a common additive as a food stabilizer, emulsifier, anticaking agent, and more. It is often found as added phosphates in food such as baked goods, baking mixes, lunch meats, sausages, ham, yogurt, cheese, frozen patties, breaded chicken, and pop. Pop is particularly high in phosphorus, often with as much as half the daily requirement in just one can. Too much phosphorus can also occur with kidney disease or low parathyroid hormone levels.

Phosphorus excess can be toxic, causing diarrhea and calcification of the organs and soft tissues, increasing our risk of cardiovascular disease and bone density loss, and interfering with our ability to absorb calcium, magnesium, iron, and zinc.

Best sources of phosphorus include:

- scallops, cod, sardines, tuna, salmon, shrimp/prawn
- mushrooms, green peas, broccoli, spinach, asparagus, squash, tomatoes, cauliflower
- soybeans, lentils, tofu
- pumpkins
- turkey, chicken, beef
- yogurt, milk
- oats
- beet greens, mustard greens, Swiss chard, bok choy, fennel.

Potassium

Like sodium, chloride, calcium, and magnesium, potassium is an electrolyte, helping to conduct electrical charges in the body. The body very tightly regulates its levels of potassium.

The main functions of potassium are:

- supports healthy bone
- plays a role in skeletal and smooth muscle function, making it important for muscle, heart, and digestive system function
- helps prevent heart attacks and strokes and may reduce elevated blood pressure
- is needed for proper water balance
- balances pH (acidity/alkalinity)

- helps move nutrients into cells and waste out of them
- is required for communication between nerves and muscles.

Hypokalemia and **hyperkalemia** are a deficiency and excess, respectively, of potassium in the body—not of kale, as you might guess from the names. Of course, because potassium is an essential component to a healthy body and we need to get it externally, as our bodies can't make it, Mother Nature has provided us with an abundance of foods rich in potassium. However, many do not eat enough of these healthy foods, and there are other things that can cause deficiency, including:

- kidney disease
- chronic digestive malabsorption conditions, such as Crohn's, ulcerative colitis
- excessive diarrhea, sweating, or vomiting
- diuretics, including blood pressure medications that are diuretics
- antibiotic use
- use of corticosteroids, antacids, insulin, laxatives, and some fungicides
- magnesium deficiency
- excessive intake of sodium.

At the other end of the spectrum, excess potassium, or hyperkalemia, is also possible. It is unlikely to occur simply through the diet, but is more common in the elderly, those with poor kidney function, those on non-steroid anti-inflammatory drugs (NSAIDs) who also have poor kidney function, severe burn sufferers, and those on ACE inhibitors or beta-blockers (both medications to lower blood pressure), chemotherapy, or potassium-conserving diuretics.

It's best not to simply start taking a potassium supplement (outside of that in a multivitamin or multimineral supplement) without guidance from a proper healthcare provider.

Best sources of potassium include:

- bananas; everyone thinks of bananas for potassium, but there are so many more options—in fact, the following are even better sources of potassium than bananas
- beet greens, Swiss chard, spinach, bok choy, cabbage, kale (of course, kale would be listed as a solution to hypokalemia!), turnip greens, romaine lettuce
- beets/beetroot
- Brussels sprouts, broccoli
- asparagus, tomatoes, bell peppers, potatoes

- celery, carrots
- fennel
- squash, sweet potatoes
- lima beans
- soybeans, pinto beans, lentils, kidney beans, dried peas
- avocado
- tuna, salmon.

Sodium

Sodium is a big topic in health, but not usually to discuss deficiencies, as it most often is with other nutrients. Instead, sodium excess as a result of too much salt is the issue most prominent. North Americans have about 3600 mg (about 1½ tsp) of sodium daily, more than double what we need (Cogswell *et al.*, 2018). While it's a necessary nutrient, we find it in excessive quantities in processed, packaged, store-bought, and restaurant foods. And that's even before we grab the saltshaker.

The reason for the profusion of salt in our foods is that it helps preserve food and enhances flavor. As mentioned in Chapter 2: How to Classify Foods Using TCM, many of us also crave salty foods, so we have to work on readjusting our sensory systems to chill on the salt intake.

The main functions of sodium are:

- controls blood pressure and blood volume
- helps muscles and nerves function properly.

Sodium and chloride are the most common ions in the fluids outside of your cells, including blood plasma, so they are essential to life. You'll recognize the combo of sodium and chloride as NaCl, or table salt.

So, is it possible to have too little sodium? Yes, it is. Called **hyponatremia**, it is most likely in older individuals, especially those who are hospitalized or in long-term care facilities because risk factors include having decreased function of the kidneys, liver, or heart. It can also happen with some kinds of cancer, underactive thyroid or adrenal glands, and for those taking diuretics, an anti-seizure medication called carbamazepine, or some types of antidepressants.

The more likely sodium imbalance issue of excess causes elevated blood pressure, puffiness, and bloating. It also increases your risk of heart disease and failure, stroke, stomach cancer, headaches, kidney disease, kidney stones, cirrhosis of the liver, osteoporosis, and aggravation of asthma. And if you think that kids can eat sodium to their heart's content, think again. Kids with a high-sodium diet are much more likely to end up with high blood pressure than kids on low-sodium diets (He, Marrero, and McGregor, 2008).

Best sources of sodium include...

Okay, so obviously salt is going to provide sodium, but since you'll want to aim for no more than 2300 mg daily if you're a healthy adult, less than 1500 mg per day if you have high blood pressure, and perhaps less if you have congestive heart failure, cirrhosis of the liver, or kidney disease, here are some natural ways you can get your 1000–1500 mg of sodium without the salt and with a better balance of potassium:

- celery
- beets/beetroot
- carrots
- spinach, chard
- artichoke
- cantaloupe
- seaweed like kombu, nori, kelp, dulse
- meats
- shrimp/prawn, lobster, crab, scallops
- dairy.

Chloride

No, this isn't the same as chlorine, which you'd use to kill germs in your swimming pool. For this answer, you could go back to your old chemistry books about elements and anions and the number of electrons. But there's no need to do that. Chlorine is a very reactive gas that combines easily with other elements. Chloride, on the other hand, is an essential mineral, representing 70 percent of the negatively charged ions in your body and acting as an important electrolyte in balance with potassium and sodium (both of which are positively charged).

The main functions of chloride are:

- balances pH
- transports carbon dioxide (waste product of respiration) out of the body
- helps with nerve conduction and muscle signaling
- maintains fluid volume outside of the cells
- combines with hydrogen in the stomach to make stomach acid (HCl), key for the breakdown of proteins and absorption of minerals and vitamin B12.

Chloride is not normally something you have to think much about when making sure you get enough but not too much. Commonly found in food, paired with sodium to make salt, deficiency is rare. Diarrhea, vomiting, or sweating profusely can cause a life-threatening condition known as alkalosis—too alkaline. Also caused by extensive body burns, water overload, and severe malnutrition, too little chloride (**hypochloremia**) can cause loss of appetite, dehydration, muscle weakness, confusion, seizure, irritability, and intense exhaustion.

Too much chloride is uncommon but can cause problems with acid-base balance and fluid retention. The issue is usually more about too much sodium.

Best sources of chloride include:

- seaweeds like kelp, nori, dulse, and kombu
- olives
- tomatoes, lettuce, celery
- rye
- salt substitutes (often potassium chloride instead of sodium chloride).

Sulfur

Sulfur isn't a mineral we think of often—usually only when we smell rotten eggs or around volcanic vents. Pure sulfur has no smell, but when combined—for instance, in hydrogen sulfide (H_2S_2)—its smell is distinctive ("awful reek" is another way to describe it). And when sulfur burns, producing sulfur dioxide, it is a toxic gas. In fact, it used to be used to fumigate buildings with infectious diseases. Did you know that the biblical word "brimstone"—as in "fire and brimstone," meaning a sign of God's wrath—is referring to sulfur?

Thankfully, the sulfur we ingest in food is not going to harm us. Instead, it is an important mineral for our bodies, as the third most abundant mineral in us. Most of the sulfur in your body is found in your skin, muscles, bones, hair, and nails, but it is key to several other organs and systems.

The main functions of sulfur are:

- helps proteins maintain their shape, thus influencing the biological activity of those proteins
- forms a key component of insulin
- is an essential part of glutathione, a vital antioxidant your body produces
- assists in the function of mitochondria to make energy for cellular activity
- aids conversion of vitamin B1 and biotin

- maintains elasticity and shape of skin, hair, nails, muscles, and bones via production of collagen and keratin
- supports liver detoxification pathways.

While sulfur deficiency has not been commonly identified as an important issue to consider, there is some evidence that deficiencies do exist, particularly for those who do not eat enough protein, as sulfur is found in the amino acids methionine (an essential amino acid that our bodies cannot produce, but that must be consumed) and cysteine. The elderly are particularly at risk because they tend to eat too little, particularly of protein, and their absorption is poorer.

Sulfur deficiency has been linked to arthritis, acne, rashes, brittle hair and nails, poor healing of wounds, depression, fatigue, and digestive issues. Supplements containing sulfur compounds can be found, including MSM (methylsulfonylmethane) for joint pain and inflammation; SAMe (S-adenosylmethionine) for depression, joint pain, and inflammation; glucosamine or chondroitin sulfate for joint pain; and DMSO (dimethylsulfoxide) for interstitial cystitis, pain, and inflammation.

While many people have allergies to sulfa drugs (sulfonamides, the early antibiotics) and sulfites (found in naturally fermented products like beer and wine or artificially added as a preservative in many processed foods), they will not have a problem with sulfur or sulfates. You won't live without sulfur.

Best sources of sulfur include:

- egg yolks
- meat
- fish, shellfish
- poultry
- milk
- garlic, onions, scallions/spring onions (yup, the watery eyes you get from cutting onions is hydrogen sulfide, as is the lovely smell from these foods)
- cabbage, Brussels sprouts, kale, lettuce, cauliflower, broccoli
- seaweed
- turnips
- nuts
- raspberries.

Microminerals
Although they are needed in smaller amounts than the macrominerals, they are no less important. Sometimes called trace minerals, they include

iron, zinc, iodine, selenium, copper, manganese, chromium, fluoride, and molybdenum.

Iron

Because you probably know someone who's iron deficient and feeling the effects of it, you might have thought this would be a macronutrient. But it's not. That just goes to show that it's not only the most abundant minerals in our body that are important.

There are two types of dietary iron, heme and nonheme. Heme iron—which makes up 40 percent of the iron found in meats, seafood, and poultry—is the best absorbed form. Nonheme iron—which makes up the remainder of that animal-source food, dairy, eggs, and all the iron in plants—is less well absorbed, so consumption of iron from those foods for vegetarians and vegans should be higher than for non-vegetarians.

The good news for the non-meat-eaters is that there are many plants rich in iron, and that a healthy vegetarian diet is often high in vitamin C, which assists the absorption of iron.

The main functions of iron are:

- forms an important part of hemoglobin, an iron-carrying protein needed to transport oxygen to your cells
- supports energy production.

The most common populations to become iron deficient are infants and young children (especially if born preterm, with low birthweight, or whose mothers are iron deficient), pregnant women, women with heavy menstrual bleeding, frequent blood donors, and those with cancer, gastrointestinal disorders, or heart failure.

The most common symptoms of **iron-deficiency anemia** include:

- fatigue
- pale skin
- shortness of breath
- dizziness
- sensation of crawling or tingling in legs
- tongue swelling or soreness
- fast or irregular heartbeat
- chest pain
- cold hands and feet
- headaches
- a craving for things that aren't food, like ice, dirt, clay, or starch.

It's a good idea to have your iron levels tested before you decide to supplement, though, as iron can accumulate in the body to toxic levels, increasing your risk for cancer and heart disease. If you have **hemochromatosis**, a genetic disease that causes an excessive buildup of iron in the blood, you'll need to watch your iron and vitamin C intake.

However, if you have healthy intestines, you are unlikely to overload on iron just from food sources.

Best sources of iron include:

From heme sources:

- organ meats
- octopus
- beef, lamb, and other meats
- poultry
- fish, shellfish.

From nonheme sources:

- spinach, Swiss chard, collard greens, beet greens, bok choy, mustard greens, turnip greens, parsley
- eggs
- dairy
- leeks, asparagus
- turmeric, cumin
- soybeans (tofu, tempeh, miso, edamame)
- lentils
- beans (navy, white, kidney, pinto, black, adzuki)
- garbanzo beans/chickpeas
- green peas, lima beans, green beans
- beets/beetroot
- kale, broccoli, cabbage, Brussels sprouts
- blackstrap molasses
- many grain products like flour, cereal, and pasta are also fortified with iron.

Zinc

Zinc's relationship status with other nutrients is very complicated. Copper intake doesn't much affect zinc, but supplementing over 50 mg a day of zinc can interfere with copper absorption. Supplemental iron may decrease zinc absorption. High levels of calcium may or may not interfere with zinc absorption. And zinc deficiency can result in vitamin A deficiency, as zinc is a component of a protein needed to transport vitamin A in the blood. Yup, it's complicated.

Zinc is a key micromineral with antioxidant properties, essential for cell growth and repair, reproduction, vision, blood clotting, sense of smell and taste, insulin use, and immune and thyroid function. We need to get zinc daily, as we have no special storage system in our bodies.

The main functions of zinc are:

- plays an essential role in immune function
- protects the body from free radical cellular damage
- is directly involved in cell division and repair, essential for growth and development
- is necessary for proper function of the reproductive system
- helps heal wounds
- is needed for proper sense of smell and taste
- is involved in blood clotting, insulin use, and thyroid function.

Because zinc is found in its most bioavailable form in meat, and because phytates found in legumes and whole grains may interfere with zinc absorption, vegetarians and vegans may need to consume as much as 50 percent more zinc than non-vegetarians. However, soaking and sprouting legumes, seeds, and grains can reduce the binding of zinc, allowing it to be more bioavailable, as can consuming more leavened grains (like bread) rather than unleavened grains (like crackers).

Other causes of zinc deficiency include gastrointestinal disease, chronic illness, pregnancy, lactation, chronic renal disease, sickle cell anemia, advanced age, and excessive alcohol consumption. Children who are exclusively breastfed beyond six months may also develop zinc deficiency, as breast milk will not provide enough zinc for infants seven months and older.

Even mild zinc deficiency can result in poor immune function, and zinc supplements, particularly in the form of syrups or lozenges taken within 24 hours of the onset of symptoms, have been shown to help reduce the duration and severity of the common cold in healthy people (Singh and Das, 2013).

If you are taking an antibiotic (particularly a quinolone or tetracycline antibiotic), take it at least two hours before or 4–6 hours after taking any zinc supplements, as they can interact in your body, reducing the absorption of both. Penicillamine, a drug for rheumatoid arthritis, should be taken away from zinc supplementation, as zinc can make the drug less effective. And because thiazide diuretics can cause you to excrete too much zinc through your urine, patients should be monitored for zinc levels if taking the medication long-term.

On the other hand, too much zinc can also impair immune function, in addition to causing toxicity symptoms of nausea, vomiting, abdominal cramps, diarrhea, loss of appetite, headaches, and copper deficiency.

Best sources of zinc include:

- oysters
- beef, lamb, liver
- spinach
- asparagus
- mushrooms (shiitake, cremini)
- sesame seeds, pumpkin seeds
- garbanzo beans/chickpeas, lentils, lima beans, black-eyed peas, pinto beans, peanuts
- cashews
- quinoa
- turkey
- shrimp/prawn, scallops
- soybeans (tofu, miso, tempeh)
- whole grains.

Iodine

Prior to the 1920s, iodine deficiency was fairly common throughout much of Canada and in many northern states, labeled part of the "goiter belt." The word "goiter" comes from the word "guttur," meaning "throat." Goiters can become quite large, and they are one of the most distinctive signs of iodine deficiency, as the thyroid (found at the front of the neck) becomes enlarged trying to produce more thyroid hormones. Iodine deficiency is still a problem in about 40 percent of the world's population, as many areas of the world have iodine-deficient soils.

The main function of iodine is:

- makes up part of the thyroid hormones triiodothyronine (T_3) and thyroxine (T_4), so is key to the proper function of the thyroid, which is in turn needed to control energy production and metabolism.

Although I've only listed one function here, a poorly functioning thyroid can have a huge impact on your health. During pregnancy, a woman's belly and breasts aren't the only things to increase in size. Her thyroid will grow by 10–15 percent if she is getting enough iodine (American Thyroid

Association, n.d.), and more if she's not getting enough iodine. If her thyroid is under-functioning (called **hypothyroidism**), she is at higher risk of pre-eclampsia, miscarriage, preterm birth, and having a stillborn or low-weight infant. It can also cause developmental deficits in her baby. Breastmilk also needs to contain enough iodine for a developing baby. Even mild to moderate iodine deficiency during pregnancy has been associated with lower IQ in school-aged children.

In adults, the most common symptoms of hypothyroidism include fatigue, weight gain, constipation, and feeling cold, though iodine deficiency is not the only cause of hypothyroidism.

Although iodized salt is widely available in North America, iodine deficiency is still possible, especially for those who do not eat iodized salt, fish, or seaweed. In addition, sufficient selenium is needed for the body to convert T_4 to the bioactive hormone T_3. Iron deficiency and vitamin A deficiency may also play a role in iodine deficiency.

And as if that weren't enough, even some of the things that are considered very healthy for you may cause iodine deficiency. These goitrogens interfere with iodine utilization or thyroid hormone production. Had I known it as a kid, I might have used the excuse not to eat my Brussels sprouts because they are a goitrogen. But then I would have also had to give up strawberries, peaches, peanuts, soybeans, sweet potatoes, and other cruciferous veggies like broccoli, cabbage, and cauliflower. Other goitrogens include tobacco smoking and some industrial pollutants.

It is also possible to go overboard with iodine. In fact, too much iodine can cause the same problem as too little. Excess-iodine-induced hypothyroidism and goiter occur because the hormone feedback signals tell the thyroid to slow down. In some areas where high seaweed consumption is not uncommon—like Japan—this has occurred, causing them to have to reduce seaweed consumption.

Best sources of iodine include:

- seaweed (kelp, wakame, nori, kombu)
- fish (cod, tuna, sardines, salmon)
- shrimp/prawn
- dairy
- eggs.

Selenium

From villain to hero, selenium was once thought to be a toxin, but was later (in the late 1950s) discovered to be an essential micronutrient and a powerful antioxidant in our bodies, especially when combined with vitamin E.

Without getting too "sciency," selenium is needed to form more than two dozen "selenoproteins"—proteins that are essential for DNA synthesis, reproduction, thyroid hormone metabolism, immune function, and more.

Available in either inorganic (selenite and selenate) form or organic (selenomethionine and selenocysteine) form, both are good sources of dietary selenium. The inorganic form is found in soil, and plants can convert it to the organic form. We store a quarter to almost half of the organic selenomethionine we use in our muscles.

The main functions of selenium are:

- makes antioxidant enzymes that help protect our cells from damage and potentially from the development of cancerous cells
- regulates cell growth and survival
- helps convert inactive thyroid hormone T_4 into active form T_4
- is necessary for male fertility—sperm production and motility
- helps regulate inflammatory and immune responses, helping to boost white blood cells.

While selenium deficiency is not thought to be common in healthy adults, there are some factors that can lead to deficiency, including (as you'll see with so many nutrient deficiencies) smoking and consuming too much alcohol. Poor absorption of selenium occurs with gastrointestinal diseases like Crohn's, ulcerative colitis, and celiac disease. Some areas of the world have also been found to have selenium-deficient soils, resulting in Keshan disease (a specific type of heart disease) in China and Kashin-Beck disease (causing joint deformities and dwarfism) in Tibet, northern and central China, North Korea, and southeastern Siberia.

Although there are mixed results, some studies have found low selenium levels to be associated with risk for various cancers, cardiovascular disease, cognitive decline, Alzheimer's, Parkinson's, epilepsy, and thyroid disease.

On the other hand, you don't want to have too much selenium. Excess chronic is called **selenosis**, and can result in hair loss, brittle nails, skin lesions, diarrhea, nausea, fatigue, garlic breath odor, irritability, neurological symptoms, and (ow!) fingernail loss. Are you nuts over Brazil nuts? Well, maybe you better mix it up a bit. Based on Brazil nuts containing 68–91 mcg of selenium per nut and a recommended upper intake limit of 400 mcg of selenium daily for adults, that's only 5–6 Brazil nuts daily to take you over the top.

Best sources for selenium include:

- Brazil nuts

- fish (tuna, salmon, cod, sardines)
- shellfish (shrimp/prawn, scallops, oysters)
- mushrooms (cremini, shiitake, portobello)
- asparagus
- mustard seeds
- turkey, chicken
- beef, lamb
- liver
- tofu
- eggs
- barley, brown rice
- sunflower seeds, sesame seeds.

Copper

Each one of us contains about as much copper as the amount found in a single penny, and a penny is only about 2.5 percent copper by weight. Yes, despite this tiny amount needed, copper is no slouch when it comes to the extent of work it does in our bodies. Copper is part of many key enzymes (cuproenzymes) that have a variety of essential functions in our bodies.

The main functions of copper are:

- helps in the production of ATP, a vital energy-storing molecule
- is needed to make the enzyme superoxide dismutase (SOD), a major antioxidant in the body
- assists in the uptake of iron into the red blood cells
- is needed for the cross-linking of collagen and elastin, required for the body's connective tissue
- is involved in several reactions essential to proper brain and nervous system function
- helps with formation and maintenance of the myelin sheath that covers nerves and is key to nerve signal transmission
- is required for the formation of the pigment melanin, needed to color the hair, skin, and eyes.

Flat-out copper deficiency is considered uncommon and is usually associated with a malabsorption issue like Crohn's, ulcerative colitis, or celiac disease, or with an inherited disease called Menkes disease or a milder form of the disease called occipital horn syndrome (OHS).

However, there is some evidence that marginal copper deficiency may be relatively common and can cause insufficiency symptoms, such as:

- iron-deficiency anemia that does not resolve with iron supplementation; this may be due to insufficient copper
- osteoporosis
- low white blood cell count
- irregular heartbeat
- bleeding under the skin
- blood vessel damage
- hair loss
- thyroid problems
- loss of pigment from the skin.

Remembering that minerals in our bodies can increase or decrease the absorption of each other, it's important not to overdo zinc over copper, as excess zinc can result in a copper deficiency. But, no, swallowing a penny is not a good solution, so check out the food options below.

A rare inherited disease called Wilson's disease can cause excessive accumulation of copper in the liver, brain, and other organs, so those with this disorder should not supplement copper. Too much copper is poisonous, and acute copper toxicity can result in nausea, vomiting, headache, dizziness, diarrhea, and even heart problems, coma, and death. If you drink well water or have copper pipes or cookware, be aware that you may be getting more copper than you think.

Best sources of copper include:

- shellfish (oysters, lobster, mussels, crab, clams, shrimp/prawn)
- organ meats (liver, kidneys, heart)
- cashews, hazelnuts, macadamia nuts, pecans, pistachios, almonds, walnuts
- sesame seeds, sunflower seeds, pumpkin seeds, flax seeds
- legumes (soybeans, lentils, navy beans, peanuts, garbanzo beans/ chickpeas, kidney beans)
- mushrooms
- beet greens, turnip greens, Swiss chard, mustard greens, spinach, kale
- sweet potato, squash
- asparagus, tomato
- grapes, pineapple, raspberries, kiwifruit
- avocado
- blackstrap molasses
- black pepper
- cocoa (yay, chocolate!).

Manganese

What does an essential trace mineral have to do with turning water to wine? Unfortunately, not much (as far as I know), but the name for manganese does come from the Greek word for magic. This mineral that you've probably not thought much—or anything—about plays an important role as part of many enzymes in your body.

The main functions of manganese are:

- helps protect mitochondria (energy producers in your cells) from oxidative damage
- plays a role in carbohydrate, protein, and fat metabolism
- is involved in blood sugar regulation
- is needed for the healthy formation of bones and cartilage
- is required for collagen production in skin, so assists in wound healing
- plays a role in thyroid hormone synthesis.

Most good sources of manganese are from vegetables, fruits, grains, nuts, seeds, and legumes, not from animal-source foods. We don't need very much manganese, and it is widely available in whole foods. However, if you eat mostly processed foods, it is possible you are lacking in the magic of manganese. Manganese deficiency can result in:

- infertility
- impaired glucose regulation
- bone abnormalities
- poor wound healing
- skin rashes
- seizures.

Manganese excess from food has not been reported, but it has been known to occur with smelters and welders who inhale manganese dust, and results in neurologic disorders, psychiatric disorders, and lung inflammation. Too much manganese has also been found in patients with severe hepatitis, post-hepatic cirrhosis, and those on dialysis.

Because iron and manganese may share common transport and absorption pathways, too much of one of these minerals can decrease the absorption of the other, and vice versa. Supplemental magnesium and calcium may also lower the bioavailability of manganese, so many bone health supplements will include all these minerals.

Best food sources of manganese include:

- oats, brown rice, wheat, rye, barley, buckwheat
- legumes (garbanzo beans/chickpeas, soybeans, navy beans, pinto beans, black beans, kidney beans, lentils)
- pineapple, raspberries, strawberries, blueberries, cranberries
- spinach, collard greens, beet greens, Swiss chard, kale, turnip greens, mustard greens, bok choy
- cloves, turmeric, cinnamon, black pepper, basil
- squash, sweet potato
- sea vegetables
- garlic
- pumpkin seeds, quinoa
- walnuts, sesame seeds
- green peas, beets/beetroot, green beans, asparagus
- broccoli, Brussels sprouts.

Chromium

Chromium is a mineral like Superman. There's the good Superman, which is the beneficial chromium found in food. Then there's the less common but bad red Kryptonite Superman, which is the toxic chromium that results from industrial pollution. We'll ignore the red Kryptonite chromium here because it's not part of our regular food cycle. I just figured you might be bored of reading about vitamins and minerals by now, thus the little (but true) side-note story.

The main functions of chromium are:

- enhances the action of insulin and glucose metabolism
- promotes the synthesis of fatty acids and cholesterol, important for brain function and other processes.

Although we don't need very much chromium, we only absorb 0.4–2.5 percent of the chromium we consume (National Institutes of Health, 2017b), so it is thought that with our modern diets that are too high in processed foods and high in sugar, chromium deficiency may be fairly common. If you eat more than 35 percent of your calories as simple sugars, you are increasing the amount of chromium that you lose through urination. Other things that increase chromium loss include infection, strenuous exercise, pregnancy, lactation, and stressful states. On the other hand, chromium absorption is enhanced when consumed along with vitamin C or foods rich in vitamin C.

There have been very few serious adverse effects from excessive intake of chromium, though it is suggested that those with kidney or liver problems, or those with anemia, should not take chromium supplements.

Best food sources of chromium include:

- brewer's yeast
- broccoli
- green beans, potatoes, tomatoes
- barley, oats
- beef, liver
- chicken, turkey
- eggs
- oysters
- molasses
- black pepper.

Phytonutrients

"Phyto" is used when we refer to plants. It comes from the Greek word for plant, *phuton*, which comes from *phuein*, meaning "come into being." So, phytonutrients are nutrients or chemicals that are found in plants. Plants have phytonutrients because, like us, they need to protect themselves from UV radiation, insects, viruses, bacteria, parasites, and other environmental factors.

Many of the phytonutrients are antioxidants, helping to prevent damage to your cells. As a result, they are often touted as anti-aging or at least promoting-healthy-aging superfoods, reducing the risk of a wide range of diseases. Some act to help regulate the immune system. Others have hormone-balancing effects. Still others kill off viruses and bacteria. The list of benefits is vast because the number of phytonutrients is large, and we are continually discovering new ones. This is one reason why trying to isolate nutrients and create a perfect, health-promoting pill is so difficult. We don't know what we don't yet know.

There are so many phytonutrients that we cannot cover them all, or even most of them, in this book, but here's a short list of some you might want to make sure you're getting. Since many phytonutrients also act as pigments to the foods in which they are found, eat lots of colorful foods (no, that doesn't mean Fruit Loops).

- Carotenoids: carrots, squash, pumpkin, papaya, melon.
- Flavonoids: blueberries, blackberries, red cabbage.
- Ellagic acid: strawberries, raspberries, pomegranate.
- Lycopene: tomatoes, watermelon, guava.
- Chlorophyll: kale, spinach, collard greens.

Probiotics, Microbiome, and Microbiota

Microbiome—a word that was coined within the last two decades—is now one of the hottest topics in health. Microbiome is defined as a mini ecosystem of microbes or microorganisms and their genes. The actual microbes in our bodies are known as microbiota, and there are over 100 trillion of them in or on us. That number is so big that it's hard to fathom. But let's try.

A hundred trillion microbiota. That's approximately ten times the number of cells in your body. "They" outnumber "you" by 10:1. So, when you say "I went to the store," what you are more truthfully saying is "We went to the store" or "They went to the store, and I tagged along."

One hundred trillion microbiota. The population of the world (in 2021) was about 7.9 billion people (United Nations, n.d.).

One Hundred Trillion Perspective

I thought it would be interesting to see how else to understand the idea of 100 trillion, so here are some ways to understand 1 trillion. Then, obviously, you'll need to times that by 100.

Let's imagine it as money. One trillion dollars would give you one million dollars to spend every day for the next 3000 years.

Or think about it in terms of time. We never feel like there's enough time! But 1 million seconds is about 11 and a half days. One billion seconds is about 32 years. One trillion seconds is 32,000 years!

What about in terms of distance? If you stack $1 trillion in $100 bills, that stack would be about 1014.5 km (631 miles) high, about two and a half times higher than the distance between Earth and the International Space Station (Kleanthous, n.d.).

All that times 100.

One hundred trillion is 100,000,000,000,000 (14 zeros).

Microbiota can be found on, in, and around our skin, mouths, eyes, genitals, and intestines, and it is this last environment that is most heavily being studied. Sometimes the gut microbiota is called "gut flora" or "intestinal flora."

But don't be afraid of these little guys. While some bacteria are pathogenic, meaning they can cause disease, many of them are either along for a free ride, causing us no harm, or are essential to our healthy survival. Microbiota are comprised of bacteria, viruses, and fungi. Most of our studies have been done on the bacteria.

We call the "good bacteria" probiotics, and the bacteria in our intestines can weigh up to 1 kg. But this is not the kind of weight you want to shed. That's because these bacteria help to:

- digest your food
- absorb nutrients like many of your B vitamins, vitamin K, folate, and short-chain fatty acids
- supply up to 10 percent of your energy through the by-products of bacterial fermentation
- support a healthy immune system
- alleviate food allergies in infants
- improve lactose intolerance
- destroy disease-causing microorganisms
- help reduce anxiety and depression
- improve insulin sensitivity, thus enhancing glucose metabolism
- control bad breath and improve oral health
- reduce the risk of colon cancer
- control inflammatory bowel disease, like Crohn's or ulcerative colitis
- manage symptoms of irritable bowel syndrome (IBS)
- shorten the duration of acute diarrhea and gastroenteritis. (Parvez *et al.*, 2006; Sanders, 2008)

Every day, it seems, we're discovering more ways that probiotics are helping us stay healthy.

You may have seen the public message advertisements "Do bugs need drugs?" The focus of this is to use antibiotics wisely and only when needed. After decades of battles against all "bugs" with the creation of a wide range of antibiotic medications, antibacterial hand washes and wipes, bacteria-killing mouthwashes, and antibacterial vaginal rinses, we've since come to realize that not all bacteria are bad. In fact, we've seen a number of "superbugs"— bacteria that are hard to destroy, as the usual antibiotics are not effective on them—created because of the overuse of antibiotics. We've also seen a rise in allergies, autoimmune conditions, and inflammatory diseases.

Because of our overuse of antibiotics and our sterile environment, we've seen a destruction of many of our valuable and healthy good bacteria, resulting in many health issues. Research has shown potential connections to these health issues (and more) (Ciorba, 2012; Clemente *et al.*, 2012; Deans, 2016; Jandhyala, 2015; Round and Mazmanian, 2009; Ursell *et al.*, 2012; Velasquez-Manoff, n.d.):

- allergies
- Alzheimer's disease

- anorexia
- anxiety
- autism
- autoimmune diseases (e.g., lupus)
- celiac disease
- constipation
- Crohn's
- depression
- gastric cancer
- irritable bowel disease
- obesity
- type 2 diabetes
- ulcerative colitis.

And probably many more.

So, what can you do? Let the bugs back in! It's okay to ingest some chemical-free dirt. Take antibiotics only when you need to. Go easy on the antibacterial products. Don't use antibacterial mouthwash. Add some good bacteria back into your body with fermented foods! Feed the good bacteria in your body with some probiotics and prebiotics.

Prebiotics

Sometimes things are named so that you can more easily understand that there's a relationship. Prebiotics are not coincidentally similar in name to probiotics. Prebiotics are non-digestible carbohydrates that are food for probiotics. It makes sense, then, that the more prebiotics you have, the healthier your probiotic population may become.

The most common prebiotics are a class of fiber called oligosaccharides. You may refer back to the Oligosaccharides section under the Carbohydrates heading towards the beginning of this chapter for more specifics on oligosaccharides. You might also note that for those on a FODMAP diet, oligosaccharides are on the "don't have" list. However, for those not needing a FODMAP diet, these prebiotics can be beneficial.

Examples of foods high in prebiotics include:

Fructo-oligosaccharides (FOS)

- Raw chicory root (sometimes ground and used as a non-caffeinated coffee substitute).
- Asparagus.
- Jerusalem artichoke (not the same as a globe artichoke).

- Leek, onion.
- Tomato.
- Garlic.
- Banana.
- Barley, rye, whole grains.
- Dandelion root.

Galacto-oligosaccharides (GOS)

- Lentils, garbanzo beans/chickpeas, hummus, kidney beans, lima beans, green peas.
- Fermented dairy products like yogurt, kefir, and buttermilk.
- Breast milk.

They might also be found added to breakfast cereals, breads, yogurt, sauces, soups, sports drinks, snack bars, and nutritional supplements.

Jerusalem Artichoke—a Misnomer with an Unforgettable Nickname

I find it interesting that the Jerusalem artichoke is neither an artichoke nor from Jerusalem. Actually a member of the sunflower family, we eat the tuber found below ground. Because *girasole* is the Italian name for sunflower, it somehow morphed into the name Jerusalem. Also, some have felt that it tastes like an artichoke. It is also sometimes called a sunchoke, simply because a farmer wanted to give it a name that was appealing.

Perhaps because it's rich in the prebiotic inulin, it has not always been pleasantly enjoyed. Work your way through this old English for the 17th-century botanist's description of this plant: "In my judgement, which way soever they be drest and eaten they stirre and cause a filthie loathsome wind within the bodie" (McGill, n.d.).

A further search on the topic of Jerusalem artichokes and I found that they are sometimes nicknamed "fartichokes." So, apparently, that botanist isn't the only one to struggle with this veggie. Having said that, many other foods also have this reputation, including cruciferous vegetables like broccoli and Brussels sprouts, and, of course, beans, beans, the musical food. However, not everyone has trouble with either those foods or with the fartichoke.

Fermented Foods

People the world over have consumed fermented foods for centuries. The oldest record of fermentation is from 6000 BC, in a historical area of the world called the Fertile Crescent (an area in the Middle East, also credited with being the origin of many other things, including agriculture, writing, and trade).

Fermented foods are made by exposing a food to bacteria and yeasts. What I hadn't known before is that there are many different types of fermentation. Lactofermentation is the kind you want for most of the good bacteria benefits, but here's a brief note on some of the types of fermentation.

Lactofermentation

Don't be afraid of lactofermented foods if you're lactose intolerant, as it has nothing to do with lactose (the sugar found in dairy). It refers to the lactic acid bacteria (found in soil and dairy milk) used to ferment the foods, resulting in lactic acid. Examples of lactofermented foods include yogurt and yogurt drinks, sauerkraut, kimchi, pickles (unless they are simply canned and not fermented), chutney, and cheese (though some are also fermented with molds).

Yeast Fermentation

This is the type of fermentation that many love most—bread and alcohol. Because yeast loves sugar, it eats up the sugar in fruits, vegetables, or grains, producing the by-products of carbon dioxide and alcohol. While the result is delicious, it doesn't contain the good bacteria that results from lactofermentation, so sorry to say, your wine or beer doesn't make a probiotic supplement.

Acetic Fermentation

Acetobacter is a type of bacteria found in our air that causes acetic fermentation. It's the type that alcohol makers want to avoid because these boozy bacteria will consume the ethanol (alcohol) to make a vinegar. While there are health benefits to vinegars, it too does not contain probiotics.

Bacterial and Yeast Mixed Fermentation

Bought yourself a bottled tea at your favorite fancy food shop and wondered about the blobby bits of floating stuff in it? If the label says "kombucha," then not to worry, those weird floating or sinking, lumpy or stringy bits are part of the SCOBY (symbiotic colony of bacteria and yeast). The yeast eats the sugars, making carbon dioxide and alcohol, which the bacteria consume to make more SCOBY and the resulting beverage or food. Because of the bacteria, you do end up with some probiotic benefits. Examples of mixed fermentation foods include kombucha, kefir, and sourdough bread.

Mold Fermentation

While we might mostly avoid moldy things, there are some foods created using molds that we do eat. Some cheeses like Roquefort and Gorgonzola are examples, but so too are tempeh, miso, soy sauce, amazake, and sake. These foods do contain bacteria, and some of them are thought to be probiotic, but it's unclear if they are all probiotic.

Fermentation Around the World

The list of fermented foods is vast. This is just a short list of some of the fermented foods found around the world. Note that some of the foods here may be traditional in more than just the country I've listed.

- Arctic: ignaq (fermented meat).
- China: douchi (black beans); doufuru ("stinky tofu").
- Ethiopia: injera (sourdough flatbread).
- Hawaii: poi (fermented taro).
- India: appam (fermented rice batter and coconut milk); dosa (fermented crepe).
- Indonesia: brem (fermented rice).
- Japan: natto, miso, and tempeh (all these are fermented soybeans); tsukemono (various pickled vegetables); amazake (fermented rice drink).
- Korea: kimchi (spicy fermented cabbage); cheonggukjang (fermented soybeans).
- Philippines: atchara (pickled unripe papaya); bagoong (fermented fish or shrimp/prawn condiment).
- South Africa: amasi (fermented milk).
- Turkey: ayran (yogurt drink).

Historically, we fermented foods because it was a way to preserve them. We didn't have grocery stores stocked with fruits, vegetables, grains, meats, fish, and dairy products year-round. We would harvest or hunt, and then enjoy the feast. But there were stretches of time (sometimes long stretches) when we wouldn't be able to get fresh food. Luckily, we figured out how to ferment, pickle, and preserve foods for future use.

Unfortunately, our clever selves have figured out that another way to preserve foods is to add chemical preservatives. Or to alter the food so much that it won't rot. Or to make a "food" that never actually existed—chemical aberrations like Cheez Whiz, Twinkies, or margarine. But that's a whole other topic!

Back to fermented foods. Even though most of us have access to fresh foods, refrigeration, and freezers, we should be including fermented foods in our diet for a few reasons other than that it preserves foods.

Additionally, we should make sure that we are getting truly fermented foods. The problem with the standard store-bought pickles or sauerkraut you'll now find in your grocery store is that they have been pasteurized and cooked using high heat, thus destroying all the good bacteria.

Some of the benefits of fermented foods include:

- Some (see above about types of fermentation) contain probiotics, beneficial bacteria.
- They can help balance the pH of the stomach, either increasing the amount of stomach acid if it's low or protecting the lining of the stomach if it's high.
- They may have a higher vitamin content.
- They can be more easily digested. (Food and Agriculture Organization of the United Nations, n.d.)

Think Fermented Foods Taste Gross?

I've tried several fermented foods that I've wanted to spit right back out (ayran and poi, for instance). And some I've not been able to get past the smell of (natto and stinky tofu). But don't be offended if those are your favorite foods. My grandmother grew up eating natto, so she likes it. I think it looks like chunky mucus and smells like rotten garbage. Nothing I'd want to eat. But the first time people try beer or alcohol, they also tend to think it doesn't taste good. Our tastes change with exposure.

My mother used to sneak yogurt into my dad's food because he doesn't like yogurt. Not knowing it was there, he didn't mind it. He still says he doesn't like yogurt. Sometimes it's also mind over matter.

Nevertheless, there are a huge number of fermented foods, all with different flavors, so I'm sure there are some that you will enjoy from the start.

Did you know that even coffee and chocolate are made from a combination of fermentation processes?

CHAPTER 4

Nutrition Tips for Common Symptoms and Illnesses

This chapter will not be a thorough listing of all possible diseases and symptoms but will cover some of the most common ones. Plus, the purpose of TCM is to get to the root cause of a symptom or disease and change the pattern creating it. So it doesn't make much sense to just treat a symptom. And since every one of us is different, even with the same symptom or disease, what works well for you might be different from what works well for another.

This book is best for long-term, everyday food choices that will help to return you to health and prevent future illnesses. However, there are some TCM food cures for common things you might suffer from, so this section targets those.

Abdominal Bloating/Pain

One of the most common symptoms I see in clinic—though not necessarily the reason why people come in for treatment—is abdominal bloating. There are many reasons for it, including irritable bowel syndrome, inflammatory bowel disease, food sensitivities, constipation, overeating, premenstrual syndrome, and just generally poor digestion.

For those who suffer from chronic abdominal bloating and/or pain, mealtimes can be a challenge, as eating often makes it feel worse. The most important thing is to figure out the cause of this symptom and address that. Are there foods that cause more discomfort? Keep a food diary to note what you're eating and how you feel afterward.

In general, choose foods that are easier to digest. From a TCM perspective, this includes foods that support the Spleen/Stomach/Earth element. Also, keep meals simple, and don't include too many ingredients in each meal. When symptoms are intense or acute, you may even want to just make congee or an equivalent. Some food options include the following:

- Soups, stews, and slow-cooked meals are generally easier to digest because they are partially broken down by the cooking process.
- Try congee (see How to Congee under Irritable Bowel Syndrome below).
- Fermented foods.
- Soaked and sprouted shoots, nuts, and seeds.
- Fennel seed—chew 1 tsp after meals or steep crushed seeds in boiling water for 10 minutes (cover with lid while steeping so beneficial volatile oils are not lost) and drink as a tea.
- Hawthorn fruit (though often used in Western herbology for cardiovascular disease, in TCM it is most commonly used for "food stagnation" from overeating, particularly for eating too much meat).
- Peppermint oil capsules are helpful for digestive cramping pain.
- Spices: many spices are carminative, meaning they help reduce digestive bloating, cramping, and flatulence. These spices include anise, caraway, cardamom, cilantro/coriander, cumin, fenugreek, ginger, orange peel, and peppermint.

Mint and Chamomile Tea for IBS

While you can certainly buy teabags of mint or chamomile, these herbs work well together to address the bloating and abdominal cramping during times of stress often associated with irritable bowel syndrome (IBS). The fresh herbs have more potency, though you can also choose dried. The volatile oils in mint are carminative, meaning they help relieve intestinal cramping and release gas to reduce bloating. Chamomile is well recognized for its use in helping to calm the nervous system. It is also anti-spasmodic and anti-inflammatory, and often recommended for use in gastrointestinal issues. Having a lidded mug or small teapot allows you to steep the herbs without letting the volatile oils escape.

- 1 tsp fresh mint leaves or ½ tsp of dried mint leaves
- 1 tsp fresh chamomile flowers or ½ tsp of dried chamomile leaves
- 1 cup water

Place the herbs in your mug. Add boiled water. Cover and let steep for 10 minutes.

Acid Reflux

See Gastroesophageal Reflux Disease (GERD)/Acid Reflux/Heartburn.

Acne

Because acne is an inflammatory skin condition associated with redness, it is often classified in TCM as a sign of Excess Heat. As a result, cooling foods that also help to cleanse the blood, support the liver's detoxification action, and restore healthy gut bacteria are often suggested. Some food options include:

- aloe vera (keep in mind that it can also act as a laxative)
- artichoke
- bamboo shoots
- burdock root (AKA gobo)
- carrot
- celery
- cruciferous vegetables: broccoli, Brussels sprouts
- cucumber
- fermented foods rich in probiotics, including kombucha, miso, sauerkraut
- foods rich in beta-carotene like carrots, pumpkin, squash, sweet potato, yam
- leafy green vegetables, including beet greens, bok choy, butterleaf, chard, dandelion greens, escarole, kohlrabi, parsley, radicchio, romaine lettuce, spinach, watercress
- omega-3 essential fatty acid (EFA) foods, like chia seeds, ground flax seeds, sesame seeds, walnuts, fatty fish
- pear
- persimmon
- seaweeds such as dulse, kelp, kombu, nori
- spirulina
- sprouts (alfalfa, clover, mung bean, radish, sunflower)
- water chestnuts
- watermelon (when seasonally available).

Burdock, Carrot, and Cucumber Salad

- 3 cups water
- 2 tbsp rice vinegar

- 2 stalks burdock root, julienned (cut into, thin strips, about 1–2" long)
- 2 medium carrots, julienned
- 1 cucumber, julienned
- 1 tbsp sesame seeds
- 2–3 tbsp sesame seed dressing (see below)

Boil 3 cups of water in a pot and add rice vinegar. Add burdock root and blanche for 30 seconds. Add carrots and blanche for another 30 seconds. Drain and set aside to cool while you make the dressing.

Toss cooled burdock root, carrots, and cucumber together with sesame seed dressing and sprinkle with sesame seeds.

Sesame Seed Dressing

- ¼ cup extra virgin olive oil
- ¼ cup seasoned rice vinegar
- 1½ tbsp of honey or maple syrup
- 1½ tbsp of sesame oil
- 1½ tsp soy sauce or tamari sauce
- 1 clove garlic, minced
- Pinch of salt

Place all ingredients in a jar and shake to mix. You can keep this in the fridge for up to 2 weeks and you'll have plenty left over.

Skin-Clearing Tea

- 1 bunch of dandelion greens
- 1 bunch of beet greens
- 1 bunch of parsley
- 4 cups of water

Boil all the greens in 4 cups of water for 15 to 20 minutes. Strain it, divide it into 4 portions, and drink 1 to 3 portions daily.

As many of you may have noticed, you may be more likely to suffer more pimples when you indulge in too much greasy, sugary, or processed food, so these are best avoided. Because acne is commonly a Heat condition, it's also best to stay away from red meats, hot spices, tropical fruits, caffeinated beverages, and alcohol.

Allergies

Of course, if you are allergic to any of the foods I'm listing here as good to treat allergies, you should continue to avoid that food, despite my general recommendations here. If you want to read more about food allergies, check out Chapter 8: Food Allergies, Sensitivities, and Intolerances.

Because the types of allergies are wide and varied—food, chemical, topical, airborne, and so forth—the general suggestions here focus on strengthening the immune system to help restore it to balance. Just as you won't want your immune system to be underactive, leaving you susceptible to infections, neither do you want your immune system to overreact, resulting in autoimmune disorders like allergies.

In TCM, your Lungs are associated with your immune system, so many of my recommended foods here support healthy lung/Lung function:

- asparagus
- bamboo sprouts
- basil
- celery
- chamomile tea
- cruciferous vegetables, including Brussels sprouts, cauliflower
- daikon radish, horseradish, radish
- fennel
- fenugreek
- fermented foods rich in probiotics, including kombucha, miso, sauerkraut
- ginger
- green tea
- honey: local unpasteurized honey may help address seasonal pollen allergies; you could also try bee pollen
- Job's tears (also known as coix seed, Chinese pearl barley, and *hato mugi* in Japanese and *yi yi ren* in Chinese pinyin; note that while it sometimes is named with the word "barley," it is not barley, and it is gluten-free)
- leafy green vegetables like arugula/rocket, Belgian endive/chicory, butterleaf lettuce, cabbage, dandelion greens, escarole, kale, kohlrabi, mustard greens, parsley, radicchio, romaine, spinach, watercress

- mushrooms, such as button, cremini, enoki, maitake, morel, oyster, portobello, reishi, shiitake
- onions, scallions/spring onions
- sprouts (clover, mung bean, radish, sunflower)
- turmeric
- turnip
- well-cooked rice (congee), oats, spelt, sweet rice, brown rice, basmati rice, rye, amaranth.

Raw Job's Tears Tea

- 1 tsp Job's tears (coix seed, Chinese pearl barley, *hato mugi, yi yi ren*)
- 1 cup hot water
- Optional: honey, cinnamon, or nutmeg

Rinse Job's tears. Steep 1 tsp of Job's tears seeds in a cup of hot water for 10 minutes. Strain and drink at least twice daily. A bit of honey, cinnamon, or nutmeg might make it more to your taste.

Cooked Job's Tears Tea

- 1 cup Job's tears (coix seed, Chinese pearl barley, *hato mugi, yi yi ren*)
- Enough water to cover
- Optional: dash of sugar, salt, honey, or cinnamon

Rince Job's tears and then put them in a pot and add enough water to cover Job's tears by about 5 cm (2 inches). Put a lid on the pot. Bring to a boil, then reduce heat to allow a slow simmer for 45–55 minutes, until Job's tears are tender and chewy. Drain the water and drink this as a tea. You can add your optional flavor. Don't let Job's tears go to waste! You can eat them as a side dish or add them to a soup, salad, or Buddha bowl.

If you're suffering from allergies, you might want to consider that some of the following foods may aggravate your allergies or even be a cause:

- alcohol
- citrus
- corn
- cow dairy

- eggs (especially chicken eggs)
- feedlot-farmed animals: ham, lunch meats, bacon, beef, pork, and organ meats
- hot spicy foods (can cause a boost of histamine release)
- nightshades (eggplant/aubergine, tomato, peppers)
- peanuts
- refined and processed foods
- soy products
- sugar
- vegetable shortening, hydrogenated fats, margarines made with safflower, sunflower, corn, soy oils
- wheat and gluten-containing foods.

Egg Substitutes

If you have an allergy to eggs or are vegan, baking can be challenging. Eggs are important for:

- binding ingredients and giving food structure
- adding moisture and flavor
- helping foods rise or puff up as the eggs trap pockets of air that can expand during heating.

You can't simply skip eggs without replacement when you're baking, so while you can find commercial egg replacers in food stores, here are some simple alternatives you can use in place of eggs. Keep in mind that baking is chemistry, so there may be some trial and error to get the exact results you want.

Each of the following replaces the equivalent of 1 egg:

- 1 tbsp ground flax or chia seeds mixed with 3 tbsp water until it's gelatinous and thick (can add a chewy or firm texture)
- ¼ cup of mashed or pureed banana, pumpkin, or avocado (note that it may change the flavor, but your baked good will be dense and moist)
- ¼ cup of yogurt (may work better if beaten before adding to other ingredients, as it can be heavy)
- ¼ cup of silken tofu (won't alter the end flavor, but tends to make your baked good heavier and denser)
- ¼ cup of applesauce (but don't add more than 1 cup to any recipe, as it can make it rubbery)
- ¼ cup of carbonated water (it obviously adds moisture, but the air bubbles in it also help your baked product to rise)

- 1 tsp baking soda mixed with 1 tbsp vinegar (works best for recipes like cakes, quick breads, and brownies to make them fluffier)
- 3 tbsp of smooth nut butter (almond, cashew, or peanut butter—even though peanuts are technically legumes—can be used in some recipes, but it will change the flavor and is heavier)
- 2 tbsp arrowroot mixed with 3 tbsp water
- 1 tbsp unflavored gelatin dissolved in 1 tbsp cold water; then mix in 2 tbsp boiling water until the mixture is frothy (keep in mind that gelatin is an animal product, so not suitable for a vegan diet; it will also make for a stiffer end product)
- 1 tbsp agar-agar powder mixed with 1 tbsp water (a good vegan option, but it results in a stiffer end product)
- 3 tbsp aquafaba (this is the liquid found in canned beans—it is an excellent substitute for egg whites)
- 1 tbsp soy lecithin powder can replace 1 large egg yolk.

Anxiety

Although there are several different types of anxiety—including panic disorder, social anxiety disorder, and phobias—and a wide range in severity of anxiety symptoms, the general symptoms include feeling panicked or uneasy, palpitations, shortness of breath, dry mouth, cold or sweaty hands or feet, muscle tension, dizziness, nausea, and problems sleeping.

TCM usually looks to the Water and Earth elements (see Chapter 6: Foods by Element) when addressing anxiety, as it is a combination of fear and worry. The Water element is related to the Kidneys and adrenal glands that pump out stress hormones. Some salty flavored foods address this issue. The Earth element is fed by sweet foods, including complex carbohydrates. Unrefined complex carbohydrates maximize the presence of L-tryptophan in the brain which aids in the formation of the neurotransmitter serotonin. Serotonin is required for calming the mind and promoting sound sleep. L-tryptophan is found in most foods, but other amino acids in high-protein foods compete with its use in the formation of serotonin, so carbohydrates are your best source.

Of course, you shouldn't go overboard on the salty or sweet foods, and you may notice you crave these foods when you're stressed, anxious, or depressed. Instead, look to find a healthy balance of whole foods that include these flavors.

Whole grains fit this category, as they are rich in B vitamins. They also contain some essential fatty acids, like the omega-3s you've probably heard about time and again as a thing you should make sure you eat. When the germ and bran of a grain is kept, you get these nutrients, and the bitter flavor of the whole grain supports the TCM Heart, helping to calm the mind. The interesting thing is that TCM and Ayurveda both use whole grains like wheat and barley (both gluten grains) as herbs and foods to help calm the mind and even improve digestion. That is, if your digestive system is not completely out of balance.

Foods rich in essential fatty acids and magnesium are also key to addressing anxiety. Essential fatty acids help improve brain function (Haag, 2003; Yehuda, Rabinovitz, and Mostofsky, 2005). Magnesium has been called "the original chill pill," as it can help decrease an overactive stress response through a number of hormonal and brain mechanisms (Deans, 2011).

Put it all together, and these are foods that can help treat and decrease your anxiety:

- avocado
- chamomile tea, which is calming and ideal for the evening
- cruciferous vegetables like broccoli, Brussels sprouts, cabbage, cauliflower, collard greens, kale, mustard greens
- green tea: contains L-theanine which helps release chemicals in the brain that promote a feeling of alertness with calmness during the day
- magnesium-rich foods, including beans (black, kidney, lima, navy, pinto, white, etc.), halibut, tuna, artichoke, dates, figs, barley, oat bran, brown rice, almonds, pine nuts, Brazil nuts, cashews, pumpkin seeds, garbanzo beans/chickpeas, lentils, broccoli, beet greens, okra, parsnips, peas, pumpkin, spinach, squash, sweet potatoes
- omega-3 essential fatty acid foods, including wild salmon, sardines, mackerel, herring, and halibut, as well as chia seeds, flax seeds (ground), walnuts
- seaweeds such as dulse, kelp, kombu, nori, wakame.

Foods that are best avoided or limited include stimulants like caffeine-containing food and beverages and processed or concentrated sugary foods.

Official Melissa Tea for Calm

I often joke with my patients that my name means someone who can both poke you and put you to sleep. It's as if my parents knew my future profession would be TCM and acupuncture, because if you've been for acupuncture, you may be familiar with the "acunap" you may enjoy on the treatment table.

Melissa officinalis, called *xiang feng cao* in TCM, is an herb more commonly known as lemon balm. The name "Melissa" comes from the Greek word *melissophyllo*, which means "honeybee," referring to the fact that bees are attracted to the flowers of this plant. "Officinalis" means that it is used in medicine.

While lemon balm is an herb that I personally don't often see used within TCM, it has been used historically for centuries. This plant belongs to the mint family, and it does have a lemon scent. It's easy to grow (even I can grow it) and, in addition to calming the nervous system, it is used as an antiviral, antibacterial, mosquito repellant, digestive, anti-inflammatory, memory enhancer, and more.

This is best if you have a lidded mug so you can let it steep without losing its volatile oils.

- 2 tbsp fresh or 1 tsp dried lemon balm leaves
- 1 cup water
- Optional: honey or maple syrup to taste

Add your lemon balm leaves to your mug, add 1 cup of boiling water, and place your lid on. Let it steep for 15 minutes or longer. Add a bit of sweetener if you like.

Arthritis

While we often associate arthritis only with the older population, there are many types of arthritis, and it can affect people of all ages. The basic diagnosis of arthritis is chronic inflammation of one or more joints. It's one of the leading causes for disability, so finding ways to manage it is essential.

Selecting foods that are anti-inflammatory and avoiding foods that are pro-inflammatory is a good starting point for all types of arthritis.

Avoid or limit these inflammatory foods:

- saturated fats: they increase inflammation—most of them are found in animal protein, which is a source of arachidonic acid, a fatty acid that promotes inflammation
- refined carbohydrates like pastries and white bread
- fried foods
- too much sugar, including that found in beverages
- feedlot-farmed animals: ham, lunch meats, bacon, beef, pork, and organ meats
- vegetable shortening, hydrogenated fats, margarines made with safflower, sunflower, corn, soy oils
- alcohol.

Enjoy these anti-inflammatory foods:

- flax seeds and flaxseed oil
- high-quality fish oil, mackerel, herring, sardines, anchovies, wild salmon, cod, halibut
- olives, olive oil and vinaigrettes made with it
- green leafy vegetables
- apples
- onions, shallots, leeks, garlic, and all related to the allium family
- berries (blueberries, raspberries, and strawberries)
- pumpkin seeds, walnuts
- seaweeds (kelp, kombu, wakame, arame)
- papaya (contains an anti-inflammatory enzyme called papain), pineapple (contains an anti-inflammatory enzyme called betaine)
- turmeric
- ginger.

In TCM, arthritis is classified as a "Bi syndrome," meaning "obstruction syndrome." The premise is basically that the joint pain is caused by something obstructing smooth movement through the joint. What's a bit trickier to explain to a non-TCM practitioner is that there are different types of Bi syndromes, each grouped by the natural element that causes the obstruction.

- Wind Bi syndrome arthritis symptoms include pain that comes and goes and that moves location (so it may be in the knees one day and hands another).
- Cold Bi syndrome arthritis causes strong, sharp, or stabbing pain in fixed locations in the joint. Heat application makes the joint feel better.
- Heat Bi syndrome arthritis shows up as joints that are red, swollen, warm to touch, and painful. A classic example of this is gout.
- Damp Bi syndrome arthritis manifests as joints that ache deeply, feel stiff and swollen, and result in a sensation of heaviness in the limbs.

It's also possible to have a combination of types of Bi syndrome. For example, a common combination is Wind-Cold-Damp Bi syndrome which results in various swollen joints that cause deep aching pain and occasional sharp pain that is worse in cold and damp weather.

Because of the different classifications of arthritis, it's important to sort out what type of Bi syndrome you experience so you can figure out your best food choices. If you're unsure, ask a Traditional Chinese Medicine practitioner what type of Bi syndrome classification you fit. If you have Heat Bi syndrome, you're best to avoid or limit foods in the Hot category (see Chapter 2: How to Classify Foods Using TCM). Of course, the reverse is true if you have Cold Bi syndrome.

Anti-Inflammatory Arthritis Elixirs

While there are different types of arthritis in TCM, these recipes are balanced in temperature and nature and contain anti-inflammatory ingredients.

Anti-Inflammatory Ginger Turmeric Green Juice

For this recipe, you'll need a juicer.

- 2 sticks of celery
- 1 large cucumber
- 1 peeled lemon
- 1" of fresh turmeric root
- 1" of fresh ginger root
- Pinch of black pepper

Process the celery, cucumber, lemon, turmeric root, and ginger root through your juicer. Mix in the pepper, as this helps with absorption of the turmeric.

Anti-Inflammatory Turmeric Ginger Green Smoothie

If you don't have a juicer, not to worry—you can use a blender for this recipe.

- 1 packed cup of spinach or kale (baby versions are sweeter and more tender)
- 1 apple, chopped
- 1 cup frozen berries of your choice
- 1 tsp ground ginger
- 1 tsp ground turmeric
- 1 cup water
- ¼ cup coconut or oat milk
- Pinch of black pepper

Blend everything until it's smooth. Add more water or coconut or oat milk if it's too thick.

Wind Bi Arthritis

Include foods like:

- green leafy vegetables, scallions/spring onions
- grapes, mulberries
- black beans
- whole grains.

Okay, not my cup of tea, but my textbooks recommend snake meat.

Cold Bi Arthritis

Include warming foods like:

- chives, leeks, mustard greens, onions, parsnips, pumpkin, squash
- cherries, pineapple, raspberries
- adzuki beans, black beans, lentils
- pumpkin seeds, sesame seeds, sunflower seeds, walnuts
- anise, cinnamon, fennel, garlic, ginger, turmeric.

Heat Bi Arthritis

Include cooling foods like:

- cabbage, celery, dandelion greens and other green leafy vegetables, radish
- cantaloupe, green apple, lemon, lime, melon
- mung beans, soybeans, tofu.

Damp Bi Arthritis

Include bland, diuretic, bitter, and drying foods like:

- alfalfa, burdock root, celery, radish, rhubarb, turnip, watercress
- cruciferous vegetables like broccoli, Brussels sprouts, cabbage, kale
- bitter melon, grapefruit
- red adzuki beans, mung beans
- amaranth, barley, hops, quinoa, rye.

Asthma

Asthma is a chronic inflammatory disease of the airways. It causes shortness of breath, wheezing, coughing, and a feeling of tightness in the chest. Although there are many possible triggers, including allergies, air pollutants, smoke, infection, exercise, and even strong emotions, food may also aggravate or improve the frequency of asthma attacks.

Choose anti-inflammatory foods that support lung health and avoid mucus-forming foods. It's also wise to limit foods containing arachidonic acids, as their metabolites can worsen asthma (Lewis and Robin, 1985).

Avoid or limit these foods, especially when you are experiencing more asthmatic symptoms:

- foods that produce mucus, including foods that trigger an immune response—avoid known food allergens and limit or avoid dairy products, wheat, pop, and processed sugar, too much salty food, and alcoholic beverages
- foods that contain high levels of arachidonic acid, such as shellfish, meat, and eggs
- inflammatory foods, including some of those listed above, plus refined carbohydrates like pastries and white bread and fried foods.

Enjoy these Lung-supporting foods:

- asparagus, bamboo shoots, Brussels sprouts, cabbage, carrots, cauliflower, daikon, greens (arugula/rocket, Belgian endive/chicory, bok choy, butterleaf, collard greens, dandelion, escarole, kale, kohlrabi, mustard greens, parsley, radicchio, romaine, watercress), horseradish, onions, pumpkin, sprouts (clover, mung bean, radish, sunflower), squash, turnip, yams
- apple, figs, lychee/litchi fruit, pear, tangerine, winter melon
- sauerkraut
- garlic, ginger, fennel, fenugreek, nutmeg, sage, thyme, turmeric
- well-cooked rice (congee), oats, spelt, sweet rice, brown rice, basmati rice, rye, amaranth, millet
- alternatives for cow's milk, such as rice milk, raw goat's milk, almond milk, hemp milk, coconut milk.

Kitchen Herb Steam Inhalation

Doing a steam inhalation is a wonderful way to decrease the smooth muscle spasms of asthma, address coughs, and help prevent or treat respiratory infections with clearing mucus. A bonus is that it can help clear the facial skin. This recipe gives a few options, and you may already have the ingredients in your kitchen. You can use just thyme or sage, or you can combine both. You can use it as a steam inhalation or you might sip it as a tea, especially if you have a sore or irritated throat.

- Handful of fresh thyme sprigs, 2 tbsp fresh thyme leaves, or 1 tbsp of dried thyme leaves
- 2 tbsp fresh sage leaves or 1 tbsp dried sage leaves
- 2½ cups water
- Optional: honey and/or slice of lemon or lime, if you want to make it as a tea

Note that these herbs are not suitable during pregnancy.

For the steam inhalation, have a large bowl and towel ready. If you're congested, have a box of tissues handy too, as you may need to blow your nose periodically. Make sure you're ready to do your inhalation once your herbs are added, as you don't want to lose the volatile oils.

Boil the water and pour it into your bowl. Add the herbs to the water and place the towel over your head, covering the bowl, so that you can inhale the steam without burning your face(!). Keep your eyes closed so that you don't irritate them. Inhale through your nose. Exhale through either your nose or mouth (through your nose is better). Breathe deeply in and out for 10 to 15 minutes or until the steam has dissipated.

If you want to make this as a tea, you can add honey and/or a lemon or lime for flavor.

Bad Breath

Yes, occasional bad breath happens to everyone. It can happen because of a garlicky lunch, from drinking alcohol or coffee, or after a night of mouth breathing. But chronic bad breath—also known as halitosis—can be a sign of digestive issues or problems in the mouth. Rather than just rinsing with mouthwash, which can destroy the good bacteria, further worsening the opportunity for bad bacteria to grow in your mouth, look to address the cause.

Keep in mind that long-standing halitosis can also be a sign of a variety of potentially serious health conditions, including chronic infections, autoimmune disorders like Sjögren's disease, diabetes (overly sweet breath), periodontal disease, or organ disease, so get yourself checked out if you're unsure.

In addition to brushing and flossing appropriately, changing what you eat can also help treat this embarrassing symptom. Many of the suggestions here are ones that are general to also improving digestion, but some are specific to preventing the overgrowth of bad bacteria in the mouth and the gut.

- Chew well.
- Limit or avoid greasy fried foods, refined and processed foods, hot spicy foods, alcohol, coffee, and sugar.
- Don't eat too much meat.
- Emphasize a variety of vegetables.
- Drink lots of water and/or green tea.
- Chew parsley or fennel seeds after meals; cloves and anise may also help.
- Include probiotic supplements or fermented foods that are rich in good bacteria such as yogurt (unsweetened), sauerkraut, miso, etc.

Crunchy Healthy-Mouth Salad

Eating raw crunchy foods helps clean the teeth. Apples and other foods containing pectin also help promote saliva production, which helps improve breath. Yogurt and other fermented foods help improve bacterial balance, reducing the growth of odor-causing bacteria in the mouth.

- 2 crispy apples (like Granny Smith), cut into large chunks
- 2 carrots,* grated or chopped
- 2 stalks celery,* sliced
- ½ cup chopped walnuts
- 3–5 tbsp plain yogurt (lactose-free or non-dairy, if you are lactose intolerant)
- Optional: sprinkle of cinnamon
- Optional: drizzle of honey (yes, this is sugar, but honey is also anti-bacterial, so just use a small amount)

Mix all together in a large bowl. When you're eating it, make sure to chew well, so you get the teeth-cleaning benefits.

* You can choose other crunchy, low-sugar foods to substitute, if you prefer.

Common Cold/Flu

Although modern medicine has been able to combat many illnesses, it can still only provide symptom relief for the common cold. Why is that? Well, viruses are tricky buggers. They have a nasty habit of mutating, changing just enough to evade pharmaceutical intervention. Even the flu shot can only be made to fend off three to four viruses among the many that may be present any given year.

Our best defense is a strong immune system that can respond quickly to the changing threats of viruses. Foods that are rich in vitamin C, beta-carotene and vitamin A, zinc, and selenium contribute to a healthy immune system. Check out Chapter 3: Foundations of Nutrition for lists of foods abundant in each of these important nutrients.

The key to not succumbing to a cold for days is to do something about it at the very beginning of an attack. Slightly scratchy throat? Nose starting to run? People around you coughing and sneezing? Don't wait. Give your immune system a supportive boost. Do all the stuff you should have been doing all along, including making healthy food choices, getting plenty of sleep, washing your hands regularly, and avoiding touching your face when you're out. And grab your immune-supportive remedies—vitamin C, echinacea, oregano oil, goldenseal, probiotics, zinc lozenges, garlic, astragalus, propolis, reishi mushroom, etc., though not necessarily all of these at once!

Since many of the remedies used to fight off colds and flus can be nasty-tasting, it's a good thing that honey is also antiviral and antibacterial because this is a simple thing you can add to ward off getting sick. Remember, however, that honey is still high in sugar, so a little goes a long way.

TCM classifies the common cold into two main categories (though there are more), based on the symptoms that present themselves. They are differentiated into pathogens that cause Heat symptoms or ones that cause Cold symptoms. Either way, TCM recommends warming up the body and allowing yourself to sweat it out under a pile of blankets, particularly at the start. Fever is your body's way to kill off pathogens and enhance the function of some immune cells, so why would you suppress your own army from defending you against attackers? Even cold-blooded animals intentionally seek warmer environments to raise their core body temperature when they are sick. And human studies have demonstrated that a rise in temperature of 1 to 4 degrees Celsius (1.8 to 7.2°F) results in "improved survival and resolution of many infections" (Evans, Repasky, and Fisher, 2015). Of course, that's not to say that a fever should be allowed to run wild, as that can be dangerous, and young children, older adults, and those with serious illness or disease will have different needs.

"I Hab a Coldt" Chicken Soup
Translation: "I have a cold."

Is it really true that chicken soup can help heal a cold? Maybe. It's helpful to keep you hydrated, the warmth may soothe a sore throat or alleviate chills, and, depending on what you add to it, it can provide nutrients like zinc and vitamins A and C to help support your immune system. Finally, it is a comfort food for many, providing some emotional reassurance when we feel unwell.

I don't know about you, but if I'm sick, the last thing I want to do is spend a lot of time cooking up a meal. If you have an Instant Pot or other pressure cooker, that's the fastest way to make a healing soup. I've also given the slow-cooker option here. Maybe you could make a batch at the beginning of cold and flu season and then freeze it for future use.

- 2 tbsp butter or cooking oil
- 1 large onion, chopped
- 2–4 cloves garlic, minced (depends on how much you like garlic and size of cloves)
- 2 medium carrots, chopped
- 2 stalks celery, chopped
- 1 tsp (or to taste) of salt
- 1 tsp (or to taste) of pepper
- 1 tsp dried oregano (1 tbsp, if using fresh)
- 1 tsp dried thyme (1 tbsp, if using fresh)
- 4 cups chicken stock
- 4 cups water
- About 2 lbs of chicken (you can use a whole chicken or pieces of chicken with bone and skin, but make sure you have at least 1 chicken breast so you can shred it and keep it in)
- 3 ounces dried shiitake mushrooms (shiitake and other mushrooms are immune supporting)
- Optional: 6–8 ounces noodles of your choice (I like egg noodles, but you could use broken spaghetti, or maybe you prefer elbow macaroni or bowtie/farfalle)

Sauté the onions, garlic, carrots, and celery in the butter or oil until the onions are translucent. With the Instant Pot, you can do this right in the pot with a push of the "sauté" button.

Add in the salt, pepper, oregano, thyme, chicken stock, chicken, shiitake mushrooms, and water.

For the Instant Pot, close the lid and set to the "soup" button for 7 minutes. For the slow cooker, place the lid on and cook on a low heat for 6–8 hours.

Once the cooking is complete, remove the chicken. Make sure to take out all the bones. Use two forks to shred the chicken (careful, it's hot!).

Add in your noodles.

For the Instant Pot, set it to "sauté" and cook the noodles until they are at your preferred softness, about 6 minutes.

For the slow cooker, cover and cook for another 30–40 minutes at the low heat setting.

Add the shredded chicken back in. Enjoy!

Wind-Heat Common Cold

The main symptom of Wind-Heat common cold is a sore throat. It also causes fever, sweating, thirst, runny nose with a yellow discharge, and a bit later a cough develops, often with dry throat or with sticky yellow phlegm. Although you do still want the fever to help kill the virus, soothing, cooling foods can help here:

- apple
- burdock root
- cabbage
- cilantro/coriander
- dandelion
- mint
- lots of room-temperature or warm water or tea.

If you have many of the Wind-Heat common cold symptoms, but not the sweating, you can include some of the ingredients in the Wind-Cold Common Cold section below to help you sweat out your cold.

Cooling Cabbage Soup

- 1 tbsp avocado or other cooking oil
- 2 medium onions, peeled and chopped
- 3 medium carrots, sliced
- 2 stalks celery, sliced
- 1 stalk burdock root (gobo), sliced thinly
- 1 medium leek, sliced thinly
- 4½ cups chicken or vegetable stock
- salt and pepper
- 1 medium cabbage, shredded
- 1 cup plain yogurt (lactose-free or non-dairy, if you are lactose intolerant)
- 1 sprig fresh parsley

Cook the onions, carrots, celery, burdock root, and leek in the oil in a large saucepan over low heat for 5–10 minutes, until they are soft.

Add the stock, salt, and pepper. Cover and bring to a boil. Then reduce heat and simmer for 30 minutes.

Add the cabbage and cook another 5 minutes, until slightly soft.

Add half the yogurt and stir for a minute until warmed through.

Serve topped with yogurt (soothing if you have a sore throat) and garnished with parsley.

Wind-Cold Common Cold

This type of common cold most often causes headaches, body aches, chills, runny nose with clear or white discharge, and cough. Warming foods that help promote sweating are usually recommended for this type of cold:

- cilantro/coriander
- cinnamon
- garlic
- ginger
- mustard greens and seeds
- scallions/spring onions.

Sweat-It-Out Cold-Fighting Tea

- 2 cups water
- ¼-inch piece of fresh ginger, thinly sliced
- 1 garlic clove, chopped
- 1 scallion/spring onion, chopped
- Pinch of cinnamon

Bring water to a boil. Turn off heat, add other ingredients, and cover with lid. Steep for 5 minutes.

Strain and drink 1 to 2 cups of the tea.

Cover up in clothing, get under blankets, and get ready to sweat out that cold.

Constipation

You likely don't think about the activity of your intestines unless you suffer from digestive symptoms. While it's not something you probably talk much about, since the body gets rid of much of its waste products via the stool, regular, complete bowel movements are essential to a healthy body. Imagine how awful it would be if your city's sewage system became clogged and backed up. Not good.

Bunged up? While it's not uncommon to suffer the occasional bout of constipation, it's considered chronic if it's ongoing for three or more months—though you likely won't want to wait that long before addressing it.

Constipation is defined as having fewer than three bowel movements in a week, straining to have a bowel movement, passing stools that are too hard and dry, and feeling as if you are unable to sufficiently empty your bowels. Many natural health providers (including me) consider it constipation if you have less than one bowel movement daily. There are many reasons why someone can become constipated, so you'll want to be properly assessed and treated if you suffer from chronic constipation. In fact, talk to your health care provider if you notice any persistent changes in bowel function.

As you can imagine, food can help or hinder how the bowels operate, so making the right food choices for you can make a world of difference.

There are many, many food cures you can find for treating constipation, including the following:

- Eat foods high in fiber from veggies, whole grains, fresh fruit, legumes, nuts, and seeds—for example, artichokes, beets/beetroot, broccoli, cabbage, cauliflower, peas, yams, barley, brown rice, oat bran, wheat bran, apples, grapes, grapefruit, figs, peaches, pears, adzuki beans, black beans, garbanzo beans/chickpeas, kidney beans, lentils, chia seeds, flax seeds, hemp seeds, sesame seeds, and walnuts.
- Veggies, veggies, veggies. Want to poop well? Eat enough vegetables. They are rich in fiber and nutrition.
- One of the gentlest but most efficient ways of ensuring regularity is to eat plenty of leafy green vegetables.
- Nearly as effective as eating the vegetables is drinking their juice—all leafy green vegetables will work. Juice green leafy vegetables or boil them in water and drink the broth.
- One vegetable you can choose (but don't eat the leaves, eat the stalk) is rhubarb. In Chinese herbology, we use rhubarb rhizome (the underground stem), called *da huang*, as a laxative. The above-ground stem of rhubarb—the part you find in rhubarb pie (yum!)—also can be used as a laxative.
- Aloe vera juice consumed on an empty stomach every morning for one to two weeks is also an easy remedy. It too is used as a Chinese herb. Called *lu hui*, it's a purging laxative that helps draw water into

the bowels, stimulates the secretion of mucus in the intestines, and increases peristalsis (wave-like muscular contractions of the intestines that move food and waste along).

- Of course, one of the most recognized constipation food cures, especially for older individuals, is prunes or prune juice. Stew a few prunes in water for five minutes. Eat the prunes and drink the juice before bedtime.
- Foods with a downward movement that may help with constipation include apple, banana, barley, cucumber, grapefruit, peach, and spinach.
- Stir 1 tablespoon of honey into a cup of warm water and drink it on an empty stomach, first thing in the morning.
- Wash 1 cup of figs. Boil the figs in 4 cups of water over a low flame for 20 minutes. Drink the juice as a tea, with a little sugar added according to taste.
- Foods that can be constipating include red meat, dairy, and processed and fried foods. Note that iron supplements may be constipating, so ask for forms that are well absorbed and non-constipating.

Lifestyle tips:

- Create a bowel routine. According to TCM, the best time of day to have your morning constitutional is between 5 and 7 a.m. If that doesn't fit your schedule, not to worry, just try to be consistent with allowing yourself the routine and enough time.
- Have a regular daily exercise/movement activity. It's important to make sure that you have enough physical activity, as a sedentary lifestyle can contribute to constipation. You might notice that dogs are most likely to move their bowels after a walk or run.
- Try abdominal massage. Using the heel of one hand, massage around your navel, moving down on your left and up on your right.
- Consider using a stool to place your feet on while sitting on the toilet. Placing yourself into more of a squat position puts your body in a better position for elimination.
- If your abdomen feels cold or if you are often cold, you may find a hot water bottle placed on your lower abdomen helps improve bowel function.
- Pay attention to whether you are eating too much or too little.

Rhubarb Jam for Constipation Relief

- 1 lb of rhubarb stalks, cut into ¼-inch pieces
- 3 tbsp honey or maple syrup
- 2 tbsp chia seeds
- 1 tbsp lemon juice

Add the rhubarb and sweetener to a medium-sized saucepan. Bring it to a boil, and then lower to medium heat. Stir it for about 5 minutes so the juice releases from the rhubarb, and then mash the solid pieces with a fork. Reduce to medium-low heat and add the chia seeds and lemon juice. Cook for about 30 minutes, stirring often. You may need to lower the temperature further, so nothing burns. When it has reached a jam-like consistency, remove it from the heat. Once the mixture has cooled, put the mixture in a lidded jar and keep it in the fridge. It can be kept for up to 2 weeks.

Cough

Coughing is a natural response when your body wants to quickly rid itself of something foreign in the throat or airway. You might develop a cough because of a cold, allergies, lung disease, acid reflux, or as a side effect of medications. As with all symptoms, it's important to pay attention to cause and address the source.

Whether you're looking for pharmaceuticals, herbs or other nutraceuticals, or foods to help stop your cough, the word you may come across to describe things that help reduce your urge to cough is "antitussive."

No matter the cause, TCM considers a cough the result of Lung Qi moving in the opposite direction from its normal course (we call it "rebellious Qi," and no, it doesn't wear a black leather jacket or drive a motorcycle). So, in addition to searching out the treatment solution to the cause of the cough—including some of the food cures listed under common cold or allergies—check out the Metal—Fall section in Chapter 6, for tips on Lung support.

- Make sure to drink lots of fluids to thin out mucus and moisturize the mucous membranes.
- Honey is both antibacterial/antiviral and soothes the throat.
- Ginger is anti-inflammatory and has antihistamine and decongestant properties.
- Licorice root can improve mucus production to soothe an inflamed and irritated throat and stop cough. It is also used to treat acid reflux.

- Lemon squeezed into hot or warm water can help ease a cough. Adding honey helps a dry, tickly cough.
- Almonds are traditionally used to help transform phlegm and alleviate cough.
- For a phlegmy cough or congestion in the nose or chest, avoid dairy as it promotes mucus production.

For a dry cough:

Asian pears (they are big and round, rather than what you might typically think as "pear-shaped") or other pear varieties can be used.

Steamed Pears for Dry Cough

- 1 pear
- Approximately 1 tbsp of honey

Cut the top off the pear, but don't toss it. Core the pear. Pour honey into the space in the pear where the core was. Put the top back on the pear. Steam the pear until it's very soft (generally 15–45 minutes, depending on the pear type and size). Let the pear cool and then eat it and all the juices.

Easy Pear Tea for Dry Cough

- 1 pear
- 2 cups of water
- 1 tablespoon of honey

Remove the core of the pear and cut it into chunks. Bring the pears to a boil and then simmer for 5 minutes. Add the honey and drink the pear tea and eat the pear chunks.

For a dry cough with thick yellow phlegm that is hard to cough up:

Daikon for Yellow Phlegm Cough

- 2 daikon radishes
- 1 cup water chestnuts
- 1 tsp honey

Juice the daikon and water chestnuts. Warm 1 cup of the juice and add 1 tsp of honey. Put the remainder in the fridge. Have 2 to 3 cups per day.

Crapulence

I came across this word from one of my TCM textbooks (sometimes you learn English from TCM textbooks because someone translated and used a less commonly known word). Because I hadn't known what the word meant and because I know that most of us have suffered from it at some point in our lives, I had to add it to the list of symptoms to treat. And, no, it doesn't mean diarrhea or something else directly (maybe indirectly) related to excrement.

Crapulence refers to sickness or feeling unwell from eating or drinking too much. It comes from the Latin word for intoxication. In other words, it could be a hangover. It could also refer to the TCM term "food stagnation."

The first and most obvious recommendation for this symptom is simply: don't overeat or get drunk. But if you have, here are some food recommendations that may help. Despite what you may want to think, neither a greasy meal nor hair of the dog (i.e., more booze) is a good idea to treat a hangover. Both will only very temporarily make you feel better but will ultimately make things worse.

- If it's a hangover you're treating, water is your best friend. Rehydrate your poor body.
- Hawthorn berries are a TCM herb (*shan zha*) used to address food stagnation, particularly from the overconsumption of meat or greasy, oily, fried foods.
- Mung beans.
- Leafy greens.
- Ginger, mint.
- Dried orange peels (TCM herbs *chen pi* and *qing pi*).
- Miso and other fermented foods and drinks.
- Congee (see How to Congee under Irritable Bowel Syndrome below).
- Persimmon (I first learned of this fruit when I lived in Japan. It was a number-one recommendation for treating hangovers, but is delicious—as long as it's ripe—for any occasion).
- Eggs are rich in taurine and cysteine, amino acids that can help with detoxification and liver support.
- Make sure to get enough fiber to help normalize bowel movements.

Hangover Quick Beverage Recipes

If you have a bad hangover, you don't likely feel up to making anything complex with ingredients you have to go shopping for. Plus, "hair of the dog"—where you drink more alcohol to offset your current hangover—isn't a healthy approach, so here are some quick recipes to help you get through the day.

Hangover Smoothie

You can swap out ingredients based on what you have on hand.

- ½ cup leafy greens like spinach, kale, or dandelion greens to provide you with lots of nutrients and support your overwhelmed liver
- ½ banana or avocado to add smooth, rich texture, while also providing you with plenty of potassium and other minerals and vitamins
- ½ cup of frozen or fresh berries, cherries, mango, papaya, or pineapple for their vitamin C, antioxidants, and flavor
- Juice of 1 lemon or lime
- 1–2 cups coconut water or regular water to help with rehydration
- 1"-piece of fresh, peeled ginger or ¼ tsp powdered ginger to help with nausea and digestion
- Optional: protein powder, especially if you are not having other sources of protein on your hangover day

Blend your choice of ingredients and adjust to the thickness you like.

Hangover Tea

In TCM, we generally prefer to recommend warming foods when trying to ease digestion, so since a smoothie is consumed cold and often uses frozen ingredients, you may prefer a warm, comforting tea.

You may be able to talk with your TCM practitioner about an herbal formula that includes herbs like *ge gen* (kudzu root); *chen pi, zhi shi,* or *qing pi* (various kinds of oranges and orange peels); and *pu gong ying* (dandelion), or you can make some simple teas with things you might already have on hand.

- 1 tbsp fresh or 1 tsp dried mint leaves to help settle your stomach and soothe your pounding head
- 1"-piece of fresh ginger root or ¼ tsp dried ginger powder to help with nausea and calm your roiling stomach

- Green tea, matcha, or oolong tea for their L-theanine which helps give you energy while keeping you calm
- Pu-erh tea, a fermented tea that is rich in antioxidants and that can help ease your digestion while helping to improve your mental focus

Diarrhea

Just like constipation, occasional bouts of diarrhea are common. It might be caused by eating something that disagrees with us, such as making a big dietary change, having greasy or fried foods, or too much spicy food. Food poisoning is another unpleasant cause of diarrhea (not that there's any pleasant cause!).

Chronic diarrhea may be associated with celiac disease, Crohn's, ulcerative colitis, proctitis, irritable bowel syndrome (IBS), or various other malabsorption disorders. Diarrhea might also be caused by emotional turmoil and stress.

When assessing issues associated with diarrhea, questions about frequency, urgency, and the presence of cramping or pain are important, as well as whether there is blood, mucus, or undigested food in the stool. Because dehydration and malnutrition can result from chronic diarrhea, it's essential to hydrate well and make sure there aren't any nutritional deficiencies.

- Eat small meals regularly to make it easier to digest.
- Focus on cooked foods. Although some enzymes will be destroyed, cooking helps break the foods down, making them more easily digested. Soups, stews, slow-cooked meals, steamed vegetables or fruit, and roasted vegetables are examples of suitable cooking methods.
- Some foods that may help with diarrhea include adzuki beans, barley, carrot, chicken, eggplant/aubergine, garlic, leek, millet, mung beans, persimmon (under-ripe), pineapple, rice, scallions/spring onions, sweet potato, and umeboshi plum.
- Ginger is recommended again. Is there anything that ginger is not good for? It can settle an upset stomach, promote the release of gastric juices and enzymes for digestion, relieve cramping, decrease inflammation, and help kill pathogens. Don't overdo it, however, as in large quantities it can promote bowel movements.
- Steep black tea for ten minutes and drink three cups per day until diarrhea subsides.
- Blackberries are astringent, so blackberries or blackberry tea is a tasty remedy for both adults and children.

- Because apples are a good source of a fiber called pectin, they can be used to bulk up stool and slow diarrhea. Note that they are also suitable for treating constipation.
- Fermented foods like yogurt provide probiotics (good bacteria), making it useful for improving digestion and destroying bad bacteria.
- Chamomile tea or lemon balm tea both calm the nervous system and reduce intestinal cramping.
- Avoid spicy, greasy, fried, and processed foods. Also eliminate caffeine and alcohol.
- A relatively bland diet is best, especially for acute diarrhea.
- Check out How to Congee under Irritable Bowel Syndrome.

Homemade Rehydration Drink

If you're suffering from either acute or chronic diarrhea, you might become dehydrated, and you shouldn't just rely on feeling thirsty as a sign to rehydrate. Left untreated, dehydration can lead to fatigue, headache, irritability, dizziness, and reduced or dark-colored urination. These are symptoms that you might be able to resolve on your own by rehydrating with the following recipe. Make this big amount that you can sip over the day.

- 4 cups water
- 1 tsp sea salt or Himalayan salt
- Juice of 2 lemons
- 3 tbsp honey

Mix well and sip over your day.

Seek emergency care if you are experiencing any of the following:

- fainting
- nausea or vomiting
- fever
- seizures
- irregular, rapid, or weak heart rate
- dizziness that doesn't go away after a few seconds
- not urinating for more than eight hours
- difficulty moving or walking
- feeling unusually tired or confused.

Flatulence

There aren't a lot of health issues that are the butt (pun intended!) of many jokes. This, however, is one of them, though there are gastroenterologists and researchers (their area of study is called flatology—not making that up) who study this full-time. Not being one of those people, I had to do my own research, and I found out that it's normal to pass gas 10–20 times a day, on average. I also found out way more about flatulence than I ever thought I would, including many nicknames—windy pop or fluff (that's what we called it when we were kids), colonic calliope, noisy bottom burps, backdoor trumpet, bean bombers, fanny halitosis, poofume, and trouser cough.

Did you know that flatulence is mostly a combination of five gases? Those are nitrogen, oxygen, carbon dioxide, hydrogen, and methane (though not everyone produces methane, so those who don't won't be able to create "blue angels"—i.e., light their flatulence on fire). The first two gases are swallowed when talking, chewing, and from drinking fizzy drinks. The last three are produced in the gastrointestinal tract as part of digestion. The part that creates the smell that makes people cringe is a combination of volatile sulfur compounds.

Most of the intestinal gases (flatus) are a by-product of fermentation by bacteria in the gut as they digest the foods that we have a hard time digesting on our own. Beans ("the musical fruit") are the most notorious food for causing gas, as they contain sugars that we have a hard time breaking down. Note that there are things you can do to make eating beans easier on you and the ones you spend time around (see below). Other foods that you might want to watch out for when you go on a date, before an important meeting, or before going on a long bus or plane ride include:

- artichokes, asparagus, broccoli, Brussels sprouts, cabbage, cauliflower, celery, corn, cucumbers, green peppers, onions, peas, potatoes, radishes
- apples, apricots, bananas, peaches, pears, prunes, raisins
- whole grains and bran, pasta
- dairy products
- beans, lentils
- packaged foods made with lactose, like cereal, breads, salad dressing
- foods with sugar alcohols, like sorbitol, xylitol, maltitol, mannitol, erythritol, and isomalt; these are often found in sugar-free foods for diabetics
- wine, beer, carbonated drinks.

Foods that are the most likely to create the dreaded gas smell include:

- alcohol, coffee
- asparagus, cabbage, cucumbers, onions, radishes
- prunes
- beans, lentils, nuts
- chicken, eggs, fish
- dairy products
- garlic
- highly seasoned foods.

Flatulence is often associated with bloating and sometimes with belching, cramping, and changes in bowel movements, so while it may be an amusing topic (I hope I made you giggle at least a little), it can also be a sign of some major digestive issues that should be properly addressed.

- Eat more slowly and chew your food well to make it easier on the rest of your digestive system.
- Eat smaller, more frequent meals.
- When making big dietary changes, such as starting to include more legumes or even vegetables to your diet, do so slowly so your body can adjust.
- Soak beans overnight before cooking them, and make sure to rinse them well.
- Fermented foods are generally more easily digested. Examples include tempeh, miso, soy sauce, yogurt, kefir, sauerkraut, and sourdough.
- Include these foods that may help to reduce flatulence: anise, basil, black pepper, caraway, carrots, cilantro/coriander, cumin, dill, limes, lemons, papaya, parsley, peppermint, pickled vegetables, sauerkraut, seaweed, and turmeric.

Simple Remedies for Gassy Guts

- After meals, you can chew on fresh ginger slices in lime juice or on fennel seeds to reduce gas.
- Steep 1 tsp of anise, basil, bay leaf, cardamom, cilantro/coriander, dill, fennel, mint, oregano, rosemary, sage, or turmeric in hot water and drink after meals.

How to Eat Legumes

- When choosing a legume, consider that some are easier to digest than others:
  - most easily digested: adzuki beans, lentils, mung beans, peas
  - harder to digest: black-eyed peas, black beans, garbanzo beans/chickpeas, kidney beans, lima beans, pinto beans
  - hardest to digest: soybeans (unless processed or fermented, as in soy milk, miso, sprouts, soy sauce, tempeh, and tofu).
- Soak legumes prior to cooking for 24–48 hours. Soaking softens the skins of the legumes, begins sprouting, and gets rid of phytic acid. It promotes shorter cooking times, makes nutrients more available for absorption, and decreases the gassiness that legumes can cause. Even better is to change the water a few times during the soaking process. And some suggest using very warm water. Make sure to discard the soaking water.
- Some find that adding apple cider vinegar, lemon juice, or baking soda to the soaking water can be helpful.
- Cook legumes with kombu seaweed to make it easier to digest and help improve the flavor and nutrient profile. Add one large piece of kombu to the pot of water and beans prior to bringing to a boil. Remove the kombu after cooking is complete.
- Adding ginger, fennel, or cumin prior to cooking beans can also decrease gas.
- For the first 20 minutes of boiling, keep the lid off the pot to allow steam to rise.
- Scoop off and get rid of the foam that comes to the surface when boiling legumes.

Table 13: Cooking Chart for Legumes

Legume (1 cup dried)	Soaking time (hours)	Cooking time (minutes)	Yields (cups)
Adzuki beans	8–12	45–60	3
Black beans	8–12	1–3 hours	3
Black turtle beans	8–12	60–90	2¼

cont.

Legume (1 cup dried)	Soaking time (hours)	Cooking time (minutes)	Yields (cups)
Black-eyed peas	8–12	60	2
Cannellini (white kidney) beans	8–12	45	2½
Fava/broad beans	8–12	45	1⅔
Garbanzo beans/chickpeas	12–19	2–3 hours	2
Great Northern beans	8–12	90	2⅔
Green split peas	–	45–60	2
Kidney beans	8–12	60	2¼
Lentils	–	15–30	2
Lima beans	8–12	60–90	2
Mung beans	8–12	60	2
Navy beans	8–12	45–60	2⅔
Pinto beans	–	1–2 hours	2⅔
Soybeans	10–12	3–4 hours	3
Yellow split peas	–	60–90	2

Note: Table 13 shows minimum cooking times, but cooking them for longer makes them easier to digest, especially for larger beans.

Gastroesophageal Reflux Disease (GERD)/Acid Reflux/Heartburn

Gastroesophageal reflux disease (thankfully shortened to GERD) is a common chronic digestive problem that involves the stomach, the esophagus (the tube between your mouth and your stomach), and the sphincter between those organs (called the lower esophageal sphincter). The stomach has a thick mucus lining that helps to protect it from the stomach acid that is important to your digestive process. The esophagus doesn't have this same protective lining, so if the sphincter is unable to do its job of keeping the stomach acid from moving back upward, you may notice symptoms.

Heartburn, or acid reflux, is the most common symptom of GERD. While most have experienced heartburn at some point, that doesn't necessarily mean you have GERD. Maybe you overdid it at the neighbor's BBQ. Or you got fired up to take part in a hot wings competition. Or maybe you splurged on a slice of cheesecake right before bedtime. Heartburn is a descriptive name (it doesn't actually involve the heart) for the sensation of warmth, heat, burning, or discomfort that can start in the upper abdomen and spread upward, maybe into your throat, leaving a sour taste in your mouth. It can interfere with sleep because it is often worse when you lie down (gravity when you're standing makes it harder for the acid to move upward).

GERD is diagnosed if you have chronic, frequent, or severe symptoms. And heartburn or acid reflux isn't the only symptom of GERD. Other symptoms include belching, bad breath, inflammation of the gums, tooth enamel erosion, and chest pain (make sure that it's not other causes, as heartburn can mask actual heart problems).

Some people are diagnosed with "silent reflux," medically called laryngopharyngeal reflux (LPR) or extraesophageal reflux, where the upper esophageal sphincter allows acid to creep upwards. When this happens, the acid affects the larynx ("voice box") or pharynx (throat), causing problems with swallowing, a feeling of something stuck in the throat, throat clearing, a chronically sore throat, laryngitis, hoarseness, chronic cough, postnasal drip, wheezing, or frequent upper respiratory infections.

While antacid ads might simply encourage you to keep their pills on hand so you can fully indulge in the all-you-can-eat buffet or fast-food joint, the first step to managing the symptoms is to stop the behavior that leads to the problem. This is along the same line as "Doctor, it hurts when I poke myself in the eye." Doctor replies, "So stop poking yourself in the eye."

However, it's not simply a matter of taking a pill to suppress stomach acid production. Not only can too much stomach acid cause GERD, but insufficient stomach acid can counterintuitively also cause acid reflux symptoms. There is controversy in this regard, with some saying that insufficient stomach acid is the leading cause of acid reflux and others in disagreement. However, it is worth recognizing that too little stomach acid results in poor digestion, a buildup of bacteria, and gas bubbles that can rise into the esophagus, carrying stomach acid with them and weakening the lower esophageal sphincter. We tend to produce less stomach acid as we age. Prolonged use of proton pump inhibitors (PPIs) or antacids, chronic stress, and stomach surgeries such as gastric bypass surgery can also reduce our natural production of stomach acid.

Either way, what's key is figuring out triggers and reducing them, improving digestion, and decreasing the irritation and damage caused by acid being in contact with tissue.

Things that are prone to causing heartburn and aggravating GERD include:

- greasy, fried, hot spicy, heavy foods

- carbonated beverages, coffee, chocolate, garlic, onions, tomatoes, citrus (try to figure out your triggers)
- large meals
- lying down shortly after eating (allow at least a few hours between eating and reclining)
- tight-fitting clothes, which can increase pressure on the sphincter
- alcohol and smoking, as both weaken the sphincter
- certain prescribed medications, which can also weaken the sphincter
- hiatus hernia
- being overweight
- pregnancy
- stress
- possibly a genetic link.

Other than reducing or eliminating your triggers, you might also benefit from trying a few other things.

- Licorice root is one of the best natural remedies for preventing acid reflux. If you have high blood pressure, make sure you pick up deglycyrrhizinated licorice root chewable tablets. Chewing it well to mix it with saliva about 20 minutes before meals makes it more effective. You can also take it before bed, if heartburn at night keeps you up. If you don't like licorice flavor, it does come in other flavor options.
- Fermented foods are rich in good bacteria that can support digestion and may help with GERD and acid reflux.

Got-GERD Remedies

- Ginger is one of those foods that is good for a ton of health conditions, especially those of a digestive nature. Either add ginger to your food or make a ginger tea to drink after meals.
- Aloe vera juice before meals can be helpful, though be mindful that aloe can also act as a laxative.
- Chamomile tea sipped before bed will not only help ease heartburn but also support restful sleep.
- As mentioned previously, licorice root can be helpful to soothe GERD, and it can be taken in pill form. It's also available as a tea, though caution should still be taken about consuming too much, if you have high blood pressure.
- If you've been told that you have low stomach acid and suffer from

GERD, then remedies like apple cider vinegar or pickle juice can help regulate stomach acid levels and stimulate digestion. For pickle juice, only sip a small amount, as it's also high in sodium.

Gout

Jolted awake because it feels like your big toe is on fire? Unless your toe is actually on fire—in which case, you should extinguish it—you may be suffering from gout.

Gout is a type of arthritis caused by an accumulation of uric acid crystals in the joint(s), and sometimes you can even see them as nodules under the skin. It results in joints that are swollen, red, and often warm to the touch. Gout was once considered a disease of royalty and the rich because it was seen in those who overindulged in meat, seafood, and alcohol. This is because those foods are rich in a chemical compound called purines.

Purines are found in all natural foods, so even those on a low-purine diet cannot (and should not) avoid intake of purines altogether. Purines are the building blocks of DNA (remember the double-helix blueprint for genetic makeup that you learned in basic biology), so they are awfully important. The problem with purines comes when our livers don't sufficiently break them down, resulting in the formation of uric acid crystals in our joints or stones in our kidneys.

Not everyone with high levels of uric acid in the blood will end up with gout or kidney stones. However, if you have ever suffered the pain of gout or kidney stones, you know you want to avoid it happening again, so avoid (or at least limit) foods too rich in purines. If left untreated, severe gout can cause joint deformity.

Foods that are rich in purines include:

- animal organ meats: liver, spleen, kidney, heart, lung, sweetbread
- game meat
- meat (limit to 4–6 ounces daily), especially for red meat
- shellfish
- anchovies, fish roe, haddock, herring, mackerel, sardines, trout, tuna
- alcohol, especially beer
- foods and drinks made with high-fructose corn syrup (e.g., soft drinks, baked goods, and even some condiments, dressings, prepackaged sauces, frozen pizzas, yogurt, cereal, and cereal bars)
- supplements with yeast or yeast extracts
- gravy.

Beneficial foods:

- lots of water to help flush uric acid
- lots of vegetables—although some are higher in purines (e.g., asparagus, cauliflower, mushrooms, peas, and spinach), research has shown that these foods do not result in more frequent gout attacks
- cherries, especially tart cherries—a classic remedy for treating and preventing gout and osteoarthritis, borne out in research (Bell *et al.*, 2014; Kuehl *et al.*, 2012)
- adzuki bean congee
- bitter gourd
- cabbage, kale, lettuce, watercress
- celery or celery juice
- celeriac
- green apple
- lemon, lime
- wheatgrass.

The most common diagnosis for gout in Traditional Chinese Medicine is termed "Damp-Heat," so herbs and foods that help treat that are drying and cooling.

Anti-Gout Juice

- 2 green apples
- 6 celery stalks
- ¼ cabbage

Juice all ingredients. If you generally tend to be cold, add a thumb-sized piece of fresh ginger to the juicer.

Anti-Gout Tea

- 1 bunch parsley
- 4 cups of water
- 1 tbsp celery seed

Crush the parsley and add 4 cups of boiling water and celery seed, steeping for 10 minutes. (Do not take if pregnant, as it can stimulate smooth muscle contractions (Fang, 1998).)

Hangover

See Crapulence. Yes, you read that right.

Headache

There are a multitude of reasons for headaches, including a cold, sinus congestion, fatigue, eye strain, nutritional deficiency, hormonal imbalance, muscle tension, jaw or teeth issues, head injury, high blood pressure, low blood pressure, allergy, food sensitivity, blood sugar imbalance, toxic overload, hangover, caffeine withdrawal, migraine (see Migraine section below—a migraine is more than just a bad headache), and even brain tumor. For that reason, it's hard to say precisely which foods are best suited to address headaches.

Red Flags for Headaches

Note that although headaches are common, they are not to be taken lightly, especially if they are severe, interfere with your daily activities, occur as the result of a head injury, last several days, or wake you from sleep. You should also seek attention if:

- your headache is severe and is in just one eye, and that eye is red
- you also have a fever, stiff neck, and nausea or vomiting
- you also have loss of balance, confusion, memory loss, problems moving your limbs, slurred speech, or a change in your vision.

However, TCM diagnoses headaches, not necessarily (or solely) by the above conditions, but also by the pattern of a combination of details regarding the headaches:

- Where on your head does it hurt?
  - Top/vertex
  - Sides/temples

- - Front
  - Back of head/occiput
  - Whole head
- What is the quality of sensation of the headache?
  - Dull, heavy
  - Sharp, stabbing
  - Tight, band-like
  - Pressure from inside
  - Empty
- What is the frequency/timing?
  - Continuous
  - Intermittent
  - Time of day
  - Time of month
  - Before or after meals, sleep, exercise, etc.
  - Changes in weather
- What aggravates it or improves it?
  - Pressure
  - Lying down or standing up
  - Exertion
  - Cold or heat
  - Damp or dry atmosphere
  - Light
  - Sound
  - Menstrual cycle
  - Sleep
  - Stress
  - Holiday
- What other signs and symptoms are associated with it?

If your headache is easily connected to another health condition addressed in this chapter (e.g., allergy, cold or flu, or high blood pressure), check out foods for that condition.

In general, healthy eating habits can help alleviate or prevent many types of headaches.

- Prevent blood sugars from rising and dropping too much by eating regularly, avoiding excess sugar, and including foods rich in fiber, protein, and healthy fats.
- Avoid foods that are common causes of headaches, like food

preservatives and color and flavor additives. MSG and artificial sweeteners are common headache triggers.

- Other foods that may be associated with causing headaches include alcohol (of course, if you drink too much, but for some, even a small amount can bring regret), aged cheese, cured meats, fermented foods, beans, and dried fruit.
- If you've ever felt the pangs of an "ice cream headache," you know that it's caused by eating very cold foods, especially when you are warm. Want to avoid these kinds of headaches? Eat or drink more slowly!
- Coffee may instigate or alleviate headaches. Quitting regular caffeine intake suddenly can also cause withdrawal headaches.
- Magnesium-rich foods may help by dilating blood vessels, relaxing tight muscles, and calming the nervous system. (See Magnesium in the Minerals section in Chapter 3 for magnesium foods.)
- Make sure you are well hydrated! Dehydration is a common, and easily remedied, cause of headaches.
- Because there are so many possible types of and causes of headaches, it's difficult to make recommendations of specific recipes. However, many folks find smelling or applying topical peppermint essential oil to be helpful.

B.H. and A.H. (Before Headaches and After Headaches)

We've all suffered from headaches from time to time, and we're usually able to point to a cause. But some of us know what it's like to experience chronic head pain. I know. From childhood through until I started studying TCM, I experienced near daily headaches. I normally attributed them to low blood sugar or to drops in barometric pressure. But though my head hurt regularly, I rarely thought about it. The headaches were mild, and I had grown accustomed to them. So during my first week of TCM school when I attended the student clinic and was asked "What can we treat for you?" I answered, "Nothing. I'm healthy." When they pushed further to how I was feeling at that moment, I hesitantly told them that I had a headache, but that it was no big deal. They questioned me about frequency, and with my answer that it was nearly daily, they knew what they wanted to treat. Long story short, I did acupuncture, Chinese herbs, and followed their TCM food cure recommendations, and guess what? Rarely do I ever get headaches now. You really don't know how good you can feel until a symptom you've lived with for years and years goes away.

Heartburn

See Gastroesophageal Reflux Disease (GERD)/Acid Reflux/Heartburn. Also called acid reflux, reflux, acid regurgitation, acid indigestion, and gastroesophageal reflux (minus the "disease"), heartburn is a symptom, but not the same as gastroesophageal reflux disease (GERD), which is a more severe and long-lasting condition. However, the remedy suggestions are the same here.

Hemorrhoids

Although most people don't talk about it, by about age 50, between half to three-quarters of people have experienced hemorrhoids (also known as "piles"). Literally a pain in the butt, other symptoms include itching and bleeding. Hemorrhoids are distended blood vessels (similar to varicose veins) that can be internal or external. Internal ones sit inside the rectum and are typically painless, though they may bleed. Problems are worse if they prolapse (protrude out of the anal canal), as they can become more irritated and infected. External hemorrhoids are ones that are positioned under the skin around the anus. These ones tend to be more painful.

Hemorrhoids are typically associated with constipation, but obesity, pregnancy, a sedentary lifestyle, and poor diet are also potential causes for an increase in pressure on the veins in the rectal and anal areas.

Improving regular healthy bowel movements is one of the best ways to address hemorrhoids:

- Make sure to eat plenty of fiber. This includes leafy vegetables, peas, artichokes, broccoli, squash, yams, sweet potatoes, pumpkin, Brussels sprouts, berries, figs, prunes, avocados, whole grains, nuts, seeds, and legumes.
- Some TCM food cures for hemorrhoids include persimmon, eggplant/aubergine, red soybean soup, having 1–2 figs on an empty stomach first thing in the morning, and eating yams or sweet potatoes.
- Drink lots of fluids through the day. Dehydration can worsen constipation.
- Do your best to create a regular bowel habit that gives you enough time, so you don't have to strain and hurry.
- Go when you feel the urge. Try not to hold it for a more convenient time as stool can build up and create more pressure.
- Regular exercise also improves regular bowel movements.
- See the Constipation section above for more healthy bowel movement tips.

Topical Options
Sitz Bath

From the German word *sitzen*, meaning "to sit," a sitz bath is a warm bath for the perineum (the area between the anus and the vulva or scrotum). You can buy a shallow tub that is made to fit over the toilet seat or you can fill your tub or a basin with a few inches of warm water. The directions for use are simply to sit with the affected area immersed in the water for 10–20 minutes after bowel movements, or at least a few times a day. Dry the area afterward by gently patting with a towel or using a hair dryer. Do not rub or scrub, as that will further irritate the tissue.

Witch Hazel

After cleaning the hemorrhoids with warm water, dab them with witch hazel. As an astringent and anti-inflammatory, it may provide some relief.

Aloe Vera

Apply pure and/or fresh aloe vera to reduce itching and inflammation.

Epsom Salts and Glycerin

Mix 2 tablespoons of Epsom salts with 2 tablespoons of glycerin. Put this on a gauze pad and apply it to the hemorrhoid area, leaving it on for 15–20 minutes. Repeat this every 4–6 hours until pain is reduced.

High Blood Pressure/Hypertension

Hypertension is defined as blood pressure being chronically elevated with readings of 140/90 mmHg or higher. So, what are those numbers actually measuring? The first number is called systolic pressure, and it measures the amount of pressure on the artery walls when the heart pumps, pushing blood through your arteries. The second number is diastolic pressure, and it is the amount of arterial pressure between pumps, when the heart is not pushing blood.

Optimal blood pressure (BP) is 120/80 or lower (see Table 14), though it can also go too low (see the Low Blood Pressure/Hypotension section for more on that). Don't panic if your blood pressure isn't perfect, as normal blood pressure is defined as less than 130/85 mmHg.

Understanding Blood Pressure Readings

Table 14: Blood Pressure

Systolic	Diastolic	Condition
Less than 120	AND less than 80	Normal
120–129	AND less than 80	Elevated
130–139	OR 80–89	Hypertension, stage 1
140 or higher	OR 90 or higher	Hypertension, stage 2
Higher than 180	AND/OR higher than 120	Hypertensive crisis (go to emergency)

Source: AHA (2023)

How to Take Your Blood Pressure

If you have a history of issues with your blood pressure, it's a good idea to purchase a decent blood pressure monitor so that you can check it at home. Remember, hypertension isn't necessarily something you can feel.

Because your blood pressure can change under various conditions (including "white coat syndrome," where it tends to be higher simply because your doctor testing your blood pressure can make you nervous), there are tips to improve accuracy.

Make sure to select an effective BP monitor device and a cuff that properly fits your arm.

Don't exercise, eat, smoke, chew tobacco, or have caffeine or alcohol for 30 minutes prior to taking your BP. Remember that coffee or other caffeinated beverages can increase your BP for several hours.

Take your reading in the morning (or at least at around the same time each time you take it), as BP tends to rise in the afternoon and evening.

Find a quiet place. Or at least somewhere relatively quiet. Kids or animals (or spouses or friends) jumping on you or jackhammers noisy in the background while you are trying to take your BP may raise your reading.

Make sure that your sleeve isn't constricting your measurement arm.

Sit up straight on a supported chair with your feet flat on the ground (don't cross your legs, and if you have to pee, go first!).

Sit and relax for at least 5 minutes with your measurement arm resting on a table or other surface at heart level.

Place the cuff around the upper arm, one inch above the bend at your elbow. Make sure that the artery marking on the cuff is pointed along the brachial artery, just to the inside of the center line of your arm when your palm is facing up. Ensure the cuff has just enough room that you can fit two fingers between it and your arm—not too much, not too little, Goldilocks just right.

If you have a manual monitor, place the stethoscope head at the inside of your elbow, so you can hear a heartbeat over the brachial artery.

Follow the directions for use if you have a digital monitor and press the buttons as instructed to get readings.

For a manual monitor, use the cuff pump to increase pressure against the arm. Pump quickly and increase until you reach 30 mmHg above your expected systolic reading. Then stop pumping and listen through the stethoscope. Slowly release the pressure valve so air from the cuff starts to leak out. At first, you shouldn't be able to hear a heartbeat. If you do, stop the reading, rest for a minute, and start over, this time pumping another 30 mmHg more. Note the pressure reading at the point that you hear the first heartbeat. This is the systolic pressure. Continue to slowly deflate the cuff. Note the pressure reading at the point that you stop hearing the heartbeat. This is the diastolic pressure. Confused or find this too hard to do? Then get a digital automated or semi-automated device.

Take three readings with one minute or more of rest in between.

Consider keeping a recorded diary of your blood pressure so you can show your doctor.

Note that stress and pain can increase blood pressure.

There are two types of hypertension: primary (or essential) and secondary. Most cases of hypertension fit in the first category, and it occurs slowly over time with no identifiable cause. Secondary hypertension can occur because of a number of health conditions, including kidney disease, obstructive sleep apnea, thyroid problems, and alcohol abuse, or medications, such as birth control pills, cold remedies, decongestants, and pain relievers.

Because we usually can't feel our blood pressure, unless it is very high or low, it's important to make lifestyle choices that help manage BP. If we don't, persistent high blood pressure can cause a heart attack, heart failure, stroke, or arterial aneurysm.

One of the first recommendations in lowering elevated blood pressure is to watch how much salt you eat. All salts contain high amounts of sodium and chloride (NaCl), whether it is refined table salt or kosher, fleur de sel, Himalayan, sea, or other salt. The latter types of salt in this list also have trace amounts of other minerals, but that doesn't escape the fact that they are still high in sodium, which is the concern for hypertension. We've long recommended avoiding too much sodium, but there is also evidence that we don't want to have too little either. Problems with hypertension have been found with levels too high and too low (O'Donnell, Mente, and Rangarajan, 2014).

The thing is that salt makes food taste better and it acts as a preservative (see the section on Salty Flavor in TCM in Chapter 2: How to Classify Foods Using TCM). If you are eating a lot of processed foods or eat out a lot, then chances are you are getting a lot of salt, and you may need to cut back. Another balancing point to excess sodium is to increase your potassium intake (and no, it's not just bananas that are rich in this mineral—see the Potassium section under Minerals in Chapter 3).

Healthy food choices that can help address high blood pressure include the following:

- Limit your sodium intake to less than 2300 mg daily. That's about 1 teaspoon. Remember that many foods already contain salt, and it's not just about what you add from your saltshaker (see the Sodium section under Minerals in Chapter 3). Foods that are canned, cured, smoked, or (obviously) salted will also contain more sodium.
- Eat more whole, fresh food and fewer processed, packaged foods. (A "no duh" recommendation, I know.)
- Also, very important for a health cardiovascular system is avoiding trans fats. If you see "hydrogenated" or "partially hydrogenated" oil as one of the ingredients on a food you intend to eat, think again (see the section Trans Fatty Acids—The Ugly in Chapter 3).
- Avoid alcohol (NIAAA, n.d.).
- Nuts, seeds, and fatty fish like sardines, mackerel, halibut, cod, and salmon are rich in essential fatty acids that can help manage blood pressure.
- TCM food cures for high blood pressure include eating mung beans, Chinese radish, celery (can also be taken as a juice), chrysanthemum flowers (often used to make tea), mushrooms, and bitter gourd.

Exercising regularly, managing stress, and maintaining a healthy weight are also foundational ways to help treat hypertension.

Fermented Garlic

Garlic is widely recognized for its heart-healthy benefits—it helps lower elevated blood pressure and cholesterol—but its powerful taste and smell aren't for everyone. Thankfully, fermenting or pickling garlic helps soften the intensity of both. It also makes the garlic easier to digest.

As with any fermented food, fermented garlic contains probiotics that are beneficial to our health. Fermenting will, however, take longer to prepare than pickled garlic, and it can also have strong odor as it is in the process of fermenting.

- 5 to 8 whole garlic bulbs
- 1 tsp fine sea salt or Himalayan salt (don't use iodized salt)
- 2 cups filtered, non-chlorinated water
- 1 16-ounce jar

Peel enough garlic cloves to fill the jar.

In a small bowl, mix the salt in the water until it is dissolved.

Add the water to the jar to cover the cloves, but not all the way to the top (or it will overflow as it ferments).

Put the lid loosely on the jar and let it sit at room temperature.

Open the jar once a day to release the pressure that builds as the garlic ferments.

Ideally, you'll let the garlic continue to ferment for one to two months. You'll notice that bubbles will form in the brine, which will turn a golden-brown color.

When the garlic is ready (choose your version of "ready" by taste), tightly lid the jar and keep it in the fridge. Use within two months.

Quick Pickled Garlic

- 6 medium-sized heads of garlic
- 1 cup filtered water
- 1¼ cup apple cider vinegar or white vinegar
- 1 tbsp sea salt, Himalayan salt, or any non-iodized salt
- ½ tsp black peppercorns
- Optional: you can also add in herbs and spices like dill, bay leaf, rosemary, cilantro/coriander, mustard seed, and/or cumin. You may also choose to add hot chili peppers or red pepper flakes.

Peel the garlic.

Place the peppercorns and any herbs or spices into the bottom of a 16-ounce (1 pint) jar.

Put the garlic cloves into the jar, packing the cloves in tightly and leaving a ½ inch of space at the top.

In a medium-sized saucepan, add water, vinegar, and salt.

Heat on medium heat, stirring periodically while it comes to a boil and the salt has dissolved.

Pour the hot mixture into the jar, covering the garlic cloves.

Screw on the lid and let the jar cool.

Once cool, place the jar in the fridge and let it marinate unopened for three days to one week.

Consume within two months.

Infertility

I would have preferred to classify this as food recommendations for fertility rather than infertility because although the causes of infertility are many, there are some general recommendations that can be made to support fertility. However, since this is a listing of symptoms and diseases, "infertility" it is labeled, but fertility support is what I'm offering here.

Of course, fertility for men and women is different, but from a TCM perspective, supporting the TCM Kidneys is a key part. If you think about the shape of your kidneys, they look like a bean, the starting point for a plant to grow. Thus, TCM practitioners will often recommend nuts, seeds, and legumes, the starting point of a plant. From a nutritional standpoint, it makes sense.

Legumes, nuts, and seeds are rich sources of protein and fiber, which help stabilize blood sugar levels, resulting in better weight management. Because obesity can disrupt fertility (Hollmann, Runnebaum, and Gerhard, 1996; Pasquali, Patton, and Gambineri, 2007; Wang, Davies, and Norman, 2002), maintaining a healthy weight for both sexes can help improve chances of conception and a healthy pregnancy. Nuts and seeds are also rich in essential fatty acids (EFAs). Foods that are rich in EFAs, in particular the omega-3 fatty acids, have been shown to help with fertility for both men and women (Saldeen and Saldeen, 2004).

Eating clean is another important factor for fertility. Our world is filled with synthetic ingredients, chemicals, and toxins. Many of these have been found to be disruptive to our hormones and may be causing infertility, miscarriages, and/or developmental disorders (Golden *et al.*, 1998; Marques-Pinto and Carvalho, 2013; Pflieger-Bruss, Schuppe, and Schill, 2004).

Want to increase your fertility?

- Eat your veggies! Get a variety, including leafy greens and brightly colored vegetables.
- Eat nuts, seeds, and legumes (see above for why).
- Eat enough and don't overdo the exercise. Being underweight can also contribute to infertility (Rich-Edwards *et al.*, 2002).
- Avoid trans fats (for reasons more than fertility, of course).
- Increase monounsaturated fats (e.g., olive oil) and polyunsaturated essential fatty acids (e.g., nuts, seeds, and fatty fish like sardines, mackerel, herring, cod, salmon, halibut).
- Eat more plant-based proteins than animal-based.
- Don't eat too much sugar.
- Get enough fiber. It helps regulate bowels, but also supports the management of blood sugar levels, maintenance of a healthy weight, and removal of toxins.
- Choose iron-rich foods. That can include meats, but choose grass-fed, organic, and/or free range. Other iron-rich foods include dark leafy greens (spinach, kale, collard greens), dried fruit (prunes, raisins), legumes (garbanzo beans/chickpeas, beans, lentils), and artichokes. For better iron absorption, eat them with vitamin C-rich foods like citrus fruits, guava, kiwifruit, papaya, strawberries, bell peppers, dark leafy greens, thyme, parsley, broccoli, Brussels sprouts, and cauliflower.
- Soaking fruits and vegetables in a water-vinegar mixture for 20 to 30 minutes followed by rinsing in clean water can remove many of the pesticides if organically grown vegetables or fruits are unavailable.
- Xenoestrogens (synthetic estrogen-like compounds) are found in plastic containers, so choose glass containers to store leftover food. At the very least, do not heat any foods in plastic.
- Choose liver-cleansing foods: artichoke, dandelion greens, arugula/rocket, beets/beetroot, Brussels sprouts, broccoli, cabbage, turnip root, daikon radish, radishes, kohlrabi, Swiss chard, watercress, parsley, mung beans, apple cider vinegar.

For women, one of the main elements for fertility is regulating the menstrual cycle.

Seed Cycling

One of the easy-to-implement recommendations for hormone balancing that some nutritionists and naturopaths recommend is seed cycling. The idea is that specific seeds can help regulate hormones related to the follicular and luteal phases.

Day 1 to Ovulation (7 Days Before Next Period)
Take 1 tablespoon each of freshly ground flax seeds and pumpkin seeds daily.

Ovulation to Next Period
Take 1 tablespoon each of freshly ground sunflower seeds and sesame seeds daily.

Insomnia
Ongoing problems with sleep are a major health issue. Suffer from insomnia? Then you risk all manner of illnesses and conditions, from ADHD to zoster (shingles). Your time spent sleeping is when your body can repair, restore, and replenish. Without enough rest time, your brain can't function properly, causing issues with memory, concentration, and decision making. You'll have a harder time managing your emotions, getting along with others, and coping with change. Having a tough time maintaining a healthy weight? If you're not getting enough sleep, that might be contributing.

For some, lack of sleep is a choice. We're busier than ever, it seems, continuously stimulated by digital media. We know that, over time, those very electronic devices need to be recharged more and more frequently. They don't seem to hold their charges effectively anymore. Yet we push our own biology, expecting that the four to six hours that we managed to get by on during our 20s should still be able to sustain us into our 30s and beyond. No matter your age, if you're not getting enough sleep (somewhere between seven to nine hours nightly for most) because you aren't allotting enough sleep time, then get more sleep. Period.

If your lack of sleep is not by choice but caused by insomnia—you can't fall asleep, you wake frequently through the night, you wake during the night and can't return to sleep, or some combo thereof—you'll likely need to try a few things to fix your situation. These are just some of the potential causes of or contributors to insomnia:

- Some medications can cause or aggravate insomnia, so talk to your pharmacist or health care provider if you suspect your medication is causing insomnia.
- Stress ("can't shut my mind off") is another key contributor to insomnia, so find ways to help you cope.
- Consider your caffeine intake. Caffeine has a half-life of 3–6 hours, meaning that it takes that long for half of it to clear your system. That translates to some caffeine potentially affecting you many hours beyond that. Some people are more sensitive to caffeine than others,

so you may have to quit your caffeine intake 8–12 hours before you plan to go to sleep or avoid it altogether.

- Are you looking at a backlit screen (TV, tablet, phone, computer) within a few hours before bedtime? If so, you are suppressing melatonin production, a key hormone to help you sleep. If turning off those devices makes you panic, you might consider wearing glasses that block blue light or trying out software to alter the screen display over the day.
- Is your room dark enough? Do you have a lot of electronics in your bedroom? Are your mattress and pillow right for you or is it time to replace them? Is your room too hot or too cold? Do you need earplugs?
- Do you have an erratic sleep schedule? If you're a shift worker, a parent, or a caregiver, you may not have much choice about going to bed and waking at a regular time. But if you do have control over bedtimes and wake times, make sure to get on top of that.
- Have you ever cared for a young child or an active animal? Then you know that getting enough physical activity during the daytime (but not too late) helps improve sleep at night.
- It's also wise to create a wind-down routine, more than just brushing your teeth.
- Perhaps you're taking sleep medication, but you're still tired during the day. You may have built up a tolerance. Sleeping pills may also be causing side effects of behavioral changes, poor sleep quality, daytime sleepiness, and even hallucinations. Plus, if you stop taking sleep medication, you may end up suffering from a rebound effect (insomnia worse than ever), at least until your body readjusts.

We have an epidemic of under-slept, over-tired people, propelling themselves through the day with caffeine and sheer will. So, let's look at some food options to help with sleep. From a TCM perspective, nighttime and sleep are Yin elements, so insomnia results in a depletion of Yin.

- Make sure that you drink enough water or fluids throughout the day. Chamomile tea is calming and ideal for the evening. Green tea contains L-theanine which helps release chemicals in the brain that promote a feeling of alertness with calmness during the day, but don't have it too late because of the caffeine.
- Limit sugar and sugary foods as they cause sugar highs and lows and put stress on your body.
- Avoid or limit greasy, fried foods, hydrogenated and poor-quality fats (margarine, shortening, refined and rancid oils), intoxicants (e.g.,

alcohol, a depressant), highly processed or refined foods, and spicy foods (they are stimulating).

- Eat fish like wild salmon, sardines, mackerel, cod, halibut, and herring at least once or twice per week, as these supply the essential fatty acids DHA and EPA, important omega-3 fatty acids that feed the brain and thus help to regulate emotions.

- Green veggies are rich in magnesium, which can help relax tight muscles and calm the nervous system. Magnesium also helps calcium work properly in the heart and nerves. Steam, blend, stir-fry, and cook in soups, stews, and slow-cooked meals.

- Try eating more vegetables including beets/beetroot, spinach, cabbage, turnip root, daikon radish, radishes, kohlrabi, cauliflower, broccoli, Brussels sprouts, romaine lettuce, onions, asparagus, alfalfa, celery, lettuce, cucumber, watercress, parsley, Swiss chard, artichoke, dandelion leaves. Include brightly colored veggies: winter squash, yam, pumpkin, carrot, peas, sweet potato, broccoli, kale.

- Spices: ginger, turmeric, marjoram, cumin, fennel, rosemary, mint; especially dill and basil as they have a calming effect.

- Foods that are rich in the mineral silicon improve calcium metabolism and strengthen nerve tissue: cucumber, celery, lettuce, barley gruel, oatstraw tea.

- Fruits: strawberries, dark grapes, blackberries, raspberries, lime, grapefruit; small amounts of peaches, cherries. Mulberries and lemons calm the mind. Tart cherries contain melatonin, so may also help with restoring a restful sleep cycle.

- Unrefined complex carbohydrates (e.g., brown rice, whole-grain pasta, whole-grain bread) maximize the presence of L-tryptophan in the brain, which aids in the formation of the neurotransmitter serotonin. Serotonin is required for calming the mind and promoting sound sleep. L-tryptophan is found in most foods, but other amino acids in high-protein foods compete with its use in the formation of serotonin, so carbohydrates are your best source. Include a variety of gluten-free grains such as quinoa (actually a seed, but prepared like a grain), millet, and amaranth.

- Yin-supportive foods include millet, barley, wild rice, black beans, kidney beans, lima beans, adzuki beans, fish, tofu, miso, coconut milk, walnuts, sesame seeds (black or regular), alfalfa sprouts, artichoke, asparagus, cabbage, cucumber, green beans, peas, sweet potatoes, water chestnuts, yams, zucchini/courgette, apple, apricot, avocado, lemon, lime, mango, melon, pear, persimmon, pomegranate, watermelon, seaweed, coconut oil, olive oil.

There are many folk and natural remedies for helping with sleep, including a warm glass of milk, chamomile tea, a warm bath (add Epsom salts and some lavender oil for extra relaxation), and some unusual ones like sniffing the fumes of a chopped onion (I've never gotten sleepy after cutting onions, but maybe you do?).

Here are some teas you might try.

Chrysanthemum and Goji Tea

Because nighttime and sleep are Yin in nature, choosing foods that calm Yang energy and nourish Yin helps calm the nervous system. Chrysanthemum flower (*ju hua*) calms Liver Yang and clears Heat, and its bitter flavor goes to the Heart. Goji berries (*gou qi zi*) nourish the Blood and Yin.

When I was in training at TCM hospitals in China, I noticed that many of the TCM doctors were drinking this tea. While I placed this recipe here for insomnia, it will not make you sleepy, but it can be helpful to calm an overstimulated nervous system. It's also an excellent remedy for red, irritated, and tired eyes (no, don't pour it on your eyes; you still drink it).

- 3–4 chrysanthemum flowers
- 1 tsp goji berries
- 1 cup hot water
- Optional: honey to sweeten

Steep the flowers and berries in the hot water for 3 to 5 minutes. You can take out the flowers when you drink it or just drink around them. You can eat the berries when you're done with the tea. You can also do more than one steep of this tea.

Pretty Little Rose Tea

Mei gua hua is a Chinese herb that is used in TCM to soothe the Liver Qi, move Blood to relieve stasis, and regulate menstruation. But several of my Chinese patients have told me their family uses it to help calm the nervous system, address anxiety, and improve sleep. If you are feeling irritable and stressed, and feel tension and tightness in your chest and ribs, then this easy tea might do the trick. Plus, it has a nice light flavor, and it looks pretty.

- 10–12 *mei gua hua* rose buds
- 1 cup hot water

To get more surface area for gaining benefits from this tea, break off the green stem and leaves from the rose buds and place both in your pot or cup. Add hot water and steep for 3 to 5 minutes. You can re-steep this tea a few times, if you like.

Lettuce Tea

If you don't have any of the ingredients listed above, you are likely to have (or can at least easily purchase) some lettuce. When you poke the stem of a lettuce leaf, you may notice a white milky fluid comes out. This has been called "lettuce opium" because it looks like that from an opium poppy, and it helps with inducing sleep.

- 3–4 large lettuce leaves
- 1 cup water
- Optional: 2 sprigs of mint or some honey

Put your water and lettuce in a pot. Place a lid on the pot and simmer the lettuce leaves for 15 minutes. Add honey and drink. Or remove from heat and add your mint. Let it sit for another 5 minutes before drinking. The honey or mint are added because the tea can be bitter-tasting.

Irritable Bowel Syndrome (IBS)

A diagnosis of IBS is really a "diagnosis of exclusion." That is, all the tests—blood, scope, ultrasound, stool sample, whatever else—come back normal. But you know you don't feel "normal." IBS is a functional digestive disorder that causes chronic, episodic abdominal pain, bloating, cramping, gas, and problems with bowel movements. IBS-D is characterized by diarrhea, IBS-C involves constipation, and IBS-M is a mix of constipation alternating with diarrhea.

Although there may not be any measurable tools to assess IBS, it can be a debilitating health issue, significantly affecting a person's quality of life.

There can be many different triggers that aggravate the symptoms of IBS, from stress or specific foods to potential hormonal issues or intestinal bacteria imbalance. Because there is no one cause of IBS, food suggestions can vary widely, and some recommendations can be found in the Diarrhea and Constipation sections above.

If food sensitivities seem to be a potential cause, check out Chapter 8: Food Allergies, Sensitivities, and Intolerances. In particular, some find the FODMAP diet (covered in that chapter) to be helpful.

Because stress often triggers IBS episodes, stress management is also key. From a TCM perspective, "Overactive Liver attacking the Spleen" is often at least one of the patterns. Choose foods that strengthen the Spleen Qi and soothe the Liver Qi. These include the following:

- soups, stews, slow-cooked meals, which are easier to digest as the food is partially broken down already
- yams, sweet potatoes, pumpkin
- peppermint tea or enteric-coated peppermint capsules
- basil, black pepper, cardamom, cilantro/coriander, cumin, dill, fennel, ginger, licorice root, marjoram, mint, rosemary, turmeric
- sprouted foods
- fermented foods.

Other tips include:

- Focus on chewing and enjoying your food while eating, rather than multitasking and feeling stressed or rushed.
- Eat smaller portions more frequently.
- Try chamomile or other calming tea.
- Meditate or practice breathing exercises, tai chi, qi gong, yoga, or other breath-focused, stress-reduction practice.
- Consider probiotics.
- Keep a food diary to see if you have any particular food triggers.

How to Congee

Yes, I think congee is so good that it should also be a verb!

Congee is also known as "rice water" or "rice gruel," and it's a common breakfast food in China that is very modifiable, and it certainly doesn't need to be restricted to a morning meal. Although most congee is made with rice, it can also be made with other grains like millet or barley.

Congee is recommended for a wide range of digestive issues, as it's easy to digest and you can mix it with other ingredients that help improve your condition. If you are trying a low-FODMAP diet, check the FODMAP chart in Chapter 8 to see which foods you should not include when adding items to your congee.

- 1 cup rice or other grain
- 8 cups water or stock
- ½ tsp salt

Cooking in a Pot

In a large pot, add all the ingredients and bring to a boil. Then reduce heat to a simmer and cook, stirring occasionally, for about an hour, until the congee is creamy or at the consistency you like.

Cooking in a Slow Cooker

Add all ingredients to a slow cooker and cook on high for about 4 hours, stirring occasionally.

Note that it will continue to thicken as it cools.

It's best to cook it on low temperature for longer and better to use too much water than too little.

You can add all kinds of ingredients to congee, including:

- vegetables like cabbage, carrots, celery, leek, mushrooms, onions, radishes, spinach, taro, and water chestnut
- fruit like apples, bananas, berries, dates, dried fruit, pears, plums, and umeboshi
- nuts and seeds like almonds, cashews, chestnut, chia seeds, flax seeds, hemp seeds, pecans, pine nuts, poppy seeds, sesame seeds, sunflower seeds, and walnuts
- meats like chicken, eggs, fish, and shellfish
- legumes like adzuki beans, kidney beans, lentils, and mung beans
- black pepper, cinnamon, fennel, garlic, ginger, mustard seed, nutmeg, and pickle.

Ochazuke

When I was a kid, my mom used to make a simple recipe called ochazuke when we were sick. Similar in idea to congee, but even easier to make, it's a Japanese recipe that would always make my sister and me feel better, even if we could eat nothing else.

- Over-cooked white rice
- Green tea (note that green tea is energetically cooling)

Pour the green tea over the rice, making it as soupy or as solid as you like. We would add umeboshi (pickled special kind of apricot that is sometimes called a plum) and sometimes a bit of chicken on top.

Joint Pain

Although there are many causes for joint pain, see the Arthritis section for recommendations.

Kidney Stones

Some argue that passing a kidney stone is as painful as childbirth. I can neither confirm nor deny. Regardless, what's clear is that it can be horrifically painful, and no one wants to hug and care for the "birthed" kidney stone.

Kidney stones are hard, stone-like pieces that can be as small as a grain of sand or as big as a golf ball. The small ones can pass with little to no problem, but if one gets stuck, you'll know it! Sharp pain in the back, lower abdomen, side, or groin is a common symptom, and it can come and go in waves. Pain can also occur when urinating, and there may be blood in the urine or urine may be cloudy. Other symptoms include an inability to urinate, problems urinating, frequent urges to urinate, nausea, vomiting, fever, or chills. If any of those latter symptoms is happening to you, put down this book and go get yourself checked out.

Most kidney stones are a combination of calcium and oxalate, though they can also be calcium combined with phosphorus or they can be uric acid stones, cystine stones, or struvite stones. The type of stone can help you determine what specific dietary measures to take.

If you've had a kidney stone, unless you make some dietary changes, you're likely to get another. So, time to make those changes.

- Drink lots of water. You need that to dilute the things in your urine that may lead to kidney stones. Have at least eight cups of water per day, more if you're sweating.
- Juices from celery, pomegranate, basil, or wheatgrass are said to help reduce kidney stones.
- Watch your sodium intake. Eating too much sodium causes calcium to be lost in the urine. Remember that a lot of commercially processed and canned foods have a lot of sodium.
- Limit animal proteins. Meat, eggs, poultry, dairy, and seafood all boost uric acid levels.
- If you have calcium oxalate stones, limit high-oxalate foods like beer, beets/beetroot, berries, chocolate, coffee, cranberries, French fries, nuts, pop, rhubarb, soybeans and soy milk, spinach, sweet potatoes, wheat bran.
- Continue to eat calcium-rich foods. I know it sounds contradictory, but calcium from food doesn't increase your risk for calcium stones.

From a TCM perspective, Damp-Heat is a common diagnosis for kidney stones, so you'll want to avoid foods that aggravate this condition, while using cooling foods and foods that drain excess Dampness. Some of these foods include:

- corn silk (you can add it to hot water and drink it as a tea)
- parsley (promotes urination)
- radish (cooling).

Lemon Water

Because lemon contains citrate, a salt in citric acid that binds to calcium, it can help stop stone formation (St Pete Urology, 2022). If you're prone to kidney stones, try drinking lemon water. Just be mindful that the citric acid can also wear at the enamel on your teeth, so don't brush your teeth right after you have this. Instead, wait for 30 minutes so that the enamel that has softened from the acid can recover before you brush your teeth. You can also rinse your mouth with water after having the lemon water or use a reusable straw (because you care about our planet!) to drink the lemon water, so it doesn't have as much contact with your teeth.

- 2 lemons
- ½–1 cup water (depending on how much pucker you like)

Squeeze out the juice of 2 lemons and add to water. Drink this daily.

If you already have kidney stones, you'll need more treatment. Lemon juice may help to dissolve or break down the stones and olive oil will help them move out.

- ¼ cup lemon juice
- ¼ cup olive oil

Mix the ingredients and drink it in the afternoon, but also make sure to drink plenty of water and lemon juice throughout the day.

Apple Cider Vinegar Kidney Stone Remedy

- 2 tbsp apple cider vinegar
- 1 cup water

Mix the apple cider vinegar in the water and sip this throughout your day.

Low Blood Pressure/Hypotension

I often hear people say they have low blood pressure when they have a reading of something like 105/65 mmHg, but technically the reading for low blood pressure is below 90/60 mmHg. There is also more than one type of hypotension: absolute and orthostatic.

Absolute hypotension is when the resting blood pressure is below 90/60 mmHg.

Orthostatic hypotension, also called positional hypotension, is when your blood pressure drops at least 20 mmHg for the systolic (top number) and 10 mmHg for the diastolic (bottom number) and stays that low for at least three minutes after you move from sitting to standing. This can happen because when we sit or lie down, the heart doesn't have to pump as hard to move the blood. But when we stand, gravity causes the blood to temporarily pool in the legs. It takes a moment for special cells, called baroreceptors, near the heart and neck arteries to sense that the blood pressure is low and signal the heart to pump faster and harder and to narrow (vasoconstrict) the blood vessels to increase the blood pressure. If these cells don't do their job, the blood pressure doesn't normalize quickly enough.

So, what about if you're one of those people who gets lightheaded or dizzy when you get up too quickly? This is very common, and if it's occasional, mild, or doesn't last long, it's likely nothing. But it's worth a bit of an investigation if it happens more frequently. What is your blood pressure? Are you dehydrated or overheated? Has it been a while since you last ate (low blood sugar), or have you been drinking alcohol or taking drugs? Are you on medications for treating high blood pressure? Are you taking antidepressants, muscle relaxants, or drugs used to treat Parkinson's disease or erectile dysfunction? Do you have a disease, like diabetes, that causes nerve damage? Are you anemic? Have you been on bed rest? Are you pregnant (it's more common in the first and second trimesters)? Were you standing still for an extended period of time? Are you over the age of 65? All these things can cause orthostatic hypotension. If you notice your blood pressure drops after you eat, you might have postprandial hypotension, which is more common in older adults.

It's possible to have low blood pressure and not know it, but symptoms include dizziness, light-headedness, fatigue, weakness, problems focusing, confusion, blurred vision, fast and shallow breathing, nausea and vomiting, fainting, falling, and even agitation or behavioral changes. It might also alter your heartrate, you could look paler than usual, or you might notice you're urinating less volume. Obviously, getting blood to your brain is a pretty important task for your body, so some of these symptoms are more serious than others. Persistent low blood pressure can increase your risk of falling, or of having a stroke, deep vein thrombosis (DVT), or heart issues. And you should certainly seek medical attention if you have fainted, have black stools, chest pain, an irregular heartbeat, shortness of breath, or a high fever.

Whether you have hypotension by diagnostic definition or just have a tendency toward lower blood pressure and find yourself mentally checking the boxes of issues listed above, low blood pressure is symptom of something going on, and listening to your body helps you prevent bigger issues from happening.

Healthy things you can do to keep your blood pressure up if you have hypotension:

- Eat regular, small meals high in fiber, protein, and good fats to keep your blood sugars stable.
- Make sure you're well hydrated. Of course this makes sense. Your blood is a liquid, and if you are dehydrated, you may not have enough blood volume to help regulate your blood pressure.
- If you do have hypotension, it also makes sense to do the opposite of some of the things you would do to treat hypertension. One of those things is to have salt. This could be to add a pinch of salt when you're cooking or include some salty foods like pickles, olives, seaweed, or soy sauce (see the section on Salty Flavor in TCM in Chapter 2: How to Classify Foods Using TCM).
- If you have pernicious (low vitamin B12) or iron-deficiency anemia, you may also be more prone to low blood pressure. While the TCM version of blood is more than the "red stuff," check out the sections on Liver Blood Deficiency and Heart Blood Deficiency in Chapter 6: Foods by Element to learn how you can build blood.
- Foods that help with both low and high blood pressure because they support a healthy heart include leafy greens, nuts, legumes, and fatty fish. Ditto for avoiding or limiting processed foods and alcohol.
- Wear compression stockings, as they help reduce the pooling of blood in the legs. When I turned 50, my friend gave me a pair of compression stockings for travel. It was a bit of a fun age joke, but also turned out to be a really practical and helpful gift.
- Rise slowly. For real. If standing up quickly after sitting for a bit makes you dizzy, then don't do it! I mean, yes, stand up. But stand slower.

Licorice Tea

When many of us think about licorice, we think about the candy. But licorice root, the herb, is not the same. Red licorice candy doesn't contain actual licorice, and black licorice may actually contain artificial flavor or anise oil because it has a similar taste. Plus, licorice candy contains sugar. So, if you want to get the benefits of licorice root, choose the real deal.

Licorice root, called *gan cao*, is a very common herb in TCM. We use it in many formulas for its own properties but also to "harmonize" the mixture of herbs used. However, when used on its own in larger quantities, it comes with warnings (af Geijerstam *et al.*, 2024). If you've ever been recommended to take licorice root for acid reflux, then you've taken the deglycyrrhizinated version of licorice, called DGL for short. But if you want to increase blood pressure, then you'll want to take the regular keep-the-glycyrrhizic-acid version of licorice root.

Just keep monitoring your blood pressure so you don't head yourself into high blood pressure territory.

- 1 tbsp chopped licorice root
- 2 cups water
- Bring the water to a boil in a small saucepan and add the licorice root. Boil the mixture for 10 minutes.
- Optional ingredients to add to the boiling water:
- A cinnamon stick (*gui zhi*) if you want help regulating your blood sugar, you have a cold, or you have poor circulation
- 3 chopped black or red dates (*da zao* or *hong zao*) if you have iron-deficiency anemia
- Honey, if you simply like honey, though licorice is already sweet

Menopausal/Perimenopausal Symptoms

Perimenopause is the time leading up to the end of menstruation, and it may last for up to ten years, meaning you could hit perimenopause even as early as your late thirties (though that is considered early) to early forties. Menopause is defined by the end of the period for a full year, and it typically happens during the late forties to mid-fifties.

When we think of perimenopause and menopause, we often think of it similarly to how we think about disease—the symptoms. But in TCM, this is recognized as a stage of life that we call the "second spring." Spring is nature's time to bring new life—flowers bud, trees re-leaf, and animals give birth. The first spring is when we may bear children, while the second spring is a time when women may find a shift in their creative energies, discovering new creative passions or skills.

According to TCM, reproductive function is controlled by the energetic system of the Kidneys (capitalized as it represents more than the physiological functions of the physical kidneys). When women are young, the Kidneys have enough blood for fertility. Before age 35, it's said that a woman is more Yin (moist, receptive, passive), but after that her Yang energy begins to express itself and she becomes more animated about her passions, more assertive, and more confident. This may or may not hold true for you but is a generality. This hot Yang energy consumes some of the Yin energy, causing dryness, hot flashes, anxiety, night sweats, and palpitations.

So why do some women suffer "the change" worse than others? A lot of it has to do with a woman's basic health prior to and during menopause. The most common causes of menopause symptoms are lifestyle and diet, with the number-one factor being overworking. Overwork drains energy from the body, causing a faster decline in Kidney Qi.

The good news is that, if you are a woman, you know the basic timeline of hormonal shifts to come. In fact, if you know when your mother hit perimenopause and menopause, yours will likely arrive around the same age. This means that you can prepare well in advance, making the transition smoother.

If you're already in the midst of sheet-changing night sweats and the like, you can still follow these recommendations to reduce the symptoms.

To support Kidney Yin, include the following foods:

- millet, barley
- mung bean and its sprouts
- kidney beans, black beans, and other legumes
- string beans
- melons
- water chestnuts
- spirulina
- seaweeds
- black sesame seeds.

Additionally, especially when you are struggling with hot flashes, night sweats, dryness symptoms, anxiety, and insomnia:

- avoid stimulants like caffeine
- steer clear of sugar, alcohol, greasy foods, and spicy foods
- see Chapter 2: How to Classify Foods Using TCM for a list of cooling foods like celery, cucumber, and watermelon.

And, because a decrease in the amount of estrogen produced by the ovaries is part of the menopausal process, many women find that including foods rich in phytoestrogens—plant compounds similar to, but milder than, our own estrogen—can be helpful. While these foods may not be suitable for all, they can be helpful for those experiencing some of the challenges (or horrors, depending on the severity!) of perimenopause and menopause. They include:

- soybeans, tofu, soy milk, tempeh, miso (see box for more about soy products)
- alfalfa, carrots, yams
- apples, pomegranates
- barley, hops, oats, wheat germ
- lentils
- flax seeds, sesame seeds.

Is Soy Healthy?

Go online and search "Is soy healthy?" and you'll find an ongoing debate. In short, the answer is, yes...and no.

The Good

- Soy is a good source of protein, calcium, magnesium, and B vitamins. It is also rich in zinc and iron, but they are poorly absorbed.
- Phytoestrogen compounds may help manage some hormonal balance issues, reducing menopausal and perimenopausal symptoms.
- Helps support bone health by stimulating the production of bone growth cells (Khalid and Krum, 2016).
- Supports heart health in perimenopausal and menopausal women, as estrogen is cardio-protective (Iorga et al., 2017).
- While many with a history or fear of breast cancer have been told to limit soy, it may actually have some protective benefits against breast cancer. Because phytoestrogens bind to the same receptors that our more powerful estrogens use to enter the cell, the milder estrogenic action on the cells actually helps reduce breast cancer risk (Korde et al., 2009; Shu, 2009; Wu et al., 2008).
- As a side note, soy may also help to protect against prostate cancer (Bilir et al., 2017; Daures et al., 2017).

The Bad

- Unless otherwise stated as "non-GMO" and/or "organic," soy products and the soy ingredients found in many foods (it's commonly used as an inexpensive way to boost protein content) are likely genetically modified. You may not consider GMO as fitting in "The Bad" category, but it is, at the very least, a relative unknown.
- Soy is a common food allergen.
- Opposite to the evidence above, soy may increase the growth of breast cancer cells (at low doses, though it appears beneficial at high doses), and it may inhibit the effect of the breast cancer treatment drug Tamoxifen (de Lemos, 2001). I know, it's confusing. That's biology; that's nature.

Making it Better—Fermenting Soy

Because soy is rich in phytic acid (also known as phytates), "anti-nutrients" that decrease the absorption of iron and zinc, food preparation methods that decrease phytic acid are beneficial. Keep in mind that lots of foods are high in phytates, including all other legumes, nuts, and seeds.

Traditionally, soy has been widely consumed in Asia for a long time. But it has often been consumed in fermented form:

- tempeh
- miso
- natto
- soy sauce (though many commercial soy sauces are not made properly, so do your research)
- fermented soy milk or powder
- soy yogurt.

If you have menopausal symptoms, but still tend to feel cold, be lethargic, have to urinate frequently and the stream is clear, have edema, and experience a lack of sexual desire, you may need to support your Kidney Yang energy as well. Try adding some warming foods such as:

- walnuts, fennel seeds
- ginger, onions

- quinoa
- chicken, lamb.

Watermelon Hydrating Smoothie

If you've been needing to change your pajamas in the middle of the night because you sweat through them or if you have been struggling with dryness symptoms, you may be happy to have a recipe to help you cool off and rehydrate. This Yin-nourishing recipe is a start, though it's probably better for hot-weather months. Note that TCM principles don't generally recommend everyone who's sweating lots or feeling hot choose icy, cold foods. But this may give you some temporary relief. You can also skip freezing the watermelon in advance and just use cut watermelon, in which case your smoothie will be more like a juice.

- 1 cup frozen cubed watermelon (you'll need to prep this in advance)
- 1 cup coconut water
- 2 tbsp lime or lemon juice
- 10–15 fresh mint leaves

Combine all in a blender and blend until smooth.

Menstruation Issues

This is a big category of possible issues, so I certainly can't cover them all, but we'll consider a few key imbalances. Fibroids, endometriosis, and polycystic ovarian syndrome (PCOS) are possible causes for menstrual issues, painful cramping, and/or heavy bleeding, so don't skip out on seeing a gynecologist for a proper exam.

Before diving into the problems, let's look first at the basic menstrual cycle.

Menstrual Cycle

- Menarche (the first period) starts between age 8 and 15, with an average age of 12.
- The menstrual cycle is 28 days, but can vary from 21 to 35 days for adults and 21 to 45 days for teens.
- Periods last for 3–7 days.

- The first day of the period is called "day 1."
- Menopause usually starts sometime between age 45 and 55.

Although a woman's cycle can vary in length, the first part (before ovulation—the release of an egg) is called the follicular phase and the second part is called the luteal phase. Ovulation occurs about 14 days before the period, regardless of the length of the menstrual cycle, so it will be around day 14 on a 28-day cycle, but on day 7 of a 21-day cycle, and on day 21 of a 35-day cycle.

Menstruation and hormone release is managed by messages between brain (hypothalamus and pituitary gland) and ovaries.

Follicular Phase

Follicle-stimulating hormone (FSH) sends signals to the fluid-filled pockets called follicles on one of the ovaries to ripen an egg. Estrogen levels rise to help rebuild the lining of the uterus. This lining is important for providing nutrients to a developing egg if it is fertilized by sperm.

Ovulation

Estrogen levels peak as the follicle matures, causing luteinizing hormone (LH) to surge, stimulating an egg to be released from its follicle on an ovary about 14 days before the next period. Some women can feel ovulation as a bit of low back or lower pelvic pain, called *mittelschmerz* (German words for "middle" and "pain"). Some notice a bit of spotting.

For those who don't have these symptoms and who have irregular periods, ovulation can also be noted by checking vaginal mucus. At ovulation, the mucus becomes the consistency of egg white—clear and slippery. It's also possible to tell ovulation by a slight increase in basal body temperature (BBT). BBT is measured with a thermometer used either orally or vaginally. Temperature is taken every morning around the same time, after at least three hours of sleep, before rising from bed (keep the thermometer at your bedside). Once charted for a month or more, it's possible to see if there's a regular pattern. Ovulation kits can also be used.

Fertile Window

The time when a woman can become pregnant lasts about six days because sperm can live for about five days and an egg lives about one day. Thus, the fertile window starts five days before ovulation and lasts until one day after. If the ovum (egg) is fertilized by sperm, it continues down the fallopian tube and attaches to the lining of the uterus.

Luteal Phase

The luteal phase is preparation for pregnancy.

After ovulation, the ovarian follicle that released the egg forms a temporary structure called the corpus luteum. The corpus luteum excretes progesterone and small amounts of estrogen to cause the lining of the uterus to thicken in preparation for a fertilized egg.

If the egg is not fertilized, estrogen production drops rapidly and can fluctuate until the start of the next period. The corpus luteum dies and stops producing both progesterone and estrogen, causing the uterus to shed its lining—the next period.

Random Facts

- Did you know that the uterus is normally about the size of a pear, but doubles in size in preparation for pregnancy or the next period?
- The more fluid and watery cervical mucus that is found during ovulation allows the sperm to swim more easily toward the egg. After ovulation, the mucus becomes thicker and stickier again.
- Stress can affect the menstrual cycle, causing missed or late cycles, irregular periods, changes in length of menstruation, missed ovulation, and worsening PMS symptoms.
- Changes in weight, being underweight or overweight, hard exercise, and use of the birth control pill can also change the menstrual cycle.

Premenstrual Syndrome (PMS)

When people talk about PMS, they're most often referring to the mood changes that happen prior to and at the beginning of women's periods, as can be seen by some of the humorous (unless you're currently experiencing PMS) definitions:

- Psychotic Mood Swings

- Pass My Shotgun
- Pardon My Sobbing
- Pack My Stuff
- Potential Murder Suspect.

Other symptoms include bloating (Pass My Sweatpants, Puffy Mid-Section), food cravings (Provide Me with Sweets, Perpetual Munching Spree), and skin breakouts (Pimples May Surface). Breast tenderness, low back pain, lower abdominal cramping, headaches, and bowel changes are some more of the charming indications of the arrival of Aunt Flow.

Of course, as with everything TCM, everyone is different, and a diagnostic pattern of imbalance should be determined for treatment. However, one of the most common patterns is "Liver Qi stagnation attacking Spleen." Liver Qi stagnation causes irritability, breast tenderness, and sometimes headaches or migraines. Liver attacking the Spleen causes bloating, loose stool, fatigue, and worry, and sweet cravings are frequently added to the symptoms. When Heat is added to the stagnancy, pimples or rashes, constipation, and heavy menstrual flow can occur. Menstrual cramps occur when Qi and Blood are unable to flow smoothly. TCM Kidneys are also closely involved with menstruation, and deficiency here can result in low back pain, joint pain, cravings for salty foods, fatigue, anxiety, and an exacerbation of the other imbalances.

If you're suffering from PMS, don't address it only when you are suffering. Your best bet is to make sure you're eating healthily all month, with plenty of the following foods:

- leafy green vegetables
- cruciferous vegetables like broccoli, Brussels spouts, cauliflower, radish, and turnip, in addition to several of the leafy greens—these foods contain a compound called indole-3-carbinol, which may help decrease "bad" estrogen metabolites, help prevent some types of cancer, and support liver detoxification
- fiber—make sure to get plenty of it
- foods rich in omega-3 essential fatty acids, including fatty fish, nuts, and seeds.

To support healthy activity of the physical liver and TCM Liver, include the following foods:

- artichokes, asparagus, bamboo shoots, beans (green, Italian, wax), beets/beetroot, broccoli, Brussels sprouts, cabbage, cauliflower, celery, cucumbers, daikon, eggplant/aubergine, greens (arugula/

rocket, Belgian endive/chicory, bok choy, butterleaf, collard greens, dandelion, escarole, kale, kohlrabi, mustard greens, parsley, radicchio, romaine, watercress), horseradish, onions, peppers (green, red, yellow), radish, sprouts (clover, mung bean, radish, sunflower), squash, tomatoes, water chestnuts

- apples, blackberries, cherries, dark grapes, plums, raspberries
- millet
- sauerkraut
- basil, bay leaf, cumin, dill, fennel, ginger, lemon balm, marjoram, mint, rosemary
- spirulina, barley grass, wheatgrass, chlorella, and other chlorophyll-rich greens.

Vitex (chaste tree berry) and evening primrose oil can also help.

Dysmenorrhea (Menstrual Cramps)

Patients often tell me that they think their intense menstrual cramps are just a normal part of being a woman and having a period. I respond that, while common, severe cramping is not normal. It's a sign of hormonal imbalance, and yes, there's a better solution than gulping back lots of anti-inflammatory painkillers every month.

Menstrual cramps are contractions in the uterus, caused by prostaglandins, chemicals our bodies produce to heal damaged tissue but that also help regulate the menstrual cycle, control ovulation, and induce labor. Although it's normal for the uterus to contract during a woman's menstrual cycle, if it contracts too strongly, pain occurs as it presses up against nearby blood vessels and cuts off the supply of oxygen to the muscles of the uterus.

Dysmenorrhea can be primary or secondary, and it is felt in the lower abdomen and sometimes back and thighs.

Primary dysmenorrhea is cramping that is not caused by other diseases. It usually starts a day or two before menstrual bleeding or when the period starts, usually lasting for a few hours to a few days. When severe, it can be accompanied by nausea, vomiting, diarrhea, fatigue, dizziness, and even fainting.

Secondary dysmenorrhea is cramping caused by a disease or disorder of the reproductive organs. Examples include uterine fibroids, infection, polycystic ovarian syndrome (PCOS), and endometriosis.

In TCM, all pain is associated with stagnation of Qi and/or Blood. In other words, things are not moving well. Severe cramping pain can be diagnosed in TCM as Cold in the Uterus, so warming herbs are indicated. Decreasing muscular contraction and inflammation also helps reduce cramping pain.

Foods that can help manage dysmenorrhea include:

- omega-3 fatty acid-rich foods like fatty fish (sardines, mackerel, herring, wild salmon, cod, and halibut) and nuts and seeds (ground flax seeds or flaxseed oil, hemp seeds, chia seeds)
- cinnamon tea: steep a cinnamon stick in 2 cups of boiled water (cinnamon bark is the Chinese herb *rou gui*, and the twig is *gui zhi*)
- ginger (the Chinese herb *sheng jiang*)
- scallions/spring onions, onions, chives
- orange peel (the Chinese herbs *chen pi* or *zhi shi*)
- saffron (the Chinese herb *hong hua*)
- foods rich in magnesium to help reduce muscle cramping and tension:
  - dark leafy greens
  - beans (black, kidney, lima, navy, pinto, white, etc.)
  - garbanzo beans/chickpeas, lentils
  - halibut, tuna
  - artichoke
  - figs
  - barley, oat bran, brown rice
  - almonds, pine nuts, Brazil nuts, cashews, pumpkin seeds
  - broccoli, okra, parsnips, peas, pumpkin, squash, sweet potatoes.

Evening primrose oil, vitex (chaste tree berry), cramp bark, chamomile tea, and valerian tea can also be helpful, as can regular exercise (think again about moving Qi and Blood—i.e., getting the circulation going), and, of course, a heated pad over the lower abdomen or lower back.

Period Irregularities

There are a slew of medical terms relating to the period because the period can be early, late, irregular, frequent, infrequent, non-existent, heavy, light, long, or short. And because the body is complex, it's important to get a proper assessment from a health professional if you want to sort out how to address it. From a Western medicine perspective, that usually means hormonal testing, physical exam, and other tests. From a TCM perspective, diagnosis is sorted into Excess, Deficiency, a combination of Excess and Deficiency, and also related to organs causing and affected by the imbalance.

In other words, it's not easy to make food recommendations that are general to treating these issues. But if you have nutritional deficiencies or a TCM diagnosis from a qualified practitioner, you can follow the recommendations in Chapter 2: How to Classify Foods Using TCM, Chapter 3: Foundations of Nutrition, and Chapter 6: Foods by Element.

It also helps to understand a bit more about the main period problems.

Amenorrhea (No Periods)

To some, amenorrhea might seem like a blessing. No periods? Hooray! But no. Unless you are under the age of 15, in menopause or perimenopause, taking medication to suppress the period, and pregnant or breastfeeding, missing more than six (some say three) periods in a row can signal that you have some work to do on your health.

The problem with not having a period is that it indicates that something may be imbalanced hormonally, and it's not just menstruation that could be affected. In addition to potential complications with fertility, amenorrhea that is caused by low estrogen levels can put you at a higher risk of osteoporosis and cardiovascular disease.

So, why might a person experience amenorrhea? Low body weight, eating disorders, obesity, rigorous athletic training, stress, thyroid malfunctions, pituitary tumor, polycystic ovary syndrome (PCOS), premature menopause, and structural issues like uterine scarring can all cause periods to stop.

Menorrhagia (Heavy or Long Periods)

Abnormally heavy or prolonged periods are defined as soaking through more than one tampon or pad every hour for several consecutive hours and/or having a period for longer than a week. Some women need to double up with both tampons and pads, need to wake through the night to change sanitary protection, and need to alter daily activities to accommodate the heavy bleeding. Many experience fatigue and shortness of breath caused by anemia from the blood loss.

Causes of menorrhagia include a number of hormonal imbalances, including obesity, polycystic ovary syndrome (PCOS), insulin resistance, endometriosis, thyroid problems, uterine fibroids, uterine polyps, uterine or cervical cancer, and having an intrauterine device (IUD).

To help manage the pain that often comes with heavy or long periods, check the Dysmenorrhea (Menstrual Cramps) section above. If anemia is a problem because of heavy bleeding, eat iron-rich foods such as:

- beef, lamb, and other meats
- poultry
- fish, shellfish
- spinach, Swiss chard, collard greens, beet greens, bok choy, mustard greens, turnip greens, parsley
- eggs
- dairy

- leeks, asparagus
- turmeric, cumin
- soybeans (tofu, tempeh, miso, edamame)
- lentils
- beans (navy, white, kidney, pinto, black, adzuki, garbanzo/chickpeas)
- green peas, lima beans, green beans
- beets/beetroot.

Metrorrhagia (Irregular Bleeding)

Bleeding that's not associated with a regular period, either light or heavy, and with or without menstrual cramping, is called metrorrhagia. There are many possible causes, including uterine or vaginal cancer, endometriosis, miscarriage, ectopic pregnancy, infection, fibroids, polyps, and blood-clotting disorders. An intrauterine device (IUD), hormone therapy, and blood-thinning medication may also cause irregular bleeding.

While the amount of blood can be very small and result in what is commonly known as spotting, it can also be relatively heavy and result in anemia, in which case it can help to eat the iron-rich foods listed above in the Menorrhagia (Heavy or Long Periods) section above.

Because the reasons for menstrual issues are so varied, it's difficult to recommend any specific recipes, but one that helps support the liver (both the anatomical liver and TCM Liver), Kidneys, and Spleen may be helpful.

Green Smoothie

One of the nice things about smoothies is that they are very modifiable. This one contains kale for the Liver, chia seeds for the Kidneys, ginger for the Spleen, avocado for the uterus, soy milk for hormone balancing (see the "Is Soy Healthy?" box in the Menopausal/Perimenopausal Symptoms section above), and cinnamon for blood sugar balancing. But play around with the ingredients to make it to your taste, texture preference, and health benefits.

- 1 cup kale (stalks removed)
- ¼–½ avocado (depending on the size and how thick you want your smoothie)
- 1 tbsp chia seeds
- 1" piece of fresh ginger, peeled
- ½ tsp cinnamon
- 1 cup soy milk (or substitute for another milk alternative)

Blend all ingredients together and enjoy.

Migraine

While people often state that they have a migraine when they have a bad headache, headaches and migraines are not synonymous. Migraines are caused by an instability in the way that the brain handles sensory information. Migraines vary from person to person, and while the key symptom for most is a headache, other symptoms include visual disturbances, light sensitivity, sound sensitivity, sensitivity to smells, nausea, and vomiting.

We think that migraines are caused by abnormal brain activity that affects some chemicals, nerve signals, and blood vessels in the brain. It appears that migraines are commonly hereditary and that certain genes can trigger this faulty wiring.

There are as many as four stages to a migraine, though not everyone has all the stages:

1. prodrome
2. aura
3. migraine attack
4. postdrome.

Some people experience symptoms a day or two before a migraine. Known as a migraine prodrome, this can include food cravings, changes in appetite, mood changes, poor concentration, fatigue, weakness, frequent yawning, constipation or diarrhea, cold extremities, increased thirst and urination, and neck stiffness.

In addition to this, some migraineurs get auras shortly before the start of their migraine. Those with visual auras may notice zigzag or wavy patterns, flashing lights, or blind spots. It looks to some like a kaleidoscope, but so much less fun. Others notice loss of coordination, tingling or numbness, inability to concentrate, confusion, uncontrollable movements, hearing sounds not present, and difficulty speaking.

A migraine attack is often when the headache comes on, and this stage can last from a few hours to a few days. Some migraineurs do not experience the headache stage. While one-sided headaches are common with migraines, they may be felt on both sides and include stiffness of the neck and shoulders. The symptoms can be so severe that they leave a person incapacitated.

Although it's a relief to get through the attack stage, sufferers frequently experience the fourth stage, a "migraine hangover," also called a postdrome, that leave a person feeling exhausted, lightheaded, dizzy, and weak.

There are many potential triggers to a migraine, including some over which we have little power, like weather changes. Some women notice migraines related to their menstrual cycles, so they can do their best to prepare and perhaps reduce other stressors that can aggravate migraines during that phase of their cycle. Hormone-balancing treatments can help with this type. Stress, sleep disturbances, and vigorous exercise triggers still others.

Because migraines can also be triggered by specific foods, keeping a food diary along with a migraine diary may help point out some of the foods best limited or avoided. Common food triggers include:

- aged cheese
- aged, smoked, dried, fermented, or pickled meats, especially pepperoni, salami, and liverwurst
- alcohol
- aspartame and other artificial sweeteners
- caffeine (conversely, suddenly stopping caffeine can also trigger a migraine, while drinking a strong cup of coffee at the start of a migraine may actually help abort it)
- chocolate
- citrus fruits
- dairy products
- food dyes and preservatives
- ice cream and other frozen foods
- monosodium glutamate (MSG)
- sugar and excess sweet foods (watch for hidden sugars in muffins, some cereals, etc.)
- fava or broad beans, sauerkraut, pickles, olives, and fermented soy products (i.e., miso, soy sauce, teriyaki sauce). These are high in tyramine, an amino acid produced from the natural breakdown of the amino acid tyrosine. Tyramine can cause blood vessels to dilate, and this may be what starts the migraine chain-reaction in some people.

Eating a healthy diet of whole foods without artificial colors or flavors, preservatives, or additives is always a good idea, but in the case of migraines, it can mean the difference between a good day and a few days needing to stay in a dark, quiet room, with a bucket beside your bed.

Magnesium supplements are often prescribed for migraine sufferers, so eating foods rich in magnesium is also very helpful. Foods that are rich in magnesium include:

- dark leafy greens and cruciferous vegetables, including arugula/rocket, beet greens, spinach, Swiss chard, kale, broccoli, cauliflower, and Brussels sprouts
- pumpkin seeds, sesame seeds, sunflower seeds
- Brazil nuts, almonds, cashews
- quinoa, buckwheat
- oats, brown rice, millet (these grains are also gluten-free)
- lima beans, garbanzo beans/chickpeas, black beans, navy beans, pinto beans, kidney beans.

Anti-inflammatory foods may also help, including the following (note there is some overlap with the magnesium-rich foods):

- apples
- artichoke
- berries (blueberries, raspberries, and strawberries)
- broccoli, beet greens, okra, parsnips, peas, pumpkin, spinach, squash, sweet potatoes
- brown rice, oat bran
- figs
- fish oil, mackerel, herring, sardines, anchovies, wild salmon, halibut, cod
- flax seeds and flaxseed oil
- ginger
- onions, shallots, leeks, garlic, and all related to the allium family
- papaya, pineapple
- pumpkin seeds, walnuts
- seaweeds (kelp, kombu, wakame, arame).

Migraine-Treating Teas

Alternatively, you may simply want to make a nice tea that can help prevent or treat migraines.

Some options include:

- peppermint tea (particularly noted to treat headaches)
- lavender tea (not just for smelling, it can calm your overwhelmed nervous system and treat headaches)
- chamomile tea (treats headaches and may help you sleep off your migraine)
- ginger tea (anti-inflammatory and helps with nausea)

- turmeric tea (anti-inflammatory)
- black or green tea (the caffeine may help treat your migraine, but be aware that it can also be a trigger)

Muscle Cramps and Spasms

Have you ever woken in the middle of the night with your lower leg screaming at you and causing your foot to be stuck in an awkward position while you grit your teeth and try to use your fingers to find a release spot in your calf muscles? Or maybe you can recall a time on the school playground when, during a skirmish, someone kneed you in the thigh and you yelled out, "Charley horse!"? Or perhaps, while out for a jog, you got a stitch in your side that made you double over until it passed?

Then, like most people, you've experienced a muscle cramp or spasm. Experiencing this every now and then, usually caused by something you can easily pinpoint, is not a big problem. But if you go through muscle cramps with frequency, then it's time to take action.

Involuntary, painful muscle contractions that last for a few seconds to several minutes can occur in any muscle, from the voluntary skeletal muscles that control your movement to the involuntary muscles of your heart, bowels, uterus, blood vessel walls, bladder, and more.

Causes of muscle spasms include:

- vigorous exercise, overuse of muscle, and injury
- dehydration
- pregnancy: can decrease the body's supply of calcium and magnesium, which can lead to cramps
- being in one position or sitting or lying in an awkward position for a long time
- exposure to cold temperatures
- insufficient potassium, magnesium, or calcium in the blood
- chronic alcoholism
- withdrawal from medications and addictive substances that have sedative effects
- medical conditions, such as multiple sclerosis, thyroid disease, circulation problems, or kidney disease
- some medications, including antipsychotics, birth control pills, diuretics, statins, and steroids
- age: can also make muscle cramps more common as muscle mass shrinks and the remaining muscle becomes more easily stressed.

From a TCM perspective, the Liver and Gallbladder are responsible for the tendons and ligaments of the body, while the Spleen and Stomach rule the muscles. Nourishing these systems, therefore, is important to prevent ongoing muscle cramps. Additionally, I usually recommend supplementing with a well-absorbed form of magnesium, such as magnesium glycinate (bisglycinate).

Select foods that are rich in the minerals magnesium, potassium, and calcium, which are anti-inflammatory and support the Liver/Gallbladder and Spleen/Stomach, such as:

- leafy green vegetables
- onions, shallots, leeks, and garlic
- asparagus, bamboo shoots, beans (green, Italian, wax), beets/beetroot, broccoli, Brussels sprouts, carrots, cauliflower, celery, cucumbers, dandelion, daikon, eggplant/aubergine, horseradish, kohlrabi, peas, pumpkin, radish, sprouts (clover, mung bean, radish, sunflower), squash, sweet potatoes
- sauerkraut
- seaweeds like arame, dulse, kelp, kombu, nori, and wakame
- olives, olive oil
- apples, avocado, berries, cherries, figs, plums
- fish oil, anchovies, cod, halibut, herring, mackerel, sardine, and wild salmon
- legumes
- flax seeds, flaxseed oil
- almonds, Brazil nuts, cashews, pine nuts, pumpkin seeds, walnuts
- barley, brown rice, millet, oat bran
- ginger, turmeric
- blackstrap molasses
- apple cider vinegar
- basil, bay leaf, cumin, dill, fennel, ginger, lemon balm, marjoram, mint, rosemary
- spirulina, barley grass, wheatgrass, chlorella, and other chlorophyll-rich greens.

Relax Muscles Smoothie

Aren't we fortunate that there are so many foods that are rich in magnesium, potassium, and calcium? What's great about smoothies is that you can swap out ingredients, including other magnesium-rich foods like cashew, pumpkin seeds, kale, Swiss chard, or arugula/rocket or anti-inflammatory foods like berries, turmeric, figs, walnuts, papaya, or pineapple. Plus, making sure that you're well hydrated is key to trying to minimize muscle spasms and cramps.

While I know most smoothies include ice, in TCM, we prefer recommending room-temperature or warm drinks over icy cold. However, if you want to add ice to thicken your smoothie, you can. You may also choose to thicken it with more banana, avocado, or by adding in yogurt.

- ½ to ¾ cup spinach (big handful)
- 1 medium apple
- 1″ piece of fresh ginger
- 1 tbsp hemp seeds, chia seeds, or ground flax seeds
- 1 cup oat, hemp, rice, or almond milk
- ½ avocado or ½ banana
- Optional: ice

If you have a very powerful blender, you may not need to chop up your ingredients much and you can keep the skin on your apple. If your blender is not that strong, you may need to chop things up more.

Nausea and Vomiting

Word of warning: skip this paragraph if you're currently nauseous. You probably know the feeling. You start to salivate, and you feel the need to swallow hard while your stomach feels like it's rising. If the queasiness progresses, then you may start to retch and eventually vomit. It's an awful sensation that has a pile of interesting names, from barf to technicolor yawn and puke to blow chunks. Sorry if that made you feel nauseous. I know how triggering this topic can be.

Nausea and vomiting can be a great defense method for the body if something offensive has entered it and needs to be removed quickly. Food poisoning is an example of this. In fact, emetics (substances that cause vomiting) are sometimes employed in a medical setting, such as addressing a drug overdose or poisoning.

Unfortunately, there are several other reasons we can experience these symptoms, including:

- flu or other pathogenic infection (virus, bacteria, parasite)
- morning sickness during pregnancy
- motion sickness
- side effect of medications like chemotherapy

- migraine
- middle ear infection
- Ménière's disease
- vertigo
- and many digestive disorders.

In TCM, the Stomach energy should always travel downward, so nausea and vomiting are diagnosed as "Stomach energy rising" or "Rebellious Stomach Qi." It certainly does feel like the stomach is rebelling! While there are some simple remedies you can try to address the symptoms, if you're experiencing frequent nausea and/or vomiting, you should get help to sort out the reason. It's also important to rehydrate because vomiting can cause a depletion of fluids and vital electrolytes.

Simple Home Remedies to Address Nausea

- Ginger is the most recognized remedy. It can be purchased in tea bags, you can slice fresh ginger into hot water and drink it as a tea, or you can find ginger candies. If you find the ginger too spicy, you can have it with a bit of honey.
- Try sucking on an ice cube or frozen fruit.
- Keep foods simple and relatively bland. Have clear liquids like broth.
- Eat smaller meals, more frequently.
- Sparkling mineral water or soda water sipped slowly may help settle the stomach.
- You may have a family recipe that you find helpful. For me, the ochazuke that I mentioned in How to Congee in the Irritable Bowel Syndrome section above is one such recipe. For others, it's a chicken noodle soup. Miso soup, bone broth, or vegetable broth are other options commonly cited.

A Story of a Boat Ride and Tips to Manage Nausea

I'm one of those lucky people who rarely gets nauseous. I can read when I'm a passenger in a car. I can go on virtually any amusement park ride. I even like the feeling of my stomach rising when I'm on one of those rides that drops quickly. So I had no concerns about getting on a boat to do a Galapagos Islands tour.

My sureness about my stomach, however, was tossed out the window (and almost over the side of the boat) on day one of the boat trip. Our engine broke, so we needed to be towed. That meant a very rocky ride, and almost all of us were sick shortly after eating dinner. With that memory fresh in my mind, a couple of days later I needed to board a much smaller boat (they called it a ferry) that was supposed to carry a maximum of 11 people. We had 11 passengers, four crew members, and a pile of heavy scuba tanks when we started out on very rough waters. About halfway through the trip, which is supposed to take two to three hours, we came across another ferry (i.e., power boat) with broken motors and a full load of people. Our load then doubled as we took them aboard. Unfortunately, stopping our boat to make the transfer meant we were bobbed about for a good 20 or so minutes, leaving most of the passengers already turning green and many of them filling barf bags. I was lucky to have a spot pretty much hanging off the back of the boat. Although it was a bit precarious, it meant I had some access to fresh air and a horizon to look at, so I was one of the few to keep my cookies down. Over the next two hours of travel, I got to think a lot about ways to avoid nausea and vomiting, so here are some of the things I learned.

- Look to the horizon if it's motion sickness you're dealing with. That means, don't go below deck, as you're probably more likely to get sick. If you're in a car, sit in the front seat or the middle back seat and look to the horizon of where the car is going.
- Try to find a way to breathe in fresh air. Especially if there are strong smells around you (even more so if others are vomiting—think of the scene in the movie *Stand by Me*).
- If fresh air is unavailable and there are nauseating smells bothering you, choose something that smells better. Thankfully, on that boat in the Galapagos, we passed around a little tin of Tiger Balm that really helped. Peppermint oil, lemons or any citrus or citrus oil, or lavender oil may also help.
- Place a cool cloth at the back of your neck. I had the cold spray of water on me when I was on that boat, and I think that helped.
- Occupy your mind. Thinking about being sick makes you feel sicker. I found a mantra/song to sing over and over in my mind; one that reminded me that everything was going to be alright.

- And, of course, there's the TCM acupressure point *Neiguan*, also known as P6 or PC6. The point is located 3 finger widths (often incorrectly and annoyingly described as 2 finger widths; acupuncturists know that our measurement is "2 cun"—pronounced "tsun"—which is 3 finger widths!) up from the inside crease of the wrist, between the tendons. Apply firm pressure to this point. You can alternate sides you press, or you can wear the anti-nausea bands found in many pharmacies.

Prostate Issues

The prostate is a walnut-sized gland under the bladder of men. The function of the prostate is to produce the fluid called semen that nourishes and transports sperm.

Rather than repeat myself for nutritional recommendations for each of the different types of prostate issues I cover here, I'll first introduce the conditions, then make food recommendations at the end of the section.

Benign Prostatic Hypertrophy (BPH)

Even if they've managed to be ignorant of its presence for most of their lives, about half of men aged in their 50s and about 90 percent of men over the age of 80 will have to take notice when the symptoms of benign prostatic hypertrophy (BPH) arise. These symptoms include interrupted sleep because of an urge to urinate, frequent and sudden urges to urinate, weak or dribbling urine stream, need to strain to urinate, trouble starting urination, the need to stop and start urinating several times, and a feeling that the bladder is full even after urinating.

The good news is that BPH is not cancer and does not cause cancer, though it can occur at the same time as prostate cancer.

The bad news is that BPH can continue to get worse if the prostate continues to grow. And, if the bladder cannot effectively empty, BPH can lead to more frequent bladder infections, bladder damage, and even kidney damage.

Prostatitis

Prostatitis is, simply put, inflammation of the prostate. There are four types of prostatitis:

- chronic prostatitis/chronic pelvic pain syndrome (CP/CPPS)

- chronic bacterial prostatitis
- acute bacterial prostatitis
- asymptomatic inflammatory prostatitis.

Chronic Prostatitis

Also called chronic non-bacterial prostatitis, this is the most common type of prostatitis, with symptoms of difficulty with urination, sometimes pain with urination, pain with ejaculation, sexual dysfunction, and pain in the bladder, testicles, penis, and perineum (area between the scrotum and anus).

The cause is unknown, but it's suspected it might be a past infection or small injury that caused the inflammation to be triggered and keep recurring.

Chronic Bacterial Prostatitis

This type of prostatitis can come and go with symptoms of a frequent urge to urinate, especially at night, and sometimes a burning sensation during urination. It can also cause painful ejaculation and pain in the bladder, testicles, penis, and perineum.

Often associated with frequent urinary tract infections, it's caused by a persistent bacterial infection, and it can be difficult to treat.

Acute Bacterial Prostatitis

As stated in the name, acute bacterial prostatitis is caused by a current bacterial infection and has symptoms of pain with urination and ejaculation, burning sensation with urination, pain in the bladder, testicles, penis, and perineum, and problems with draining the bladder. A main distinguishing factor from other types of prostatitis is its sudden onset and fever and chills.

Asymptomatic Inflammatory Prostatitis

If this is the type of prostatitis you have, then lucky you. It was likely only discovered when you were being checked for something else because, as the name implies, it doesn't have symptoms. Better yet, it usually doesn't require treatment.

So, now to the food part.

Because the prostate is related to reproductive function and has a strong impact on urinary health, TCM often links prostate health to the health of the TCM Kidneys and TCM Urinary Bladder. Thus, foods that support these TCM organs are generally recommended for prostate health.

These include:

- nuts

- seeds (especially pumpkin seeds)
- legumes
- barley
- cornsilk (it's a diuretic—i.e., makes you urinate)
- figs
- lychee/litchi
- pomegranate
- seaweed
- watermelon
- winter melon.

For BPH, studies report that the isoflavones and flavonoid compounds in soy help to both treat and prevent BPH (Garg *et al.*, 2013; Geller *et al.*, 1998). See the "Is Soy Healthy?" box in the Menopausal/Perimenopausal Symptoms section above for more about soy.

For prostatitis, it's important to help manage the inflammation, and the following foods may be helpful in that regard (also listed in the Arthritis section above):

- flax seeds and flaxseed oil
- high-quality fish oil, mackerel, herring, sardines, anchovies, wild salmon, cod, halibut
- olives, olive oil and vinaigrettes made with it
- green leafy vegetables
- apples
- onions, shallots, leeks, garlic, and all related to the allium family (also helpful if there is an infection)
- berries (blueberries, raspberries, and strawberries)
- pumpkin seeds, walnuts
- seaweeds (kelp, kombu, wakame, arame)
- papaya (contains an anti-inflammatory enzyme called papain), pineapple (contains an anti-inflammatory enzyme called betaine)
- turmeric
- ginger.

Pumpkin Seed and Sun-Dried Tomato Pesto

Pesto is the besto. While pesto originates in Genoa, Italy, and was originally made of pine nuts, olive oil, basil, garlic, and parmesan cheese, the word "pesto" comes from the Genoan word *pestare* which means "to crush" or "to mash." So, pesto is more about a way to prepare the food, not specifically the ingredients. This pesto doesn't contain any of those ingredients but, like its ancestor, is delicious to top on crackers, vegetables, or pasta, or it can be used as a dip.

- ¼ cup pumpkin seeds, toasted
- ½ cup oil-packed sun-dried tomatoes, drained
- ⅓ cup extra virgin olive oil
- Optional: 1 tbsp capers

You can either place all the ingredients in a food processor or chop them all up and mix together.

Skin Diseases (e.g., Eczema, Psoriasis)

With skin as the largest organ of your body, it's no surprise that skin issues are often quite complex, with many different diagnoses and causes. In TCM, the Lungs govern the skin. In fact, we often see people with lung issues like asthma and allergies also suffering from eczema. The TCM Lung's elemental partner, the Large Intestines, may also play a role. If there is improper elimination through the bowels, toxins may accumulate and exit through the skin instead. It's not uncommon to see people with Crohn's or colitis also dealing with skin problems. As organs that filter out toxins from the blood, the liver and kidneys may also be involved. Finally, impairment of the digestive organs—the TCM Stomach and Spleen—can further complicate issues.

While the TCM patterns of imbalance are quite varied, some common TCM diagnoses for skin issues like eczema, acne, psoriasis, and rashes include Damp-Heat, Toxic-Heat, Blood-Heat, Blood Deficiency, Yin Deficiency Heat, and Wind-Heat.

The intention of this section is not to teach how to diagnose a skin condition either from a TCM or a conventional disease approach, but instead to help outline some ways that symptoms can direct some foods that may be helpful (or harmful).

Some simple ways to consider TCM patterns with their symptoms include considering the following (note that this is not a complete listing):

- Wind: itchiness is the main symptom; location of skin issues tends to move around.
- Damp: puffiness or swelling, raised bumps, weeping of skin, blisters.
- Heat: redness, inflammation.
- Dryness: scaling, flaking, dry skin.

- Toxins: irritation, inflammation.
- Blood deficiency: pale spots, dryness.
- Blood stagnation: purplish spots, darkened areas or nodules.

Although dietary recommendations vary based on the condition, TCM diagnosis, and an individual's constitution, here are some general recommendations:

- Avoid processed, greasy, and fried foods.
- Limit sugar.
- Limit or avoid stimulants like caffeine and intoxicants like alcohol.
- Limit hot spicy foods like cayenne and hot spices and foods like garlic, ginger, clove, nutmeg, and cinnamon, especially if you have a lot of Heat signs.
- TCM would also have you avoid shellfish (bottom-feeders higher in toxins) and tropical fruit like pineapples and mango (high in sugar).
- Limit or avoid dairy if you have Dampness signs.
- If you have a lot of Heat signs, include cooling foods like cucumber, watermelon, winter melon, cabbage, dandelion greens and other leafy greens, and aloe vera.
- Include mung beans—said to help with detoxification.
- Eat foods rich in beta-carotene like carrot, squash, sweet potato, pumpkin, peas.
- Spruce up your diet with sprouted foods like alfalfa sprouts, pea sprouts, soy sprouts, and sprouted seeds, legumes, or grains.
- Seaweeds are rich in skin-benefiting nutrients, and according to TCM, their salty nature makes them also suitable for helping to break up masses like nodules, cystic acne, and boils.
- Blood-cleansing foods include gobo root (burdock root), dandelion root and greens, and red clover blossoms.
- Foods rich in essential fatty acids can help heal skin, so include flax-seed oil, hemp seeds or oil, chia seeds or oil, or borage oil.
- Make sure you're getting enough fiber and that your intestines are eliminating well.
- If you suspect food sensitivities or allergies, seek the help of a health professional who can guide you.
- Consider probiotic supplements and/or fermented foods to support the good bacteria that are needed for a healthy digestive system, immune system, and so much more.
- Hydrate well!

Food with "Bad" Skin

Remember the earlier chapter about choosing foods based on their appearance? Sometimes we do judge a book by its cover. Well, it's food for thought that TCM generally recommends you avoid pineapple, durian, and other "ugly skin" foods if you're struggling with a skin condition. Durian is quite hot in nature, so that alone may be part of the problem for those with red, irritated skin diseases.

Dandelion Tea

They're a pretty yellow, they're easy to grow, and they have many health benefits. So why are dandelions so hated by many? I get that they can take over your garden, but the next time you have to do some weeding, collect those dandelions instead of composting them. Dandelions are known as the herb *pu gong yin* in TCM, and they are used to clear Heat and Toxins, treat urinary tract infections, clear the eyes, reduce abscesses and nodules, and promote lactation. From a Western herbalist perspective, dandelions are used to support liver health, as an anti-inflammatory, to help regulate blood sugars, as a diuretic, and to support digestion. Just make sure that the ones you use have not been sprayed with pesticides and that you clean them well (no one wants to be consuming dog pee, I assume). By clearing Heat, reducing Dampness, and supporting both the TCM Liver and the physical liver, dandelion is a good herb for many skin disorders, especially where there is redness, pus or weeping, hard nodules, and inflammation.

- 6–10 dandelions with flowers and leaves
- 1 cup water
- Optional: honey

Bring water to a boil and add dandelions. Lid the pot and let steep for 10 minutes. Strain and add honey to taste, as dandelion is bitter.

Snoring

Snoring is one of those symptoms that in and of itself may not seem a big deal. But snoring can, in fact, be life-threatening. And not just because your sleeping partner is seriously sleep deprived and has had enough. Snoring can cause sleep disturbances for the snorer too, such as with sleep apnea—a condition in which the person stops breathing intermittently through the night. Sleep apnea is a serious condition that, left untreated, can result in a heart attack, stroke, high blood pressure, type 2 diabetes and other metabolic disorders, cancer, glaucoma, daytime sleepiness and fatigue, cognitive dysfunction, and depression. This isn't really that surprising, of course, as you know the importance of sleep—and breathing! If you suspect sleep apnea, get assessed via a sleep study.

Snoring is caused by vibration of the soft tissue at the back of the mouth or nose when an obstruction in the passageway creates turbulent air. Reasons for the obstruction include:

- thicker or floppy soft palate, enlarged tonsils, elongated uvula, large tongue base, deviated septum—surgery is likely the best option for these conditions
- nasal congestion caused by a cold, allergies, sinusitis
- being overweight, which causes extra mass at the neck and throat area, thus narrowing the breathing pathways
- too much alcohol, which relaxes the muscles in the throat too much, making obstruction more likely.

In TCM, the most common cause of snoring is stagnation from Dampness or Phlegm, so a key nutritional approach is to avoid Damp-inducing foods, including:

- sugar
- alcohol
- dairy products
- processed foods
- greasy and fried foods
- wheat
- too much raw, cold food.

Some foods that can be helpful include:

- bitter foods that dry Dampness, like arugula/rocket, asparagus, celery, kohlrabi, bitter melon, amaranth, barley, rye, chamomile, fenugreek, and mustard seed (see the Bitter Foods section in Chapter 2 for more options, but skip the coffee, alcohol, beer, and wine bitter foods—sorry!)
- pungent foods that can help clear obstructions, like fennel, garlic, onions, pepper, ginger, peppermint (see the Pungent Foods section in Chapter 2 for more options)

- foods that decrease inflammation and support a healthy respiratory system, like mushrooms, green leafy veggies, basil, ginger, and turmeric.

More "No Snore" Options

- Maintain a healthy weight.
- If you only snore when you're on your back, try to force yourself to sleep on your side. One way to do that is to get a pair of pantyhose or tights and place a tennis ball inside one of the legs. Tie the tights around your waist so that the tennis ball sits at your back. If you roll onto your back while sleeping, you'll feel the ball and automatically roll back onto your side (or wake yourself up in discomfort and roll onto your side).
- If you're congested, do a saline nasal rinse before bed. You can use the traditional Ayurvedic neti pot or some modern version you can find in your local natural health store or drug store.
- If you have allergies, use an air purifier to remove inhaled irritants in your sleeping quarters.
- Try aromatherapy of eucalyptus or peppermint to help open your sinuses.
- Quit smoking.
- Look for alternatives to sleeping medications and antihistamines, as they can overly relax the muscles of your throat, allowing for more obstruction of the air passageway.
- Get acupuncture! My favorite acupoints to do are on either side of the nostrils. I love these points for two main reasons. One (the most authentic reason), because it works quickly at helping to open the sinus pathways. Two (a selfish reason) is that it's entertaining for me when patients have these points in and the needles wiggle like whiskers if the patient talks or laughs (don't worry, I tell them this reason, which is how I get to see most of them laugh).

Urinary Tract Infection (UTI)

The medical world has a lot of abbreviations that the average person doesn't know. For example, ACU stands for "ambulatory care unit," though for me it's an abbreviation for "acupuncture." I looked up my initials, MC, and found that it's short for "metacarpal bone" or "medical certificate"—these are okay—but also "mass casualties," "medullary carcinoma," and "molluscum contagiousum"—not good. UTI, however, is one that a lot of women know because they are relatively common, and, for some women, recurrent.

A urinary tract infection is an infection in any part of the urinary system—the kidneys, ureters (tubes between kidneys and bladder), bladder, and urethra (tube from bladder to exit of the body). UTIs most commonly affect the bladder and urethra, and it becomes much more serious if the kidneys become affected, so don't wait to treat a UTI.

Symptoms of a UTI depend on what part of the urinary tract is infected. If the infection is in the urethra, symptoms are likely to be a burning sensation with urination and a discharge. Infection in the bladder can cause frequent and painful urination, lower abdominal discomfort, a sensation of pelvic pressure, and blood in the urine. Higher up, an infection of the kidneys can be felt as back and side pain, nausea, vomiting, a fever, shaking, and chills. Other symptoms of a UTI include pelvic pain, feeling a persistent urge to urinate, urine that's cloudy, urine that has a strong smell, or urine that's red, pink, or cola-colored (signs of blood in the urine).

Women are more prone to UTIs because of the anatomical proximity of the urethra to the anus and the shorter distance between the urethral opening and the bladder. This is why girls are instructed to wipe from front to back. Women's risk for these infections also increases with sexual activity, the use of a diaphragm or spermicidal agents, and menopause (it's the drop in estrogen). Factors that affect both men and women include anatomical abnormalities of the urinary tract, suppressed immune system, catheter use, and blockages in the urinary tract (as from kidney stones or prostate issues).

The most common diagnosis for UTIs from a TCM perspective is "Damp-Heat." In fact, a combination of TCM's definition of Dampness and Heat is usually some sort of inflammation and/or infection. Those who frequently get UTIs should also look to boost Kidney Yin because when it is persistently weak, it allows Heat signs to accumulate and results in chronic inflammation.

Thus, during a UTI or if you're prone to getting UTIs, avoid or limit foods that cause too much Dampness and/or Heat, such as:

- sugar
- dairy products (except yogurt which, though it may increase Dampness, may help restore the balance of good bacteria to ward off bad bacterial growth)
- processed and refined foods
- greasy, fried foods
- alcohol.

In between UTIs, if you chronically get UTIs and also have dry skin, dry hair, dry mouth; need to drink a lot of fluids; suffer with a sore lower back or knees; tend to get night sweats or hot flashes; feel generally too warm; and are often constipated, choose foods that support Kidney Yin:

- lima beans, mung beans, yellow soybeans, tofu
- seaweeds
- almonds, cashews, flax seeds, hazelnuts, hemp seeds, poppy seeds
- clam, cuttlefish, mussel, oyster, perch, scallop, squid
- apricot, avocado, banana, blackcurrant, blueberry, cantaloupe, grapefruit, kiwifruit, lemon, lime, orange, pear, persimmon, plum, strawberry, tangerine, watermelon
- alfalfa sprouts, asparagus, celery, potato, string bean, sweet potato, yam
- chicken egg
- ghee, yogurt
- kamut, millet.

Foods that can be helpful to relieve Damp-Heat include foods that are neutral or cooling in temperature and foods that help to drain, dry, or transform Dampness. You can check back to Chapter 2: How to Classify Foods Using TCM, and here are some key ones, many of which are also antibacterial:

- cranberries are the most recognized food to treat UTIs—if you get a cranberry juice, make sure it doesn't have added sugar
- blueberries may also be helpful
- anise, basil, cilantro/coriander, cinnamon, clove, dill, nutmeg, oregano, parsley, peppermint, rosemary, sage
- alfalfa, celery, fennel, turnips
- onions, chives, scallions/spring onions, leek (cousins of each other from the allium family)
- amaranth, barley, and rye are bitter grains that can help to drain Dampness
- foods that are also used as Chinese herbs to drain Dampness include Job's tears (also known as Chinese pearl barley, *yi yi ren*) and adzuki beans (*chi xiao dou*)
- fermented foods rich in good bacteria, including yogurt, kefir, sauerkraut, and kombucha, especially if you take antibiotics.

The most important nutrition tip is to make sure to drink plenty of water.

Job's Tears Tea

Job's tears, also known as coix seeds and *hato mugi*, are sometimes called pearl barley, but they are not barley. They are, however, a commonly used Chinese herb called *yi yi ren* which is used to strengthen the Spleen, reduce Dampness, and treat Damp-Heat. By doing so, it may support digestion, treat diarrhea, and help with urinary tract infections.

- ½ cup Job's tears
- 6 cups water
- 1–2 tsp honey
- Juice of 1 lemon

Rinse Job's tears and drain well. Add water and Job's tears to a deep pot and bring to a boil. Reduce heat and simmer for 30–45 minutes. Add honey to taste. If you're drinking it hot, squeeze in the lemon juice and enjoy. If you're drinking it cool, let it cool before adding in lemon so that you don't cook off the vitamin C.

Varicose Veins and Spider Veins

One common health complaint I hear from patients comes in the form of "Oh, it's not my main health issue, but can you also help with my varicose/spider veins?" Varicose veins look like bulging, twisted ropes, purple or blue in color. They can occur in any vein, but most commonly affect the ones in the legs because blood needs to travel against gravity all the way back to the heart. The body does this using a few mechanisms. Muscle contractions in the legs pump blood through elastic veins, while a series of valves within the veins open for the blood to flow toward the heart and close to stop blood from flowing backward.

For many, the cosmetic unsightliness of varicose veins is enough of a problem; for others, that's a minor inconvenience next to the other symptoms that can arise, including a feeling in the legs of aching, tiredness, heaviness, cramping, throbbing, restlessness, tingling, or itchiness. Lasting discoloration around the veins can occur, along with the development of dry, itchy venous eczema. Worsening swelling should not be ignored because long-term fluid buildup in the tissues can cause ulcers, while poor circulation may also increase the risk of deep vein thrombosis (DVT), which can result in a pulmonary embolism (blood clot blocking a major blood vessel in the lungs).

Aging causes wear and tear on the valves and a loss of vein elasticity, allowing the blood to pool more and create varicosity. Women get hit harder in this category (not fair!) because hormonal changes (premenstrual, pregnancy, and menopause), as well as birth control pills and hormone replacement medications, tend to relax the vein walls. Hormones—ugh.

While another common cause is heredity (another thing you can blame your parents for!), there are some risk factors you can influence. Keep a healthy weight to prevent added pressure on the veins, and avoid sitting or standing still for too long. While experts say that sitting with crossed legs doesn't cause varicose veins, if you have varicose veins already, it may further aggravate circulation, as can wearing high heels and clothing that is tight around the waist, groin, and thighs. Conversely, wearing compression stockings can help move the blood from the feet, ankles, and calves back up toward the heart.

Spider veins are basically the same as varicose veins, but are milder, showing up as smaller red, blue, or purple twisting blood vessels. They most often show up on the legs and face. Prolonged or excessive dilation of the blood vessels in the face, as caused by too much sun exposure, excessive alcohol consumption, extreme heat, and rosacea can all cause spider veins on the face.

Of course, the TCM diagnosis varies from person to person, depending on their constitution and symptoms. Commonly, however, varicose and spider veins are caused by a weakness in the Spleen system and stagnation in the TCM version of Blood. The Spleen/Earth system regulates the muscles and connective tissue. It also helps keep the blood in the blood vessels, while helping to lift the falling (upward movement). As symptoms progress and the tissue appears purplish, pain increases, and dry eczema, ulcers, or clots occur, Blood stagnation becomes more apparent as a diagnosis.

By now it should come as no surprise that foods that aggravate inflammation—processed foods, too much sugar, trans fats, caffeine, and alcohol—are not helpful in preventing, managing, or treating varicose veins.

Foods that may help include ones that support the TCM Spleen, move blood, and decrease inflammation.

- Sweet potatoes, yams, beets/beetroot, pumpkin, and squash are all vegetables that support the TCM Spleen and are also rich in fiber and antioxidants.
- Dark leafy greens (no surprise!) are a good idea, as they are rich in vitamin E, reducing the risk for the formation of dangerous blood clots.
- Other foods rich in vitamin E include sunflower seeds, avocados, olives, and nuts.
- Citrus fruits (include some of the rind), blueberries, bilberries, blackberries, strawberries, cranberries, and cherries support the TCM

Spleen with their sweet flavor. They are also rich in bioflavonoids and vitamin C that can help strengthen the valves of the veins and the walls of the veins themselves.

- Other foods rich in bioflavonoids and vitamin C include mango, papaya, pineapple, guava, kiwifruit, red peppers, Brussels sprouts, broccoli, and red cabbage.
- Buckwheat is one of the best food sources of rutin, a bioflavonoid that helps support vascular health.
- Ginger is a great natural anti-inflammatory, and one of the top foods for supporting Spleen health.
- Fatty fish, including wild salmon, sardines, herring, mackerel, cod, and halibut, are rich in anti-inflammatory omega-3 fatty acids.
- Fiber foods like legumes, grains, vegetables, fruit, and seeds are important, as they help improve cardiovascular health and prevent constipation, which can cause bloating and straining that increases pressure on the veins in the abdomen and legs.
- Foods that help to move the blood include garlic, onion, and rosemary.
- Note that cayenne and hot spicy foods also move the blood, but be mindful if you have a lot of Heat signs like redness and dryness.

Buckwheat Milk

You've heard of soy, almond, oat, hemp, coconut, rice, and cashew milk. You may even have heard of flax, hazelnut, potato, and pea milk. But there's more! Non-dairy milks can be made from a wide range of grains, legumes, nuts, and seeds—including buckwheat. Despite its name, buckwheat has nothing to do with wheat. It's not even a grain. And it does not contain gluten. Buckwheat is a seed that, like quinoa, cooks like a grain and is rich in amino acids. As one of the best sources of rutin, a bioflavonoid that strengthens and increases the flexibility of blood vessels, buckwheat can help reduce varicose veins, spider veins, and hemorrhoids, and reduce easy bruising. Plus, it has a lovely nutty flavor that can be had plain or enhanced with vanilla, cinnamon, or other flavors.

For this recipe, you can opt to skip part 1 below, but you'll get best results by soaking your buckwheat overnight or for at least eight hours.

Part 1 (Overnight Soak)

- ½ cup raw buckwheat groats
- 2 tsp apple cider vinegar

In a large jar, combine the buckwheat and apple cider vinegar. Cover the seeds entirely with warm water, lid the jar, and let it soak for at least eight hours. Then drain and rinse the buckwheat for the next steps.

Part 2 (Make the Milk)

- ½ cup buckwheat groats (your soaked, drained, and rinsed ones *or* raw or lightly toasted ones)
- 1½–2 cups water
- Pinch of sea or Himalayan salt
- Large piece of cheesecloth or a nut milk bag
- Optional flavors: ½ tsp vanilla extract, ½ tsp cinnamon, 1 tsp cacao powder, 2 tbsp honey or maple syrup

Blend the buckwheat groats and water on high in a blender until smooth.

Strain the mixture through a cheesecloth or nut milk bag, making sure to squeeze excess milk through the bag or cloth.

Pour the filtered milk back into the blender and add salt and your flavors. Blend again until thoroughly mixed.

Pour into a container that can be lidded, as you'll need to shake this before each pour, as it will start to separate. Keep it in the fridge and enjoy for up to four days.

Five Elements Quiz— What Am I?

Many of us enjoy learning a bit more about ourselves and others, and how we interface based on our personality differences. Perhaps there's someone you live with who always jumps passionately on projects but fails to complete them before diving onto the next, while you are a steady plodder, frustrated with the unfinished mess. Or maybe you love the process of free-flow creativity, while your boss is constantly on you to keep to a tight schedule and structure.

"Five elements" is one aspect of TCM that offers a diagnostic approach. By answering a series of questions, such as those in Table 15, you can find out which element or elements you are most strongly associated with.

The five categories are based on TCM's five elements: Water, Wood, Fire, Earth, and Metal.

Determine Your Element(s)

By answering the following questions, you can get an idea about your areas of strengths as well as challenges, and based on that, learn things you can do to improve your health.

Do your best to answer these questions honestly. Of course, over your lifetime, your answers to these questions will change, so place emphasis on the past two years. For each line, score how true the statement is for you based on the following:

- Not true = 0 points
- Rarely/mildly true = 1 point
- Sometimes/moderately true = 2 points
- Often/strongly true = 3 points.

Place your rating number in the left column, next to each symptom or description.

Once you have finished answering each line with a number, tally up the numbers *for each* of A, B, C, D, and E. For example, if you often get headaches at the top of your head, you will rate the first symptom below as 3. If you never get frontal headaches, sometimes clench your jaw, and have mild hair loss, you will put "0" in the second line, "2" in the third line, and "1" in the fourth line. When totaling up your numbers, up to this point, you would have 0 points for "A," 1 point for "C," and 5 points for "D."

Questionnaire

Table 15: Five Elements Questionnaire

Category	Your rating	Characteristic or symptom
(D)		Headaches at the top, sides, temples, or base of the skull or behind the eyes
(A)		Frontal (forehead) headaches, often associated with worrying
(D)		Jaw pain, temporomandibular joint (TMJ) syndrome, or clenching or grinding of the teeth
(C)		Premature thinning or graying hair or hair loss
(E)		Red complexion or blush easily
(B)		Dry skin, dry hair, dry throat, or dry nasal passages
(B)		Dry and itchy skin rashes, hives
(D)		Oily skin
(E)		Easily overheat or perspire easily
(B)		Lack of perspiration even when hot or skin that is sensitive
(D)		Dizziness, light-headedness, or vertigo
(D)		Blurry vision, visual floaters, sensitivity to light, or eye disease
(D)		Red or dry eyes
(C)		Dark circles under or around eyes
(B)		Nasal or sinus congestion, runny nose, sinusitis, or sinus infections
(B)		Poor or overly sensitive sense of smell
(C)		Chronic low ringing or buzzing in the ears (tinnitus)
(C)		Poor hearing

(C)		Tooth problems: multiple cavities, weak teeth, or tooth sensitivity
(E)		Canker sores in the mouth or on the tongue
(A)		Swollen, sore, or bleeding gums
(E)		Stuttering or talking too fast
(D)		Tension or pain in neck and across shoulders
(E)		Tightness in the chest
(B)		Phlegm or congestion in the chest or throat
(E)		Racing or skipping heartbeat (or sensation of it), palpitations
(E)		Heart or blood vessel disease or issues
(B)		Asthma, chronic obstructive pulmonary disease (COPD), or other respiratory disease
(B)		Shortness of breath, find it hard to blow out candles, or fatigue with wheezing
(B)		Frequent sneezing or chronic cough
(B)		Food, chemical, and environmental sensitivities or allergies
(B)		Frequent colds or slow recovery from colds and other infections
(A)		Stomach pain, acid reflux/heartburn, indigestion, nausea, or vomiting
(A)		Bloating, gas, lower abdominal cramping or pain, slow digestion, loose stools
(A)		Excessive or poor appetite
(A)		Diabetes, metabolic syndrome, or poorly managed blood sugars
(E)		Preference for cold drinks or food
(A)		Strong like or dislike of sweet foods or starchy carbohydrates
(E)		Strong like or dislike of bitter foods
(B)		Strong like or dislike of spicy (e.g., hot peppers, cayenne) or pungent (e.g., garlic, onions) foods
(D)		Strong like or dislike of sour food
(C)		Strong like or dislike of salty food
(A)		Find it hard to either gain or lose weight

cont.

Category	Your rating	Characteristic or symptom
(D)		Pain or discomfort in the ribs, breast pain or tenderness, pain in the groin or genitals
(D)		Liver or gallbladder issues: liver cirrhosis, hepatitis, gallstones, or problems digesting fats
(B)		Constipation, hard-to-pass stools, or irregular bowel movements
(B)		Colitis, diverticulitis, diverticulosis, Crohn's, or other intestinal disease
(D)		Hernia, pain at the side of the body, or sciatica
(C)		Issues with prostate, testes, ovaries, uterus, or cervix
(C)		Urinary issues: difficulty, painful, frequent, slow, dribbling, or incontinence
(C)		Low libido, difficulties with intercourse, or infertility
(D)		Muscle cramps, restless legs, menstrual cramps, or premenstrual symptoms (PMS)
(A)		Bruising easily or heavy menstrual bleeding
(C)		Low back pain, knee pain, ankle pain, or foot pain
(C)		Puffiness, water retention, or edema in the lower legs and ankles
(E)		Varicose veins, spider veins, or issues with blood clots or poor circulation
(A)		Sinking or dropping sensation of any organ
(D)		Tremors, shaking, or tics
(C)		Osteoporosis or osteopenia
(D)		Nails split, peel, or break easily
(A)		Lumps, cysts, or abnormal bumps that are filled with fluid, mucus, hair, or oil
(E)		Symptoms that cause burning or heat sensation or that show redness
(B)		Sensitivity to changes in temperature or other environmental changes
(E)		Easily startled, feeling faint with excitement or worry
(A)		Challenges with shutting down mind, worrying, or overthinking
(A)		Challenges with grief, sadness, or letting go
(D)		Challenges with irritability, frustration, or anger

(E)		Challenges with overexcitement, nervousness, or mood swings
(C)		Challenges with fear or phobias
(E)		Vivid dreams, dream-disturbed sleep, or nightmares
(A)		Foggy-headed feeling or problems concentrating
(A)		Tiredness that leaves you feeling weighted down, weak muscles
(C)		Fatigue from overwork, overactivity, or long-term stress
(E)		Restlessness, confusion, or anxiety
(C)		Poor memory or forgetfulness
(B)		"I have been called methodical, efficient, or organized"
(C)		"I have been called a trendsetter, creative, or unique"
(D)		"I have been called strong-willed, determined, and driven"
(E)		"I have been called charismatic, passionate, dramatic, or a romantic"
(A)		"I have been called dependable, accommodating, or the peacemaker"
(D)		"I am competitive"
(A)		"I am adaptable and able to mold myself to different situations"
(B)		"I like problem solving—puzzles, mysteries, and dilemmas"
(B)		"I live and expect others to live by high moral codes and standards of conduct"
(A)		"I put the needs of others before my own"
(C)		"I enjoy solitude and need to have time to myself"
(E)		"I thrive on emotional intimacy and physical contact"
(D)		"I enjoy being in charge and dislike taking orders"
(E)		"I try to enjoy the pleasures of today, and I might not plan for tomorrow"
(C)		"I am curious and have a lively imagination"

Your Tally

A . . . .   B . . . .   C . . . .   D . . . .   E . . . .

A = Earth   B = Metal   C = Water   D = Wood   E = Fire

CHAPTER 6

Foods by Element

As introduced in Chapter 1: Basics of TCM, one of the ways that TCM practitioners can make food recommendations is via the classification of the five elements: Earth, Metal, Water, Wood, and Fire. You can determine which element best fits your current physical state by completing the questionnaire in Chapter 5: Five Elements Quiz—What Am I?

You might also select foods and lifestyle recommendations from each of the elements based on the season. In fact, just knowing which season relates to which main symptoms can help you plan in advance, perhaps reducing the severity or frequency of health issues before they arise.

For example, if you have spring hay fever allergies, rather than only treating the symptoms when the flowers start pollinating and you're feeling miserable, begin addressing them at least one to two months in advance, strengthening your TCM Lungs (the main system affected by allergies—immune system, runny or stuffy nose, clogged sinuses, sneezing, skin rashes) and supporting the TCM Liver (the dominant organ of springtime) by including some of the foods listed under Metal and Wood. You'd also be wise to pay particular attention to your food and lifestyle choices in autumn, when the Metal element—which relates to the TCM Lungs and Large Intestines—is active. If you receive supportive health treatments from a TCM practitioner, get them to help you in the fall to reduce the impact of your spring allergies.

Earth—Late Summer/Seasonal Transitions

Think of a garden full of vegetables. The soil makes you feel grounded, while the veggies will nourish you. Earth people are the caregivers, the mother hens, and the peacekeepers. They can most readily adapt to a variety of situations, molding their approach and style of communication to their environment. Dependable and sympathetic, they are the go-to person when you need support or help. Relationships are key to Earth types, and they are bothered by disharmony between others, so, asked to or not, they may try to mediate the conflict. Earth people spend a lot of time thinking, ruminating, pondering, wondering, contemplating, deliberating, and cogitating over just about everything—including, perhaps, which of these words best fits the meaning of this sentence.

The stomach and pancreas/TCM Spleen are the organs most affected for Earth folk. Thus, when things go off kilter, digestive symptoms can occur, like nausea, heartburn, indigestion, bloating, belching, flatulence, abdominal or stomach pain, diarrhea, constipation, and either excessive or poor appetite. Sweet is the flavor for this category, so problems with blood sugar regulation can occur here, including diabetes, hypoglycemia (do you get "hangry"?), sweet cravings, and problems with weight management (either weight gain or loss). But it's not only tummy troubles and belly burdens that disturb Earth types. In addition to processing food and drink, the TCM Earth element is also involved in the processing of thoughts, so disruption here causes problems with concentration, poor memory (especially short-term), worry, overthinking, and anxiety. Additionally, the TCM Spleen controls the muscles, so muscle cramps, tension, sprains, strains, and weakness are sometimes Earth issues. If you find you're bruising easily or are bleeding easily, know that one of the TCM Spleen's roles is keeping blood in the blood vessels. The Spleen is also assigned the task of keeping your organs lifted, so any prolapse (dropping or descending of an organ) includes a TCM diagnosis of Spleen Qi deficiency.

Earth weakness can cause fatigue and "Damp" symptoms in the body, like foggy-headedness, feeling weighed down, bloating, diarrhea, and puffiness.

While many of us associate the idea of fire in the stomach with heartburn or indigestion, from a TCM perspective, Stomach Fire is essential. We think of the Stomach as a cooking pot, so without some fire, there is no cooking, and thus the digestive process is greatly weakened. The concept of Stomach Fire is probably most easily understood from a physiological standpoint as stomach acid. Gastric acid—composed of hydrochloric acid (HCl), potassium chloride (KCl), and sodium chloride (NaCl)—is highly acidic, with a pH of 1. Sufficient stomach acid is needed to help activate digestive enzymes, digest proteins, and kill pathogenic microorganisms. So, yes, you want to have enough Stomach Fire, just not too much.

For most Westerners, there are four seasons to a year, so how do we reconcile that there are five elements, and each one relates to a season? By allocating a fifth season, of course. It's not random, though, as I've lived in and traveled to many places that have a season distinct enough to seem to need its own designation—late summer. It is the time of switching from the Yang warming seasons to the Yin cooling seasons. In the northern hemisphere, usually starting sometime in September and lasting four to six weeks, you can still feel the warmth of summer, but you can also sense the shift into the brisker weather of fall. Of course, the other seasons also have this transition time, so Earth also relates to those transitional times between fall and winter, winter and spring, and spring and summer.

Are you sensitive to seasonal changes with the ups and downs of temperature, barometric pressure, and humidity? For some, these unsettled transitions can cause joint pain, headaches, fatigue, mood shifts, skin issues, a weakened immune system, and more.

In all these cases, supporting the Earth element can be helpful.

- Practice some self-care; you are a better caregiver when you take care of yourself.
- Get in touch with some real earth (i.e., soil, land, dirt). Do some gardening, walk barefoot outside (carefully, though), or make a mud pie (sure, why not?). If those aren't options, you could mentally picture yourself connecting to the earth.
- Spend some daily time being present. Worriers, by definition, spend too much time thinking about the future or past.
- Learn to trust your intuition sometimes, as your mind isn't always right. Does a pros and cons list always make a decision easier to make? You list a pro reason. Then find a con. Then pro, then con. Ad infinitum, it seems.
- Chew, chew, chew your food, fully use your teeth...(sung to the tune of "Row, Row, Row Your Boat").
- Speaking of singing, according to TCM, singing is good for the Earth element. Belt it out! And if you sound as "good" as me, just tell those around you that it was prescribed for your health.
- Focus on eating when eating. You may like to multitask, but your digestive system prefers you do not.
- Keep your muscles strong. That means use them.
- Watch the sweets! Put down the candy/cake/pastry/muffin/cereal/ cookie/snack bar...you know your fix. Instead, you may choose mildly sweet foods like carrots, yams, sweet potatoes, pumpkin, squash, and rice.

There are many different TCM diagnoses that have to do with the Earth element, so specifying foods becomes challenging. However, following are some general recommendations for some of the more common patterns.

The Earth element is about processing—processing food and drink, processing thoughts. We ruminate, digest, and chew over both the things we ingest and the things we think about.

Spleen Qi Deficiency

The most common symptoms of Spleen Qi deficiency are tiredness (mental and physical), muscle weakness or fatigue, bloating, gas, soft stools or diarrhea, undigested food, blood sugar imbalance, easy bruising, varicose veins, organ prolapse, excessive worry and overthinking, and problems with concentration, focus, and short-term memory.

Help your TCM Spleen become stronger by relieving some of its burdens. Choose foods that are easier to digest. That means avoiding heavy, greasy, fried, and processed foods.

- Soups, stews, and slow-cooked meals are easier to digest because they are partly broken down by the cooking process, but still contain most of their nutrients.
- Roasted vegetables, especially root vegetables (particularly in their growing season) like carrots, parsnip, potato, sweet potato, taro, turnip, and yam, are sweet-tasting without being too sugary.
- Other Spleen-supportive vegetables include cauliflower, fennel, kohlrabi, leek, pumpkin, and squash.
- Congee is one of the traditional foods of TCM to support Spleen Qi deficiency.
- Other well-cooked grains may also be easier to digest, including oats, millet, rice, and barley (noting to avoid gluten-containing grains if you are sensitive to them).
- When you are particularly weak, small amounts of some naturally sweet foods can be helpful, including molasses, honey, syrup (the real stuff only), dates, and figs.
- Animal-source foods are often very nourishing to build Qi, but they are harder to digest for some. Cooking them in a slow cooker, pressure cooker, soup, or stew can help break down the proteins and ease digestion.
- Anchovies, carp, herring, salmon, sardines, shrimp/prawn, tuna, beef, chicken, duck, goat, goose, lamb, mutton, pork, rabbit, and turkey are all choice options.
- Soaking and sprouting nuts, legumes, and grains helps with the breakdown of nutrients. Some good options here include garbanzo

beans/chickpeas, lentils, soybeans, almonds, chestnuts, hazelnuts, peanuts, and sunflower seeds.

- Include some of the mildly warming and pungent foods and spices like fennel, leek, onion, ginger, cinnamon, cardamom, and nutmeg.
- Fermented foods like miso, tempeh, sauerkraut, kombucha, and (if you are okay with dairy) yogurt contain digestion-supporting good bacteria.
- Avoid too many raw and cold foods (see the Cooling and Cold Foods section in Chapter 2), including salads, juices, smoothies, frozen foods (i.e., eaten still frozen, such as ice cream), and iced drinks.

Spleen Yang Deficiency

In addition to the symptoms above and the recommended foods, someone with Spleen Yang deficiency will have more signs of cold—feeling cold, abdominal pain, loss of appetite, watery stools that may contain undigested food, and edema (water swelling).

In addition to following most of the above recommendations, you are best to include more of the warming foods listed in the Hot and Warm Foods section in Chapter 2, and make sure to have more cooked foods than raw foods.

Limit or avoid citrus fruits, seaweeds, tofu, raw greens, tomato, banana, grapefruit, cereal grasses (wheatgrass, barley grass, etc.), and blue-green algae (spirulina, chlorella, etc.). Although these foods are generally healthy and nutrient-rich, they are not suited for this constitutional diagnosis.

Choose rice or oats for your congee and add in warming spices and foods.

Dampness

Dampness accumulation is common with Spleen Qi deficiency, and that may be obvious with symptoms of visible swelling or water accumulation. However, more commonly, it will manifest as many of the same signs as with Spleen Qi deficiency, but more significant. These include bloating, loose stools or diarrhea, and fatigue that can manifest as foggy-headedness or feeling as if weighed down. If the Dampness sits in the joints, they will feel achy, stiff, and may appear swollen. It will also show as a swollen or puffy tongue, teeth marks (scalloped appearance) at the sides of the tongue, and possibly a thick coat on the tongue. Note that thick white patches of coating on the tongue can be a sign of oral thrush (candida), which, from a TCM perspective, is diagnosed partially as Dampness.

Dampness can be trickier to remedy, as it often combines with other factors, like Heat, Cold, or Wind, and it is cloying, sticky, and tends to hang on in the body. Left unchecked, Dampness can offer a comfortable home for pathogens like viruses, yeasts, bacteria, and parasites, or it can solidify to form cysts and tumors, so it's important to limit Damp-forming foods like too much sugar, alcohol, processed foods, dairy, and greasy or fried foods.

Foods that can help reduce Dampness include pungent foods that help stimulate the clearing of Dampness by allowing the body to sweat it out. Note that many of these foods also help to kill pathogens:

- onions, scallions/spring onions
- garlic
- ginger
- basil, black pepper, cinnamon, mustard seeds, nutmeg, rosemary, saffron, thyme.

Bitter foods can be helpful to dry Dampness, and some examples include:

- artichoke
- asparagus
- broccoli, Brussels sprouts
- burdock root
- cauliflower
- celery
- chard
- kohlrabi, turnip
- bitter melon
- amaranth, barley, hops, rye
- quinoa
- chamomile, nettles, turmeric.

Excess Stomach Fire

While having Stomach Fire is key to good digestion, too much causes problems. Heartburn, nausea, vomiting, sour regurgitation, bad breath (halitosis), strong thirst, constant hunger or poor appetite, constipation, nosebleeds, and bleeding gums are all possible symptoms of the TCM diagnosis of Stomach Fire.

- As you might imagine, hot spicy foods can contribute to this pattern, so it's best to avoid them if you are struggling with these symptoms.
- Alcohol is heating, so it's also better to limit or avoid this.
- No, ice cream is not a good option to cool down Stomach Fire. Nice try, though. Instead, go for cooling (not temperature cold, but Cold in TCM nature) and easy-to-digest foods like cooked barley, buckwheat,

or millet. Check out the Cooling and Cold Foods section in Chapter 2 to read up on cooling foods, including cucumber, spinach, and green apples.

- See How to Congee in the Irritable Bowel Syndrome section in Chapter 4, as easily digested, relatively bland foods can be soothing.
- Peppermint tea may help soothe indigestion, though you should limit or avoid it if you have GERD (gastroesophageal reflux disease), as it can relax the lower esophageal sphincter that helps prevent stomach acid from moving up into the esophagus. Do not have peppermint to relieve heartburn but consider having a cup of peppermint tea before meals to improve gastric emptying.
- Although ginger is a warming herb/food, many know that ginger is a first-pick food to help soothe nausea. It is also anti-inflammatory and can aid digestion.

Stomach Qi Uprising

Also called "rebellious Stomach," this is the pattern that causes you to upchuck (see the Nausea and Vomiting section in Chapter 4 for a few more classic nicknames). Stomach Qi should always go down. When it goes up, you'd better find a toilet or container quick. Vomiting can be the best thing to save you, as in the case of poisoning, but if your Stomach often wants to lead a rebellion, then here are some tips you may want to consider.

- The most recognized food for calming nausea is ginger. Ginger is a common herb in TCM, most often found in one of two forms: fresh ginger (*sheng jiang*) and dried ginger (*gan jiang*). The latter is warmer in property. In the grocery store, fresh ginger can be purchased as the rhizome and peeled and sliced, while dried ginger is most easily purchased as ginger powder.
- See the Downward Foods section in Chapter 2 for a listing of foods that tend to direct downward. They include banana, barley, and mung bean. Mung bean is sometimes used in TCM to help detoxify as well, so it may help if vomiting is caused by food poisoning.

Food Stagnation in Stomach

While a lot of TCM diagnostic terms are hard to understand, this pattern is—at least, metaphorically—relatively clear. Gorge at a holiday meal? Get more than your money's worth at an all-you-can-eat buffet? Win an eating competition? Then, you may be suffering from food stagnation. In fact, you might be struggling with this even if you didn't overeat, but your digestive system isn't keeping up.

Food stagnation can result in a feeling of fullness, distension, stomach discomfort, indigestion, sour regurgitation, heartburn, acid reflux, belching with foul smell, passing gas, and possibly nausea, vomiting, diarrhea, or constipation. "Why, oh, why," you ask yourself, "did I eat that?"

It's also possible to have more chronic food stagnation from a long-standing poor diet or ongoing digestive weakness or illness, and the symptoms may be much less severe (but enduring) than if it's acute.

- The first step is to not overeat. In Japan, the expression *"hara hachi bu"* means eat until you are 80 percent full. If you tend to overeat because you eat too fast, do things to slow yourself down. Eat with your non-dominant hand, put your utensils down with each bite, don't use your drink to wash down food, and make sure to sit for your meals. Eating more slowly will give your body time to tell you when you are no longer hungry. Stop then instead of waiting until you're full.
- Avoid greasy, fried, processed foods, as well as too many raw and cold foods, as they are hard to digest.
- Choose easier-to-digest foods like soups, stews, and slow-cooked meals that are already partially broken down by the heating process. If you tend to have a lot of Heat signs (e.g., red face, feeling hot), you may do better with some shakes and freshly juiced foods.
- Fermented foods like sauerkraut, yogurt, kombucha, and miso are also partially broken down and contain some good bacteria (probiotics) that can help your digestive process.
- Sprouting of grains, seeds, nuts, and legumes has many benefits. It partially helps degrade anti-nutrients—elements that can inhibit the absorption of vitamins or minerals. These sprouted foods have fewer starches than their non-sprouted varieties, so they are easier on our blood sugar levels. They are also easier to digest. Note, however, that the warmth and moisture that helps with sprouting also renders them ideal for growing undesirable (i.e., make you sick) elements, like salmonella, E. coli, and listeria.
- Spices that may help include anise, caraway, cardamom, cilantro/coriander, clove, dill, fennel, fenugreek, and ginger.

Stomach Yin Deficiency

Because lack of the cooling energy of Yin results in Heat symptoms, some of the symptoms and recommendations here are the same as for Stomach Fire. Prolonged Stomach Fire can also consume the Yin energies of the Stomach, resulting in this deficiency pattern. It's possible with this pattern to have insufficient stomach acid causing symptoms that seem like too much—heartburn, acid reflux, burning sensation in the stomach or chest—because the lower esophageal sphincter (the valve that prevents stomach acid and stomach contents from moving back up into the esophagus) doesn't close properly.

Symptoms include either no appetite or a slight hunger but with no desire to actually eat; feeling of fullness; nausea, sometimes with vomiting; dull pain or slight burning sensation in the stomach; constipation with dry stools; and a dry mouth, especially in the afternoon or at night, with a desire to drink small amounts of fluid.

Follow the food recommendations in the Stomach Excess Fire section above, and make sure to consume plenty of hydrating foods. Other foods that nourish Yin include:

- millet, barley, wild rice
- black beans, kidney beans, lima beans, adzuki beans
- fish
- tofu, miso
- coconut milk
- walnuts, sesame seeds (black or regular)
- alfalfa sprouts, artichoke, asparagus, cabbage, cucumber, green beans, peas, sweet potatoes, water chestnuts, yams, zucchini/courgette
- apple, apricot, avocado, lemon, lime, mango, melon, pear, persimmon, pomegranate, watermelon
- small amounts of honey
- coconut oil, olive oil.

Cold in the Stomach

A pattern of Cold in the Stomach can occur because of an excess Cold pathogen, such as from eating too many raw and cold foods, or from a deficiency Cold pattern resulting from chronic digestive weakness and irregular dietary habits.

As you might imagine, some of the symptoms for this pattern include feeling cold and preferring warm food and drinks. Other signs include dull or severe sharp pain in the stomach area that improves with warm compresses, vomiting of clear fluid, lack of thirst, and poor appetite. For those with deficiency symptoms, bloating, loose stools, fatigue, and pale complexion are additional symptoms.

- Soups, stews, slow-cooked, roasted, and warm foods can help ease digestive stress and weakness for this pattern.

- Ginger, cardamom, cinnamon, cloves, cilantro/coriander, fennel, and nutmeg are all warming spices that can help improve digestion.
- Avoid or limit raw and cold—either by temperature or TCM energetic temperature (see Chapter 2: How to Classify Foods Using TCM)—foods.

Metal—Fall

Picture a stack of coins, neat, organized, and precise. If you were to place a quarter in the nickel pile and someone spoke up that that really bothered them, then you are likely in the company of someone with a lot of Metal in their personality. Metal types tend to be strongly opinionated perfectionists, but they are also methodical problem solvers. They hold very strong values and morals and are often willing to come forward like a knight in shining armor, using their sharp wit to protect those ideas and people they are loyal to. Metal individuals may sometimes come across as cool and calculated, but they might in fact be quite sensitive.

The most challenged organs of the Metal person are the lungs and the large intestines. Asthma, emphysema, chronic obstructive pulmonary disease (COPD), bronchitis, and pneumonia are common issues related to the lungs. The immune system is closely associated with the TCM Lungs, so Metal types are more prone to issues with catching colds or to having an overactive immune system causing autoimmune disorders like allergies, lupus, scleroderma, Sjögren's disease, rheumatoid arthritis (RA), and multiple sclerosis (MS). In TCM, the Lungs are associated with the skin, so skin problems also fit this category, including sensitive skin, eczema, psoriasis, rosacea, acne, and many other forms of dermatitis.

Intestinal disorders that may occur here include general issues with constipation or diarrhea, but also inflammatory bowel diseases like Crohn's and ulcerative colitis, as well as diverticulitis and colonic polyps. It's also common to see the emotions of grief and sadness—sometimes somewhat hidden and suppressed—come into play here.

Weakness in the Metal element can lead to breathing problems, a chronic cough, problems with the bowels, and deep sadness or issues around letting go.

Fall is the season when the Metal elements come most into play. In the fall, the trees let go of their leaves and harvest-time prepares for winter's rest. It's interesting that with the transition into fall, many of us actually accelerate our busyness, with kids returning to school and adults buckling down at work. While this is often the rhythm of our habits, we can still use this time to go a bit inward and reflect on things and thoughts we can let go of, preparing for the rebuilding of our Yin (restorative, reflective, nourishing, quiet) energies over the winter.

Metal people can benefit from the following:

- Let go of those things that are no longer of service—stuff, ideas, beliefs, habits, routines, and perhaps even people (bye-bye once best friend who pops up only when they need something or ex who is better kept as an ex). If your tendency is the opposite of holding on, and you have a hard time with commitment, work on holding on a bit longer and waiting things through instead.
- Watch for a tendency for being over-judgmental and righteous. Unless you're an *America's Got Talent* judge. *Then* you can be "judgey."
- Breathe. Obviously, you're doing this. But are you *really* breathing? Practice conscious, slow, deep breathing. Our lungs have far more capacity than most of us are using.
- Get fresh air and enjoy some activity outdoors.
- Don't smoke!
- Support your lymphatic system with some dry brushing (use a natural bristle brush to lightly brush the skin of your whole body, using long strokes, always toward the direction of the heart), rebounding (jumping on a mini trampoline—whoopee!), or alternating hot and cold in the shower.
- Drink lots of water.
- Go for a walk or move around after eating to help support healthy bowel movements.
- Mushrooms are a great Metal element food, as they support a healthy immune system. But make sure to cook them. Hate 'shrooms? No problem. Garlic, onions, and moderate amounts of other pungent foods and spices are other options.

Because different patterns of imbalance can affect the Lungs and Large Intestines, the following are some food recommendations based on some of the more common TCM diagnostic patterns for the Metal organs.

The Metal element is about "letting go"—eliminating digestive waste, expiring respiratory waste, clearing out pathogens, and releasing things that are not serving us.

Lung Qi Deficiency

Lung weakness may be congenital (born with it) or acquired through infection, illness, exposure to toxins or irritants, sadness, grief, trauma, or overexertion. Because the TCM Lungs also include the body's physical organ of lungs, weak breathing, shortness of breath, a weak cough (either dry or with a thin, watery sputum), and a weak voice are common symptoms for this pattern. The Lungs are termed "the delicate organ" by Traditional Chinese Medicine because they are the most exposed to the external world via the nose, mouth, and skin, so they are the most likely to allow entry of viruses or bacteria. Linked to the immune system, when Lung Qi is weak, we are more prone to catch colds and flus. Because the Lungs also circulate the defensive energy (*Wei Qi*) to protect the body at the surface by opening and closing the skin pores, weakness of the Lungs can cause excessive sweating, spontaneous sweating (perspiring for no reason), and an aversion to cold temperatures.

Of course, since the TCM Lungs and physical lungs are organs of respiration, according to the ancient Daoist source *Daoyin Benjing* (*The Original Classic of Guiding the Breath*), "If we want to restore purity in the Metal [Lungs and Large Intestines], we must first strive to regulate the breath." In addition, a healthy, balanced diet is key to providing the resources the Lungs need to keep the body well.

- The flavor associated with the Metal element of the Lungs and Large Intestines is pungent or spicy. Keep in mind, however, that too much pungent food can dissipate the energy of the Lungs and too much hot spicy food can irritate the Lungs and Large Intestines.
- Eat these pungent and spicy foods in moderation: anise, fennel, garlic, kohlrabi, leek, mustard greens, onions, radish, taro, turnip, hot peppers, basil, black pepper, caraway seeds, cinnamon, cilantro/coriander, clove, dill, ginger, horseradish, marjoram, mustard seeds, nutmeg, peppermint, rosemary, saffron, spearmint, thyme, white pepper, and wine.
- Other foods that support the Lungs include asparagus, cauliflower, daikon, bamboo shoots, Brussels sprouts, sprouts (clover, mung beans, radish, sunflower), almonds, walnuts, pears (see recipe for Steamed Pears for Dry Cough in the Cough section in Chapter 4), apples, and grapes.
- Include green leafy vegetables like arugula/rocket, bok choy, butterleaf lettuce, collard greens, dandelion greens, endive/chicory, escarole, kale, kohlrabi, mustard greens, parsley, radicchio, romaine

lettuce, and watercress. But limit the quantity of raw salads, which are too cold in nature, and thus can weaken Lung Qi.

- Fermented foods like sauerkraut, miso, and kombucha are also supportive.
- Well-cooked rice (congee), oats, spelt, sweet rice, brown rice, basmati rice, rye, amaranth, and millet (especially when these grains are sprouted) are also relatively easy to digest for many, and they can support weak Lungs.
- Make room to add 'shrooms to your plate. Shiitake mushrooms, maitake mushrooms, and mushrooms in general can support a healthy immune system.

Lung Yin Deficiency or Lung Dryness

Because the Lungs are "delicate" organs, they don't handle extremes well. They are like the Goldilocks of the organs—disliking too dry, disliking too damp. Dry cough or cough with sticky phlegm or a bit of blood? Dry mouth or throat? Dry skin? Then you may be struggling with Lung Yin deficiency or a possible precursor of Lung Dryness. Lung Yin deficiency is also characterized by general Yin deficiency signs of night sweats, a low-grade fever or feeling heat in the evening, malar flush (redness of the cheeks and bridge of nose), five-center heat (feeling of heat at the palms of hands, soles of feet, and center of chest), and insomnia.

- Avoid hot, spicy foods as they will contribute to burning off fluids and contribute to more dryness and Yin deficiency.
- Limit warming and pungent herbs and spices like ginger, cinnamon, cloves, cardamom, garlic, and onions.
- Keep a lid on alcohol and cigarettes, and limit your coffee intake, as all are heating.
- Include foods that are a bit cooler and moistening like melons, green leafy vegetables, cucumber, zucchini/courgette, and eggs. Check out the sections Neutral Foods and Cooling and Cold Foods in Chapter 2.
- Nuts and seeds, like almonds, pine nuts, flax seeds, hemp seeds, sunflower seeds, sesame seeds, and peanuts (actually a legume), are moistening.
- Pears are commonly employed for treating dry coughs. See the Cough section in Chapter 4 for recipes for a dry cough.
- Honey coats and soothes a dry, irritated throat. It is also antibacterial.

Invasion of the Lungs by Pathogens (Wind-Heat, Wind-Cold, Wind-Damp)

This is most commonly an acute pattern that most people know as a cold or flu. For detailed information on this, see the section on Common Cold/ Flu in Chapter 4 for food recommendations.

Damp-Phlegm Obstructing the Lungs

As you might imagine (though you may not like picturing it), this pattern is often indicated by mucus or phlegm being coughed up. If the phlegm is yellow, green, or brown, read instead the Phlegm-Heat Obstructing the Lungs section below. If the symptoms are acute and the result of a cold, also check out the Common Cold/Flu section in Chapter 4. If the phlegm is white or clear-ish, and if the cough is chronic or lingering from an otherwise resolved cold, this is the pattern to read about.

Other symptoms include difficulty with breathing, a feeling of stuffiness in the chest, and, often, an aggravation of the symptoms when lying down.

It makes sense that the main piece of advice here is to avoid foods that create phlegm and increase foods that help to break it up. While TCM has a broader view of phlegm than the general view of tangible mucus, it does also include the actual gunky stuff that you can cough up, blow out of your nose, or feel stuck in your chest. Two key categories of herbs and foods can address this physical phlegm. Expectorants decrease the thickness (viscosity) of mucus, allowing you to cough it up to expel it from the respiratory tract. Mucolytics break down the chemical bonds in the mucus, thinning it and allowing it to be removed more easily by the body. TCM also directs you to choose foods that are easy to digest, as poor digestion also leads to more Dampness and Phlegm congestion in the body.

- Dairy is commonly associated with creating more phlegm. While studies don't necessarily find the body produces more phlegm with the consumption of milk, for many it does make the phlegm thicker and may thus feel more irritating. Plus, most adults don't digest the lactose sugars from dairy, though some have developed or inherited an ability to produce more lactase enzymes, so don't have a problem.
- Limit sugar and sweets, greasy and fried foods. Although this is generally a good idea, it is particularly useful when you have too much Damp-Phlegm.
- Daikon and other radishes help to break down mucus.
- Other pungent foods like onion, scallions/spring onions, kohlrabi, leek, turnip, mustard greens, horseradish, wasabi, garlic, and fennel can also help clear the lungs of mucus.

- Include the pungent spices of cardamom, cayenne, cinnamon, ginger, basil, clove, dill, marjoram, pepper, peppermint, rosemary, and thyme.
- Mushrooms promote healthy immune function and support the Lungs.
- Stewed or steamed pears, persimmons, kumquats, or cherries are a healthy sweet choice.
- Salty flavor is said to break up masses, so may help break up resistant phlegm. Seaweeds are an easy way to add a healthy and mineral-rich source of salt. Celery, artichoke, and pickles are other options.
- Bitter flavor dries up Dampness, so you can include cooked whole grains like amaranth, barley, rye, and the grain-like seeds quinoa and buckwheat. But it is best to limit wheat.
- Bitter vegetables like asparagus, broccoli, Brussels sprouts, burdock root, cauliflower, cilantro/coriander, dandelion greens, kale, rhubarb, and Swiss chard can also be good choices.

Phlegm-Heat Obstructing the Lungs

The phlegm observed in Phlegm-Heat in the Lungs is thicker and colored yellow, green, or brown. Yellow and green phlegm is more associated with bacterial infection, so if it lingers for a while, seek medical attention. Brown phlegm is possibly the color of old blood, so it's important to have it checked out.

The food recommendations for this pattern are very similar as for Phlegm-Damp Obstructing the Lungs, so follow the suggestions for that and include more cooling foods.

- Cooling foods that also help clear phlegm include asparagus, broccoli, button mushrooms, celery, daikon, radish, Swiss chard, seaweeds, watercress, amaranth, barley, buckwheat, millet, mung beans, grapefruit, persimmon, mint, and peppermint.

Damp-Heat in the Large Intestines

All patterns affecting the Large Intestines affect the bowel movements, as elimination of stool is the main activity of the Large Intestines.

Damp-Heat in the Large Intestines causes diarrhea with a feeling of burning or heat, mucus or blood in the stool, and often strong foul-smelling stool. There may also be abdominal pain, scanty and dark urine, fever, heaviness sensation in the body, feeling of stuffiness in the chest or stomach area, and thirst without a desire to drink.

- Light and easily digested foods should be emphasized.

- Limit or avoid spicy, greasy, fried, and heavy foods.
- Cooling foods that help clear Dampness should be included, such as asparagus, bean sprouts, bok choy, broccoli, Brussels sprouts, burdock root, cabbage, celery, dandelion greens, kale, Swiss chard, and watercress.
- Choose well-cooked grains like amaranth, barley, buckwheat, millet, and rice.
- Mung beans can help, as can adzuki beans.

Heat in the Large Intestines

Constipation with dry stools is the most common symptom of this pattern. There may also be a burning sensation in the anus and in the mouth, and the urine is likely scanty and dark.

- Avoid or limit hot and warming spices and herbs like cayenne and other hot peppers, cinnamon, clove, garlic, ginger, oregano, rosemary, and thyme. Too much hot spicy food may be one reason you have this pattern.
- Avoid foods that are listed as Hot, including lamb and durian.
- Some warming foods like pumpkin, squash, and sweet rice are fine, but make sure to include more cooling foods like alfalfa, green leafy vegetables, celery, cucumber, watercress, zucchini/courgette, prunes, cantaloupe, coconut, green apple, kiwifruit, citrus fruit, and pear.
- Make sure to eat plenty of fiber in the form of vegetables, fruit, grains, and legumes. Cooked grains to include are amaranth, barley, millet, oats, oat bran, rice, and rye. Pre-soak legumes for easier digestibility, and include kidney bean, mung bean, navy bean, and soybean.
- Other foods that can help with constipation include prunes, figs, dates, artichoke, ground flax seeds, chia seeds, hemp seeds.
- Fermented foods like kefir, yogurt, sauerkraut, kombucha, miso, and tempeh are also easier to digest and supply a good source of probiotics.

Dryness of the Large Intestines

Once again, constipation with dry stools is the main symptom, but the cause may be different. While Heat in the Large Intestines may be a more acute or temporary pattern brought on by a specific situation or overindulgence, Dryness of the Large Intestines is more likely a chronic condition caused by Yin or Blood deficiency. It is most common in the elderly and in women after childbirth.

One of my TCM teachers used to describe this type of constipation as the stool being like a boat stuck in the canal with no water to float along. That was a reprieve from the other descriptions my teachers gave about the stool, as they often used food to compare its shape or consistency—a banana, rice grains, oatmeal, blueberries, and so forth.

On that note, in the hope that I haven't destroyed your appetite, here are some foods that can help promote fluids in the body and in the Large Intestines.

- Since the main symptom is constipation, you can check out the Constipation section in Chapter 4.
- Make sure to drink plenty of fluids throughout the day.
- Choose foods that contain a lot of moisture such as melons, berries, zucchini/courgette, cucumber, peaches, and grapefruit.
- If you tend toward a lot of dryness symptoms, include Yin-nourishing foods like alfalfa sprouts, artichoke, asparagus, cabbage, mung bean sprout, pea, potato, spinach, sweet potato, tomato, watercress, yam, zucchini/courgette, avocado, banana, mango, pear, persimmon, pomegranate, watermelon, barley, millet, adzuki beans, black beans, kidney beans, lima beans, mung beans, soybeans (and their products of tofu, soybean sprouts, tempeh, and miso), sesame seeds, walnuts, eggs, fish (all kinds, but especially clams, oysters, and sardines), seaweed, coconut milk and water, and honey.
- If you also suffer from dizziness, low blood pressure, anemia, blurred vision, and pale lips or fingernails, include Blood-tonifying foods like beets/beetroot, broccoli, dandelion, fennel, leafy greens (especially dark ones like chard, kale, parsley, and spinach), red cabbage, tomato, apricot, blackberry, cherry, dark grapes, date, fig, longan, plum, raspberry, strawberry, amaranth, barley, oats, sweet rice (also called glutinous rice or sticky rice), wheat, adzuki beans, black soybeans, kidney beans, almonds, black sesame seeds, sunflower seeds, most animal-source foods (including beef, bone broth, bone marrow, crab, cuttlefish, duck, eggs, fish, liver, mussel, octopus, poultry, squid), seaweed, nettles, and molasses.

Water—Winter

Imagine a river weaving its way around and through a dense rainforest. Water-type people are determined and powerful, but also secretive and introverted. You may not always see their power and their might, but water can wear down rock. Despite this, they tend to have several fears. With their ability to be self-reflective, curious, and comfortably spend time on their own, they are often great creatives. For this reason, they are sometimes poorly understood because they seem mysterious or even eccentric, but they often don't mind that title—they may like being an enigma and thrive on being different.

The Water element organs are the Kidneys and Urinary Bladder, so common symptoms include frequent urinary tract infections, cystitis, bladder or kidney stones, incontinence, and overactive bladder. Prostate issues, low libido, and infertility are other possible Water issues. Because teeth, bones, and joints fit this category, tooth issues, osteoporosis, osteopenia, bone pain, arthritis, joint pain, and particularly low back, knee, ankle, or foot pain are potential problems. The sense organ connected to Water is the ears, so signs include frequent ear infections, hearing problems, and tinnitus (ringing in the ears). Other physical symptoms include poor long-term memory, swelling, edema, hair loss or thinning, adrenal issues, and dark circles under the eyes.

When the Water element is weak, low back or joint pain, urinary tract issues, and adrenal fatigue may occur, along with an increase in fear and anxiety that can cause a person to feel isolated.

Water people can benefit from the following:

- Work on balancing a healthy dose of fear with trusting that you'll be okay. While avoiding poisonous snakes, jumping out of an airplane without a parachute, and mystery food in the fridge is good survival planning, it's important to sometimes take a leap of faith.
- Avoid becoming too isolated. If you're home but your neighbors think you've gone on holiday because you haven't been out for days to collect your mail or newspaper, if your friend passes out from shock when you agree to go out to a party with them, or if your nickname is "The Hermit," then you need to get out more.
- Limit news and media, especially before bedtime. Bad news often sticks with us more than good, and that can become overwhelming. Consider an occasional "news fast," where you avoid it and other bad news places like the comments section of online articles and social media posts.
- Drink plenty of clean water.
- Do weight-bearing exercise to strengthen your bones.
- Don't listen to loud music with headphones and protect your hearing at concerts and Earls restaurants (why do they play their music so loud?).
- Get enough sleep and find ways to calm your nervous system when you get overwhelmed, fearful, anxious, or stressed.
- Watch your salt intake. Yes, you love it, but limit your consumption.

If you have tendonitis from using the saltshaker, you have been going way overboard.

- Satiate your salt cravings with a bit of seaweed—salty, but full of a variety of minerals too.
- Eat foods from the Water—Winter section, including nuts and seeds, soups, fish, and watery foods like melons.

While we are all born with certain constitutional strengths and weaknesses, and though all our energies tend to decline with aging, the TCM Kidneys are most closely connected to our genetic nature and to aging. Thus, those with hereditary diseases and anyone working to temper the decaying effects of time may look to bolster the Kidneys.

Some of the common patterns of imbalance for the Water element are listed here, along with some nutritional recommendations.

While all the elements are connected to birth and the process of aging, the Water element is most about what you are born with—your constitution and genetics—and how you preserve your Qi—whether you get enough restorative time and don't overstress your adrenals.

Kidney Qi Deficiency

Symptoms of Kidney Qi deficiency include urinary issues, prostate concerns, reproductive organ problems, infertility, poor memory, and weakness or soreness of the low back, knees, and ankles. Because the adrenal glands sit on top of the kidney organs, anxiety, fatigue, and salt cravings are shared symptoms for adrenal fatigue and Kidney Qi deficiency. The Kidneys' association with the ears and bones means that deficiency in this organ system can result in hearing or other ear issues and bone and joint weakness.

Sufficient Kidney Qi is also needed to help grasp Lung Qi during inspiration, meaning that weakness in Kidney Qi can result in shortness of breath and difficulty with breathing in deeply. So, while those with asthma should look to support their lungs, they may also benefit from boosting their Kidney Qi.

Having enough Kidney Qi is obviously very important, so how do we support it? Check out the shape of the kidneys. They look like beans. So guess what food might be helpful for them, according to TCM? You got it...

- Beans! Choose from all types of beans, from adzuki, black, and cannellini to kidney beans themselves. Make sure to soak them for easier digestibility.

- Other types of legumes, including lentils, peas (green, snow, snap, black-eyed), and peanuts, also support the Kidneys.

- Just as beans are the starting point for growing a plant, so too are nuts and seeds, and they too support Kidney Qi. Almonds, Brazil nuts, cashews, hazelnuts, macadamia nuts, pecans, pine nuts, pistachios, walnuts, chia seeds, flax seeds, hemp seeds, pumpkin seeds, sesame seeds, and sunflower seeds are good sources of protein, good fats, and fiber. Many of them can be soaked and sprouted for easier digestion.

- The Kidneys are the roots for our starting energy, and root vegetables are helpful to support us in this manner, according to TCM. Include root veggies like beets/beetroot, carrots, parsnip, potato, rutabaga/swede, sweet potatoes, turnips, and yams.

- Just as the previous foods are the starting point for plants, eggs are the starting point for the growth of animals, so chicken, duck, and other animal eggs also support Kidney Qi.

- Bone broth is part of a nose-to-tail use of animals reared for their meat, and it is rich in minerals and amino acids in the form of proteins like collagen.

- Seaweeds, including nori, arame, kombu, hijiki, dulse, and wakame, offer a wide array of minerals, amino acids, protective antioxidants, and fiber. They also provide polysaccharides that feed the good bacteria in your gut. Because they are a rich source of iodine and tyrosine, consumption of seaweeds may help boost thyroid function, but be mindful not to overdo them.

- The natural saltiness of seafood like abalone, anchovy, clam, crab, cuttlefish, lobster, mussel, octopus, oyster, sardine, scallop, sea cucumber, and squid can be useful here.

- Pork and duck are salty meats that can support Kidney Qi.

Kidney Yang Deficiency

Yang warms the body, stimulates action, and supports the growth of Yin. Kidney Yang deficiency results in symptoms of feeling cold and an aversion to cold, lethargy, apathy, pain, or weakness with a feeling of cold in the low back or knees, and loose or weak teeth. Because Yang energy is needed to both hold and circulate the fluids of the body, weakness here can cause issues with urination (incontinence, frequent and copious urination, or reduced urination) and edema. Since the TCM Kidneys are associated with reproductive function, low Kidney Yang can also result in low sex drive, impotence, and infertility.

Now, here's another area where TCM can get hard to understand for those not yet indoctrinated, but just take it at faith for now. Kidney Yang is required to "warm the Spleen," so when it is weak, a common symptom is "cock's crow diarrhea." This is when a person regularly has diarrhea in the early morning. If you get that, then you're like, "Oh, it has a name." If you don't, then you might be thinking, "That's a thing?"

To support Kidney Yang, many of the Kidney Qi-supporting foods listed above are helpful, though some of them are too cooling. The focus should be on including foods that are warming to boost Yang function.

- Eat mostly cooked, warm foods while limiting raw and cold foods.
- Soups, stews, slow-cooked, baked, and roasted foods are warm in nature.
- From the list for boosting Kidney Qi, limit the cooling foods—seaweeds, clam, crab, octopus, lima beans, mung beans, and tofu—but otherwise enjoy the other foods.
- Warm nature seafoods include anchovy, eel, lobster, mussel, salmon, shrimp/prawn, and trout.
- Nuts and seeds that are warming (the others are mostly neutral) are chestnuts, pine nuts, pistachios, pumpkin seeds, sunflower seeds, and walnuts.
- Your best bet for a legume that has a warming nature is black bean.
- Include warming spices like basil, cardamom, cinnamon, clove, fennel, fenugreek, garlic, ginger, nutmeg, rosemary, sage, savory, star anise, and thyme.
- Most root vegetables are warm or neutral in nature, so they can be emphasized.
- Fennel bulb, kale, leek, onion, bell pepper, pumpkin, scallions/spring onions, and winter squash are all warming vegetables.
- For fruit, blackberry, cherry, date, guava, kumquat, longan, lychee/litchi, quince, raspberry, and umeboshi plum are all on the warm side.
- Warm grains include oat, quinoa, and spelt.
- Keep in mind that not all your foods should be warm or hot, as this can tilt the balance in the opposite direction. Instead, just have more warming foods than cooling as a general principle.

Kidney Yin Deficiency (and Kidney Yin Deficiency Heat)

Kidney Yin cools and moistens the body, providing calming and nourishing energy, while supporting the development of Yang. Kidney Yin deficiency leads to symptoms of dryness and, like all deficiency syndromes, weakness. When the Kidney Yin is frail, it fails to cool the body sufficiently, leading to heat signs like hot flashes, night sweats, afternoon fever, hot palms or soles, and malar flush (redness of the higher part of the cheeks). This heat also leads to constipation, dark urine, and a tendency to be thirsty.

Just like the other forms of Kidney deficiency, Kidney Yin deficiency also causes sore low back and knees. Additionally, it can result in tinnitus (ringing in the ears), dizziness, vertigo, poor memory, and sexual dysfunctions like premature ejaculation and nocturnal emission.

The solution, of course, is to support the rebuilding of the Kidney's Yin energy. One might think that if it is recommended to eat warm, cooked foods to build Yang, then eating cool, raw foods is the best answer to increasing Yin. This isn't necessarily the case, as TCM generally still suggests avoiding eating too many cold and raw foods, as they can be hard to digest, particularly when the body is weak. Instead, TCM principles guide you toward avoiding too many hot, spicy, drying foods like hot peppers, coffee, alcohol, red wine, cloves, cinnamon, and lamb, and eating generally moistening and cooling foods.

- From the legumes and beans category, all are good, but black beans and tempeh are on the warmer side, so wouldn't sit at the top of the list to support Kidney Yin. Lima beans, mung beans, yellow soybeans, and tofu are cooling options if the Yin deficiency has led to hot flashes or other feelings of heat.
- All the seaweeds are cooling or cold.
- Nuts and seeds are helpful for supporting the Kidneys, but most of them are warm or neutral in nature. Neutral temperature ones include almonds, cashews, flax seeds, hazelnuts, hemp seeds, and poppy seeds.
- Suitable seafoods for Kidney Yin building include clam, cuttlefish, mussel, oyster, perch, scallop, and squid.
- Choosing fruits that are juicy or soft can help with the moistening effects of Yin, so enjoy apricot, avocado, banana, blackcurrant, blueberry, grapefruit, kiwifruit, lemon, lime, melon (cantaloupe, watermelon), orange, pear, persimmon, plum, strawberry, and tangerine.
- You can't easily go wrong with eating lots of vegetables, but particularly supportive ones for Kidney Yin include alfalfa sprouts, asparagus, celery, potato, string bean, sweet potato, and yam.
- Egg can support Kidney Yin, as can goat milk and cheese.
- Kamut, millet, and wheat are good grain options.
- Since most culinary herbs and spices are pungent or bitter in flavor, they tend to be drying, and many of them are warm, but that doesn't mean you can't use them. Continue to use these herbs to flavor your

foods, as you aren't likely to need too much. Cooler spices include marjoram, mint, and peppermint.

- Nettles are a good cooling herb to support Kidney Yin and Jing, so pick some to make a tea.

Kidney Jing Deficiency

While many have heard of Qi and understand it basically as energy, fewer have heard of Jing. Jing has often been translated as essence. It is said to form the material basis of the body, carry our genetic information (DNA), and support our growth and development. It is involved in the production of semen, the uterine lining and eggs, and Marrow (TCM's version of Marrow produces the bone marrow, brain, and spinal cord).

Prenatal Jing is what is passed from parents to fetus, and that nourishes the fetus during pregnancy, determining the basic constitution. It is stored in the Kidneys, and this form of Jing cannot be added to after birth; its depletion can only be slowed. After birth, Postnatal Jing is taken from the food and drink we consume and the air we breathe, and it helps support and supplement the Prenatal Jing.

Symptoms of Kidney Jing deficiency in children include problems like slow or incomplete physical or mental development. Because Jing depletes over time—sped up by overexertion, stress, sexual intemperance, substance abuse, and poor diet—aging will eventually cause Kidney Jing deficiency with symptoms of weak or brittle bones, hair graying and/or loss, poor memory, dementia, deafness, low sex drive, and infertility.

Put more colloquially, if you are looking for the fountain of youth, the closest you'll likely get is finding ways to nourish Jing. It's not sexy, but living a moderate life is one way to save your cells. Practicing qigong, tai chi, yoga, meditation, breathing exercises, or other similar routines also tops up the tank, while certain nutrient-dense foods can serve to protect, preserve, and nourish Jing.

- Foods that support the Kidneys in general, but especially the Kidney Yin, support Kidney Jing.
- Bone broth and bone marrow, fish and meat stock, organ meats (in particular, kidneys and liver), oysters, mussels, raw milk (unfortunately, not pasteurized milk), and eggs are suitable options.
- Not to worry, vegans and vegetarians, because algae (spirulina, chlorella, dulse, kombu/kelp, nori, wakame, and arame), sesame seeds, and walnuts (they look a bit like brains!) are also good choices.

Damp-Heat in the Urinary Bladder

Have you ever felt the burning, painful, urgent sensation of a urinary tract infection (UTI)? Then, you've likely had Damp-Heat in the bladder. The urine may be difficult to pass, dark in color, or cloudy. It may also contain stones that have built because of Dampness congealing. Because UTIs are almost synonymous with this pattern, flip to the description for what foods to eat in the Urinary Tract Infection (UTI) section in Chapter 4.

Damp-Cold in the Urinary Bladder

If there is cloudy, frequent, urgent, or difficult urination and a heavy sensation in the lower abdomen or pelvis, but no burning or heat signs, Damp-Cold in the bladder may be the TCM diagnosis. This can be seen with chronic non-bacterial prostatitis, interstitial cystitis, and overactive bladder. Because this is a condition of obstruction—Dampness and Cold stuck in the bladder—draining Dampness with neutral or warm foods can be helpful:

- rye, sorghum
- capers, cornsilk, onion, oyster mushroom, parsnip, pumpkin, radish, scallions/spring onions, squash, turnip
- cherry, grapefruit peel, lemon peel, orange peel, papaya
- black-eyed beans, fava/broad beans, garbanzo beans/chickpeas, kidney beans, lentils
- anchovy, eel, mackerel, tuna
- aniseed, basil, cardamom, cinnamon, fenugreek, garlic, horseradish, pepper, rosemary, sage.

Because Kidney Yang is needed to warm the bladder and help transform and excrete fluids, choose from the list of foods above that support Kidney Yang.

Urinary Bladder Deficiency-Cold

While this pattern sounds like Damp-Cold in the Urinary Bladder, the main differentiation is that the previous one is a pattern of stagnation (excess), while Urinary Bladder deficiency-Cold is mostly about Kidney Yang insufficiency (deficiency).

Symptoms include urinary incontinence, dribbling, and frequent, copious, pale-colored urine. It is also often accompanied by sore lower back and many of the Kidney Yang deficiency symptoms.

Food recommendations are essentially the same as for tonifying Kidney Yang. I swear it's not a cop-out to let me move on to the next section.

Wood—Spring

Visualize a tree, strong and determined to grow, even on top of a rock or through cement. This is the power of the Wood element. These people are classified as type A, driven, decisive, loving challenges, taking charge, and doing well under pressure. They can make powerful, but sometimes overwhelming, leaders. They can also be quite stubborn, hating to give up control and finding it hard to believe anyone else can do the job to their satisfaction.

Not all but some may use substances like alcohol, drugs (prescription or recreational), caffeine, and cigarettes to help them push farther or to calm their nerves, making them prone to problems with the liver and gallbladder, so they should avoid or limit their exposure to toxins. Tending to have tight muscles, they may suffer from tension headaches, grinding or clenching jaw pain, muscle pain (especially neck, head, and shoulders), and muscle twitches or cramps. Regular stretching can be helpful. A tree is strongest when it has some flexibility to move with the wind. Wood people can also suffer from digestive issues, especially when stressed. The natural element of Wind is associated with Wood, so symptoms of dizziness, vertigo, ringing in the ears, stroke, Bell's palsy, tremors, tics, and aversion to wind may occur. Additionally, the Wood element follows routine and order, like a military general keeping a tight schedule, so abnormal signs that occur with regularity (like waking every night at 2:37 a.m., or some such time) or the loss of routine (like irregular periods) signal a disruption in this element.

Conversely, when Wood is weak or stuck, indecisiveness, wishy-washiness, and depression (often with feelings of frustration, irritability, and anger) can occur.

Wood people can benefit from the following:

- Loosen your reins of control. Allow yourself to build trust. It's possible! Trust me.
- Balance strength with flexibility, both in personality and in physicality. Be like a strong, powerful tree that bends and yields appropriately so you don't break.
- Create regular de-stress routines. Serenity now!
- Stretch, especially the side body.
- Drop your shoulders away from your ears (they should not be too friendly with each other).
- Relax your jaw and your eyes.
- Make sure to protect your eyes from becoming dry and irritated, as can be caused by spending too much time at the computer or staring at your phone or from exposure to wind or other irritants. Use eye drops if you have dry eyes.

- Avoid or limit stimulants and intoxicants. This is a good idea for all, but especially for you. Sorry to be a party pooper, but your body will be thankful.
- Consider periodic cleanses, even just eating particularly cleanly, especially during the spring season.
- Eat lots of dark leafy greens and cruciferous vegetables—think foods that look like trees, including cauliflower and broccoli.
- Include fermented foods (sour taste goes to the Liver), such as kefir, yogurt, miso, tempeh, natto, kombucha, and sauerkraut.

Because the Wood element is such a strong and controlling one, some of the most common patterns of imbalance here involve how it overpowers other elements—Earth, in particular. While all the other Yin organs—Spleen, Kidneys, Lungs, Heart—suffer from Qi deficiency, the Liver doesn't. When it's weak, it's the Yin aspects of the Liver (Liver Yin deficiency and Liver Blood deficiency), not the Yang (Yang and Qi), that struggle.

Another unique aspect of the Wood element is the Gallbladder. While all the Yang organs are hollow, the Gallbladder is unique in that it isn't just a temporary passageway for "impure" substances. The stomach holds food that is yet to be useful energy. The intestines and urinary bladder are passageways and temporary storage for waste products waiting to be eliminated. The Gallbladder, on the other hand, is called a "curious organ" because it stores the pure substance bile which is made by the liver. It is both Yin and Yang. This is me geeking out on TCM. If you are not a TCM practitioner and that confused you, not to worry—just read on to find out what foods are suitable for the Liver and Gallbladder patterns.

> The Wood element is associated with control. Like a military general, it likes routine and order, but just as a tree should be strong and solid, it also needs to be flexible. Otherwise, it breaks.

Liver Qi Stagnation

While it is possibly true that the diagnosis of Liver Qi stagnation is over diagnosed, it's also a very common pattern in today's modern, impatient world. Someone with Liver Qi stagnation may find themselves often frustrated or irritated, though they may not outwardly display that. They may also struggle with depression, moodiness, or a general feeling of tension. Frequent sighing, pain or feeling of distension in the chest or ribcage, sensation of a lump in the throat ("plum pit Qi"), tension headaches, migraines, jaw pain, teeth grinding or clenching, tendonitis, cold hands and feet, and menstrual issues of irregular cycles, painful periods, breast tenderness, and PMS are other possible symptoms.

Feelings of stress, irritability, frustration, anger, and the impression of loss of control and wish for control can turn up the volume of any of these and the following pattern combinations, as it causes the Liver Qi to stagnate further.

When the Liver Qi stagnation overpowers and causes Spleen Qi deficiency (also called Liver attacking Spleen), additional symptoms include bloating, borborygmus (rumbling sound in the intestines), and diarrhea or soft stools. Check as well Spleen Qi Deficiency in the Earth—Late Summer/Seasonal Transitions section above.

If the Liver Qi stagnation instead attacks the Stomach, nausea, vomiting, epigastric (stomach) pain, belching, acid reflux, sour taste in the mouth, and indigestion are possible add-on symptoms. For this, see both Liver Qi Stagnation and Stomach Qi Uprising in the Earth—Late Summer/Seasonal Transitions section above.

Alternating diarrhea and constipation along with some of the above symptoms for Liver Qi stagnation is Liver attacking the Large Intestines. Focus on moving the Liver Qi and you can also address whichever is dominant—diarrhea or constipation—using the food cures by symptom. Or if constipation alternates with diarrhea, include foods from the Spleen Qi deficiency category, as these are generally foods that are easier to digest.

When choosing foods for addressing Liver Qi stagnation, it's important to both move Liver Qi and calm the Liver.

- Because the Liver does better with regular routines, set regular mealtimes. That might be breakfast, lunch, and dinner, or it could be more or less frequent meals, but do your best to make them around the same time of day, every day.
- Avoid or limit processed foods and intoxicants, as the liver doesn't need more work to filter out toxins when it is already stressed out.
- Ditto to sugar. The liver stores excess sugar as glycogen when signaled to do so by insulin. It then releases some of its stores back into the blood as sugar when glucagon tells it that blood sugar levels have dropped. Eating too much sugar increases sugar cravings, and the blood sugar highs and lows are like a roller coaster of work for the liver. Remember, too, that alcohol is high in sugar. So, while it might seem like a donut or glass of wine is the remedy to your stress, it's not. It's temporary, and the impact on a stressed-out liver/Liver is more trouble than it's worth. It's not the end of the world to occasionally follow cravings, but know it's not a long-term solution.

- To calm the mind and ease the Liver, try decaffeinated teas like chamomile, rooibos, mint, lemon balm (the Latin name is *Melissa officinalis*, so clearly, I think this is a good option), passionflower tea, or rose tea (so pretty if you get the little rose buds like TCM's herb *mei gui hua*).
- Green tea, though it contains caffeine, is also a good option for calming the mind and moving Liver Qi. It contains L-theanine, an amino acid that helps release chemicals in the brain that promote a feeling of alertness with calmness. If you are sensitive to caffeine, you can get decaf (though you'll also lose some of the healthy components in most commercially prepared decafs) or genmaicha (because it's a blend with roasted popped rice, it has fewer green tea leaves). You can also make your own less-caffeinated version by steeping the tea in hot water for 30–45 seconds and then dumping out that water. This is called the first pour. Add fresh hot water back in with the tea leaves and steep it again and drink. This is the second pour. You can also do a third pour.
- Leafy greens make the checklist once again. The Liver loves greens, so pick your faves and try some new ones too. Arugula/rocket, bok choy, cabbage, collard greens, chard, dandelion greens, endive/chicory, kale, mustard greens, spinach, and turnip greens are some examples. One of the reasons that these vegetables may fit this category is because they are rich in magnesium, a mineral that helps restrain a complex of amino acids in the brain that seem to play a role in anxiety. Magnesium also helps reduce muscle cramping. If you struggle with digestive weakness, steam or otherwise cook these veggies for easier processing for your body.
- Cruciferous vegetables also make the grade for a happy Liver. Some are already listed in the leafy green section above, but additional ones include broccoli, Brussels sprouts, cauliflower, daikon, kohlrabi, radish, rapini, and rutabaga/swede.
- Fruits that either move or calm the Liver include blackberry, cherry, dark grape, date, grapefruit, kumquat, lemon, lime, lychee/litchi, mulberry, orange, peach, raspberry, strawberry, and umeboshi plum.
- Unrefined complex carbohydrates (e.g., brown rice, whole-grain pasta, whole-grain bread) maximize the presence of L-tryptophan in the brain which aids in the formation of the neurotransmitter serotonin. Serotonin is required for calming the mind and promoting sound sleep. L-tryptophan is found in most foods, but other amino acids in high-protein foods compete with its use in the formation of serotonin, so carbohydrates are your best source.
- From a TCM perspective, the best grains to calm the Liver and move

Liver Qi include oats and rye. Amaranth and buckwheat are also good options here, and though they are often thought of as grains, both are actually seeds, so they are gluten-free.

- Almonds, flax seeds, pistachios, and sesame seeds are good nut and seed choices, but that doesn't mean you're limited to these ones, as the whole category is good for providing essential fatty acids, fiber, and protein.
- Try eating more fish like wild salmon, sardines, and herring, as these supply the essential fatty acids DHA and EPA, important omega-3 fatty acids that feed the brain and thus help to regulate emotions.
- Other seafood to support moving and calming Liver Qi include abalone, clam, crab, eel, mackerel, oyster, perch, squid, and whitefish.
- In the meat category, beef, pork, quail, and rabbit help nourish the Liver, but it's best not to overdo meats for those with Liver Qi stagnation.
- Aniseed, chive, cinnamon, cumin, fennel, fenugreek, garlic, juniper, licorice, oregano, pepper, saffron, and turmeric all move Liver Qi, but keep in mind they are all warming. For cooling herbs that still work on Liver Qi, you can choose marjoram and mint.
- Since the Liver's flavor is sour, vinegar is a fitting condiment to choose.

Liver Blood Stagnation

Since Qi is needed to move the Blood, Liver Qi stagnation usually happens along with Liver Blood stagnation, but if pain is present, it turns from dull aching to stabbing and fixed in location. For women, menstrual pain, clots in the menstrual blood, and irregular periods are common symptoms, and this pattern may be a sign of uterine fibroids or ovarian cysts. It may also be part of a TCM diagnosis for endometriosis.

- To move Liver Blood, it's helpful to include the foods that move Liver Qi, so incorporate the foods from that list too.
- Capers, leek, mustard leaf, onion, bell pepper, pumpkin, scallions/spring onions, winter squash, and turnip are all vegetables that help move the Blood.
- Note that most of the Blood-moving foods are also warm, so if you have Heat signs like feeling warm, hot flashes, night sweats, fever, constipation, and dryness, you will want to include cooling vegetables like eggplant/aubergine or neutral temperature ones such as kohlrabi or wood ear mushroom (black fungus).
- Fruit-wise, cherry, lemon, lime, lychee/litchi, papaya, peach, and rhubarb are wonderful (and delicious!).

- The sweet flavor of most grains and beans makes them mostly nourishing, but glutinous (sweet) rice, wheat germ, and black soybean can also help move the Blood.
- From the fish and meat categories, crab, mussel, shrimp/prawn, sturgeon, chicken, and chicken egg will help get that Blood to "move along, move along" (Star Wars geeks know the reference).
- Dig into your spice cupboard and pull out and use bay leaf, cayenne, chili, chive, cinnamon, dried ginger, hawthorn, nutmeg, saffron, and turmeric.

Liver Fire

If you know someone who goes red-faced, eyes bulging, cartoon-smoke-blowing-out-of-the-ears angry, then you've seen someone expressing some Liver Fire signs. They've likely had some long-standing anger, whether expressed or suppressed, associated with Liver Qi stagnation. Left stagnant, the Liver starts to accumulate Heat and can build into Liver Fire.

Liver Fire can also come from suppressing stress or trauma for a long time, from consuming too many toxins or processed foods, or from having prolonged Liver Yin deficiency.

Other symptoms include red face, red eyes, temporal (sides of head) headache, migraine, dizziness, tinnitus (ringing in the ears), hearing loss, bitter taste in the mouth, thirst, constipation with dry stools, dream-disturbed sleep, and insomnia.

Once again, you can choose foods that move the Liver Qi, as that is often part of the starting pattern. Then make sure to include some Fire-dousing cooling and moisturizing foods.

- Go green leafy veggies gonzo, and also include artichoke, broccoli, celery, dandelion leaf, eggplant/aubergine, plantain, tomato, water chestnut, and wood ear mushroom (black fungus).
- Seaweeds are cooling, so include a variety of them, in particular agar, kelp (kombu), and laver.
- Look to the list of fruits that have cooling energy. Ones that cool off an overheated Liver include blackcurrant, gooseberry, lemon, lime, mulberry, and plum.
- Nuts and seeds are generally neutral to warm in temperature, so though you can include them in moderation in your diet, they aren't going to be the main place to turn for putting out Liver Fire.
- On the other hand, there are some good seafood options, including clam, crab, and octopus.
- Meats tend to be warming and nourishing, so while they can be

included to nourish new Blood, they should be consumed in moderation to avoid adding more fuel to the Fire.

- Instead of coffee or alcohol, have a nice cup of mint or nettle tea. It may seem less enticing at first, but you'll feel so much better!

Liver Yang Rising

Very similar to Liver Fire, the stand-out emotional key here is big anger. I think this pattern could be a good threat from parents to their children who are misbehaving: "You had better listen to me or my Liver Yang will rise." This anger tends to be more explosive and shorter in duration, and it might culminate in shouting. If serious enough, it could lead to a stroke, lack of ability to speak, and sudden deafness. It can also cause headaches, tinnitus (ringing in the ears), dizziness, and insomnia. Because this pattern is more volatile, it is commonly treated either after the fact of a big health event or in prevention.

While the focus for treating Liver Fire is moving the Liver Qi and cooling things down, the main aims for addressing Liver Yang rising include calming the mind, sedating Liver Yang, and nourishing Liver Yin.

- In terms of food, most of the foods already listed to move Liver Qi, calm the Liver, and clear Liver Fire would also be suitable to address Liver Yang rising.
- Additionally, it can be helpful to select foods that tend to have a downward movement, including apple, banana, barley, clam, cucumber, eggplant/aubergine, grapefruit, kumquat, lettuce, mango, mung bean, peach, and spinach.

Liver Blood Deficiency

The TCM Liver's job is to store the Blood. Because it's the Spleen's duty to transform food into energy used to make Blood and then to keep the Blood in the vessels, and it's the Heart's role to move the Blood where it needs to go, when there are Liver Blood deficiency signs, it's important to check those other two systems to see who dropped the ball. If there are digestive issues like bloating or soft stools, boost Spleen Qi too (see Spleen Qi Deficiency in the Earth—Late Summer/Seasonal Transitions section above). If there are palpitations (feeling like the heart is racing or skipping a beat), anxiety, and dream-disturbed sleep, calm the Heart and nourish Heart Blood (see the Heart Blood Deficiency in the Fire—Summer section below).

Liver Blood deficiency can lead to dizziness, orthostatic hypotension (blood pressure drops quickly when standing quickly), blurred vision, visual floaters, numbness in the extremities, muscular weakness, muscle cramps and spasms, tics, tremors, insomnia, dry skin and hair, brittle nails, and light period flow or amenorrhea (no period).

- Animal-based foods are the richest nourishment for the Blood. Ones that are particularly guided to support Liver Blood include carp, cuttlefish, eel, mussel, oyster, squid, beef, pigeon, pork, quail, cheese, kefir, yogurt, and chicken eggs.
- But that doesn't mean you need to be a carnivore or even an omnivore to use foods to build your Blood. Non-meat options include adzuki beans, black beans, kidney beans, soybeans, tempeh, coconut, hazelnuts, peanuts, and sesame seeds.
- Blood-supporting vegetables include alfalfa sprout, artichoke, beet, Swiss chard, dandelion leaf, broccoli, fennel, kale, kelp (kombu), red cabbage, reishi mushroom, shiitake mushroom, spinach, sweet potato, tomato, and watercress.
- Avocado, cherry, date, dark grapes, lychee/litchi, and mulberry are fruits that go particularly to support Liver Blood. Other Blood-building fruits include apricot, blackberry, fig, longan, plum, raspberry, strawberry.
- Some grains that nourish the Blood are amaranth, barley, Job's tears (also called *yi yi ren*, coix seed, Chinese pearl barley, *hato mugi*), oat, quinoa, rice, and wheat germ.

Liver Yin Deficiency

Yin deficiency, in general, has symptoms of dryness (mouth, throat, eyes, nose, hair, skin), constipation with dry stools, and thirst with desire to drink in small sips. When Yin deficiency is prolonged or becomes more intense, it leads to Heat signs like a low-grade fever, feeling of heat (especially in the evening), night sweats, and malar (upper cheek) flush.

When it's the Liver Yin that's weak, additional symptoms can include blurred vision, dry and tired eyes, dizziness, vertigo, dull headache, and dull pain in the hypochondriac region (lower rib area).

- Because Blood is a Yin fluid, many of the foods that support Liver Blood also support Liver Yin.
- As is the case for supporting the Liver's health overall (and for health, in general), limit stimulants like coffee and sugar, intoxicants like alcohol, and processed foods. Avoid having too much cayenne, chili and other hot peppers, cinnamon, clove, garlic, ginger, horseradish, onions, and wasabi, as they are all quite warm and drying. Hot foods

like durian, lamb, and soybean oil should also be avoided. All these foods tend to heat the body and consume Yin energy.

- Emphasize foods that are moist and cooling, without choosing too many raw or cold foods, as too much cold can be hard to digest.
- Add artichoke, beet, carrot, cucumber, kelp (kombu), mung bean sprouts, parsley, spinach, squash, string bean, tomato, water chestnut, wood ear mushroom (black fungus), and zucchini/courgette to your menu planning list to support Liver Yin.
- Fruits that are particular to supporting Liver Yin include apple (especially green ones), avocado, coconut, grape, lychee/litchi, melons, mulberry, orange, peach, plum, and strawberry.
- Some grains that nourish Yin energy are barley, kamut, millet, spelt, and wheat.
- Black beans, hemp seeds, kidney beans, and peas are all nourishing to Yin. Flax seeds, lima beans, mung beans, pine nuts, sesame seeds, and soybeans are particularly good for Liver Yin.
- Liver Yin animal-based foods include abalone, clam (freshwater), crab, cuttlefish, eel, octopus, oyster, perch, squid, beef, pigeon, pork, rabbit, eggs (chicken, duck, pigeon, quail), cheese, kefir, and yogurt.
- High-quality oils like flaxseed oil, hempseed oil, grapeseed oil, olive oil, and sesame oil can all be used.

Cold Stagnation in the Liver Channel

Because the Liver channel passes through the groin area, Cold stagnation here causes a sensation of fullness, distension, pain, and contraction in the scrotum. For women, it can cause severe menstrual cramping that is relieved by the application of heat on the lower abdomen. For it to be diagnosed as a Cold pattern, there will also be signs like feeling cold, cold hands and feet, preference for warmth, and pale or slightly blue skin or nails.

It stands to reason that because the main problem here is too much cold, the counterbalance will be to add warming elements. This can be done, in part, with foods.

- Choose foods and cooking methods that are warmer in nature. Limit cold, cool nature foods and raw foods.
- Plant-based foods that are particularly warming to the Liver include Brussels sprouts, fennel bulb, kale, leek, onion, oyster mushroom, parsnip, blackberry, cherry, date, kumquat, lychee/litchi, raspberry, umeboshi plum, pine nuts, pistachios, and walnuts.
- Animal-based Liver-warming foods include eel, lobster, mussel, shrimp/prawn, beef, and venison.

- For spices and culinary herbs, some good options are aniseed, chive, cumin, fennel seed, fenugreek seed, garlic, hawthorn, juniper, oregano, rosemary, sage, and turmeric.

Liver and Gallbladder Damp-Heat

Liver and Gallbladder Damp-Heat is commonly given as a TCM diagnosis for candida overgrowth by natural healthcare providers because pathogens such as yeast and bacteria like moist and warm conditions to grow. Damp-Heat offers an ideal environment for these infections to thrive. However, be careful, as these diagnoses are not interchangeable.

This TCM pattern can cause bloating, nausea, vomiting, diarrhea or constipation, gas, odiferous (nicest way I could put it) stools, jaundice (yellow coloring of skin and eye whites), gallstones, dark yellow urine, vaginal itchiness and discharge, red swelling of the scrotum, bitter taste in the mouth, and fullness sensation in the chest, lower ribs, and under the ribcage. This pattern is also common in inflammatory skin issues like eczema, acne, and rashes that are red, swollen, and weeping or contain pus.

If you are diagnosed with this pattern and given Chinese herbs to treat it, be prepared for some very bitter-tasting herbs. Bitter and cooling foods are also good options.

- Go easy on your liver. Avoid alcohol, drugs, and processed foods.
- Also avoid greasy, fried, heavy foods as they are difficult to digest, and they contribute to Damp and Heat in the body.
- Sugar should also be limited as it feeds yeast and bacteria and stresses the liver and increases Dampness.
- Check the lists of foods in the Bitter Foods section and Cooling and Cold Foods section in Chapter 2 for foods that can drain Dampness and cool the excess Heat.
- Dark leafy greens and cruciferous vegetables top the list for foods that can help address this pattern of imbalance. They include arugula/ rocket, bok choy, broccoli, Brussels sprouts, cabbage, cauliflower, chard, collard greens, daikon, dandelion greens, endive/chicory, kale, kohlrabi, radish, spinach, turnip, and watercress.
- Other great vegetables are artichoke, beets/beetroot, burdock root (gobo), celery, chicory root, and eggplant/aubergine.
- In other words, eat lots of veggies. Steamed, roasted, slow-cooked, pressure-cooked, or in soups or stews make them generally easier to digest.
- Fruits are generally sweet, which means their sugar content can be contrary here, so keep them in limited quantities. However, better

options based on their TCM flavor and action in the body include gooseberry, lemon, lime, and rhubarb.

- When choosing grains, make sure to use the whole-grain form, not flour or processed forms. The outer layers provide the Dampness-draining effect via their bitter flavor. Best options are amaranth, barley, buckwheat, and rye.
- The smaller legumes tend to be helpful at draining Dampness, so choose cooling or neutral temperature small beans like adzuki, black-eyed pea, garbanzo beans/chickpea, kidney, lentil, mung, and soybean.
- Nuts and seeds are nourishing, and their oils are Yin supportive, but they can aggravate excess Dampness, so it's best not to overdo these if you have Damp-Heat signs.
- When it comes to meat and fish, it's best not to have too many, but some more suited to helping (or at least not worsening) address Damp-Heat in the Liver and Gallbladder include abalone, clam, crab, and quail.
- Avoid dairy altogether, as it strongly strengthens the Yin and can easily accumulate Phlegm and Dampness.
- While hot spices are best avoided, sprinkle in some marjoram and mint for their cooling properties. Nettle, purslane, and tamarind are your Damp-Heat clearing options. Now you're getting fancy!

Gallbladder Qi Deficiency

The Gallbladder is viewed as a pivot, neither fully a Yang organ (called *Fu*) nor a Yin organ (called *Zang*). For the TCM students and geeks, this is because the Gallbladder (along with the *San Jiao*/Triple Warmer) is *Shaoyang* ("little Yang"), and *Shaoyang* is the turning place between interior and exterior, between Cold and Hot, between Yin and Yang. Note that the Gallbladder channel travels along the sides of the body. One of my foundation TCM teachers used to remind us that the Gallbladder helps you choose whether to go right or left, swivel forward or backward.

This TCM organ is said to empower you to make decisions and feel courageous, while the Liver powers you to act on those decisions. If the Liver is like a military general, then the Gallbladder is like the general's advisor. While the expression of someone having a lot of gall is often said in a derogatory sense, it does mean the ability to take a strong stance. If the Gallbladder Qi is deficient, you might feel paralyzed in indecision, and lacking in initiative. If you find yourself overly self-critical, worried about telling others how you feel, lacking in assertiveness, unable to take a side, and fearful about the possible outcomes of many of your decisions, you may want to try to tonify your Gallbladder.

For those who have had their physical gallbladder removed, this doesn't necessarily mean you are Gallbladder deficient, as the physical little "g" gallbladder and the TCM big "G" Gallbladder are not one and the same. However, with both Gallbladder Qi deficiency and gallbladder removed, you may have a reduced ability to digest a lot of fat in one sitting. The gallbladder stores the bile the liver produces, and bile is needed to help with the digestion and absorption of fats and fat-soluble vitamins.

Gallbladder Qi deficiency can also result in issues along the channel pathway. These include headaches (especially at the temples, sides of head, and base of skull), tinnitus or hearing problems, and pain or weakness along the sides of the body. It can also share many of the same symptoms as for Liver Blood or Yin deficiency, including blurry vision, visual floaters, dizziness, and vertigo.

I know making choices is tough for those with Gallbladder Qi deficiency, so I'm going to make it easy when it comes to picking out some healthy foods. Because the Liver and Gallbladder are so closely connected, many of the same foods that are recommended for supporting the Liver are also listed here.

- To avoid draining the Gallbladder's Qi further, don't overtax the Liver with stimulants, intoxicants, or processed foods. Avoid excess sugar, coffee, alcohol, greasy fried foods, and overly processed packaged goods.
- I'll make it simple. Green vegetables are a go. Include leafy greens, broccoli, Brussels sprouts, asparagus, string beans, cucumber, and zucchini/courgette.
- Artichoke, beets/beetroot, carrots, celery, fennel, leek, oyster mushroom, parsnip, shiitake, sprouts, squash, water chestnuts, wood ear mushroom (black fungus), and seaweeds like kelp, laver, and wakame are also solid choices.
- Fruits you could choose include apple (especially green ones), avocado, blackberries, blackcurrants, cherries, dates, grapes, kumquat, lemon, lime, lychee/litchi, melon, mulberries, orange, peach, plum, raspberries, and strawberries.
- Include some fermented and sour foods like pickles and pickled vegetables, sauerkraut, tempeh, miso, lemons, umeboshi plums, Granny Smith apples, and vinegar.
- Grains like amaranth and rye make the cut, as does sourdough bread in small quantities, as these support the TCM Liver, but you might also include millet, brown rice, quinoa, buckwheat, and oats.
- Mung beans, lima beans, soybeans, black beans, kidney beans, peas, flax seeds, pine nuts, and sesame seeds are ones to include on your grocery store list.

- Choose lean meats, and you might also include some seafood like abalone, clam, cuttlefish, eel, mackerel, mussel, oyster, perch, shrimp/prawn, squid, and whitefish.

Fire—Summer

Feel yourself sitting near a fire. It can be warm and comforting, drawing you in closer. Or it can be unpredictable and fierce in its capacity to burn you. Fire-type people are passionate and dramatic, and their sense of humor, openness, and desire to make those around them happy means they are the charismatic life of the party whom everyone wants to meet. Intensely heart-centered, they are generally excellent speakers, firing people up with their energy and enthusiasm. If you hear someone laughing big, that person likely has a strong Fire element. Fire people are romantics, chasing pleasure and stimulation, and they usually don't like to be alone.

The most affected organs of a Fire type are the Heart and the Small Intestines. Fire types are more prone to heart attacks, heart failure, strokes, aneurysm, heartbeat irregularities, coronary heart disease, deep vein thrombosis (DVT), atherosclerosis, arteriosclerosis, palpitations, varicose veins, hemorrhoids, and all issues having to do with the cardiovascular system. Related to the small intestines, Fire individuals may also suffer from digestive issues.

Because fire is hot, those with a lot of fire in their system or personality may struggle with inflammation, red skin rashes, canker sores and other ulcerated sores, urinary tract infections, and a tendency to overheat. Limiting exposure to hot temperatures, hot foods, and hot tempers can help bring better balance.

TCM geeks joke that we have two hearts and no brain. This is because, in TCM terms, we discuss the physical heart that oxygenates and circulates blood and the emotional Heart whose primary emotion is joy, but that houses all the emotions. Yet we never mention the brain as its own entity. Instead, we allocate the different functions of the brain—organizing, processing, understanding, concentrating, remembering—to the various TCM organ systems. We simply don't talk about the three-pound mass of protein and fat you lodge in your skull. By TCM standards, it would be worse, then, to be called heartless than brainless.

Fire people know and respect the value of their hearts because they lead with their heart, though sometimes to their detriment. Emotionally, Fire folk are generally joyful and happy when things are good, but they may find themselves feeling anxious and struggling with manic behavior or insomnia when not doing well. When Fire is weak, a person can feel depressed, cold, weak, scattered, or easily startled.

The TCM Heart is called the king. If the king is weak, unbalanced, or under attack, the other systems in the body will be affected as they try to support their monarch.

Fire people can benefit from the following:

- Spend time with those you love, allow yourself to be a romantic, and experience the joys of laughter. But also seek time alone, nurturing your love of self, independence, and self-confidence.
- Limit or avoid stimulants like c-c-c-c-c-caffeine!
- Build some structure and routine in your life (e.g., meal and sleep/wake times) to counter the tendencies to become too flighty or...squirrel!...scattered.
- Smoking is not good for anyone, of course, but adding the fire of smoking to the Fire person is even worse.
- Avoid eating too many hot spicy foods (e.g., cayenne, hot peppers).
- If you have Heat signs, include cooling foods like melons, cucumber, mint, etc.
- Include eating bitter foods like dark leafy greens, artichoke, barley, and dill.
- Exercise your heart with some heart-pumping activities, though also include some calm, slow-moving exercises as well. It shouldn't all be hard core. Like a high school dance or wedding, DJs know how to mix it up between fast and slow.

Dysfunction of the Heart becomes obvious as excess (fires flaming) or deficiency (burnt out), and the former can easily lead to the latter. What might seem less obvious is how the Heart is connected with the Small Intestines in TCM, but excess Fire from the Heart can transmit to the Small Intestines which then passes it to the Urinary Bladder (see the Excess Heat in the Small Intestines section below for more on that).

With all the importance that the Heart carries, the TCM Small Intestines are often skimmed over in teachings. The role of the Small Intestines is to separate the "pure" from the "turbid." The pure part is what is absorbed and used as nutrients and energy for your cells. The turbid part goes to the Large Intestines and Urinary Bladder for elimination.

The Small Intestines assist the Heart psychically by helping with judgment, separating the clear from the turbid, filtering out the negative. When someone has a hard time distinguishing right from wrong, good from bad, part of the issue may be with dysfunction of the Small Intestines.

So, you can see how one organ not doing its job properly can affect a number of other systems. Let's see what happens when the Heart and Small Intestines go off kilter.

The Fire element is key to your ability to feel joy, or really any emotion. With its primary organ, the Heart, being the king organ, it may be the last element covered here, but it is obviously not the least!

Heart Qi Deficiency

Is your heart beating fast or unevenly, pounding away and making you pay attention to it? Palpitations are one key sign of possible Heart Qi deficiency. Other signs include fatigue, shortness of breath, spontaneous sweating, a pale face, and, sometimes, a deep crack along the midline of the tongue to the tip of the tongue. If the sensations are sudden and intense, you might need to go to the emergency department to have your heart checked or it could be an anxiety attack. If the symptoms are chronic of late and relatively mild or sporadic, and you've been checked out for physical heart issues, there are things you can do on your own to help support your Heart king.

Other Heart Qi deficiency signs include depression, feeling lackluster, anxiety, insomnia, being easily startled, and feeling confused or easily lost.

Heart Qi deficiency can occur because of long-term overexertion, constitutional weakness, or trauma. For those who wear their heart on their sleeve, it's easy to see how they can burn out and how a shocking event can deplete their Heart Qi.

While I interpret "eating clean" as meaning eating whole foods that are not overly processed and have few or no chemical additives, some think of it as cleansing, detoxifying, fasting, and purging. In TCM, if there is deficiency, we choose to nourish. So, while many with heart conditions may be instructed to do a detox or to fast, I would encourage clean eating that nourishes the body for those with Heart Qi, Yang, or Blood deficiency conditions.

- Each of the organ systems has a two-hour time of day when it is most strongly affected. The Heart's hours are 11 a.m. to 1 p.m., when the fiery sun is at its highest. Because this is when many of us eat lunch, pay particular attention to nourishing your TCM Heart at this meal.
- Don't overstimulate the Heart with things like coffee and sugar as the poor dear is already in distress if you feel this pattern fits your situation.
- If you're tired, consider green tea instead of coffee. Green tea can be

energizing while being less stimulating because it contains a compound called L-theanine. L-theanine is an amino acid that enhances your alpha brain waves, helping you feel both calm and alert. You could also choose to have a decaf version of green tea or choose white tea, which has a bit less caffeine. You can also do a second pour of your green or white tea, to reduce the amount of caffeine. That means letting your tea steep for 30–45 seconds and then pour out the hot water. Then pour in fresh hot water and steep, and drink the second pour.

- Other calming teas that can support the Heart Qi include chamomile, lavender, lemon balm, licorice, and rose (makes a very nice tea; the TCM herb is *mei gua hua*, tiny rose buds).
- Beets/beetroot and tomatoes with their lovely red colors are easy to remember as vegetables that can support your heart. Endive/chicory, lotus root, reishi mushroom, and scallions/spring onions are other vegetables that TCM categorizes as good for your TCM Heart or Small Intestines, but truly, a wide range of vegetables are heart friendly. Really, I'd be hard pressed to try to pick a vegetable that isn't somehow good for your heart. Veggies are rich in vitamin A and carotenoids, B vitamins, folate, vitamin C, magnesium, potassium, and a wide range of phytochemicals (plant chemicals) that can improve circulation, decrease oxidative damage, lower elevated blood pressure, keep cholesterol levels in check, and so much more.
- Like vegetables, fruits are also nutrient-rich, but just don't eat too many because they can be higher in sugar than many vegetables. Your best bet for fruit here includes apple, cherry, crab apple, red grapes, longan, pomegranate, strawberry, and watermelon.
- Because grains are good sources for replenishing Qi and Blood, and since whole grains are generally a bit bitter, many of them are supportive for the Heart Qi, including buckwheat, kamut, oats, quinoa, and wheat. Just make sure to have them as much as possible in their whole form and not overly processed or in quantities that are too large.
- Coconut is listed in TCM books as supporting Heart Qi and Blood, but I'd also include flax seeds, gingko, hemp seeds, pistachio, poppy seeds, and sunflower seeds.
- Adzuki beans would be the first legume I'd reach for to support Heart Qi, and you can also enjoy garbanzo beans/chickpeas, lentils, mung beans, and peas.
- While TCM would often recommend eating the organ that is deficient for you, in many places today, it would be tough to find that

in a grocery store. Instead, if you eat animal products, you could choose high-quality fish and meat, as they are nourishing to the Qi and Blood. Some believe that the type of life the animal experienced prior to being killed for consumption affects its Qi and thus the energy you will receive from it. If this is true (and even if it's not), then it would be better to choose animals raised well over ones in cramped, unhealthy, or indeed tortuous environments.

- Eggs are one common animal-source food said by TCM rankings to nourish the Heart.
- Herbs and spices you could include are borage, cayenne, chickweed, cinnamon, garlic, American ginseng, hawthorn, hops, oregano, passionflower, pepper, rosemary, safflower, saffron, sage, skullcap, and thyme.

Heart Yang Deficiency

Heart Yang deficiency causes many of the same things as Heart Qi deficiency. In fact, they are often combined. A key additional sign is feeling cold, even if there is sweating. The tongue is usually pale and swollen instead of thin.

It is often combined as well with Kidney Yang deficiency, so the lower back may be sore and there is usually swelling (edema) in the legs.

- In addition to choosing foods that support the Heart Qi, choosing warming foods will help tonify the Yang.
- You should avoid cold foods like ice cream and cold drinks, but in addition, limit your intake of raw foods, smoothies, and juices, as these too are cold in nature.
- Get your cooking game on to bring the warming nature into your foods with soups, stews, slow-cooked or pressure-cooked meals, and all the variants of cooking.
- If you're craving a salad, first, good on you! Next, make it a warm, cooked salad. It doesn't all need to be cooked, but pick and choose which of the following items you want to include, so the bulk of it is on the warmer/cooked side: steamed greens, roasted veg, steamed or baked fruit, cooked legumes, lightly pan-fried nuts or seeds, or a sprinkling of cooked meat or fish.
- Some of the warmer vegetables you can include are Brussels sprouts, kale, mustard greens, cilantro/coriander, capers, leek, onion, scallions/spring onions, fennel bulb, parsnip, winter squash, pumpkin, and bell peppers. Mushrooms are another good choice. They are usually warm or neutral in nature.
- Steaming or baking fruit warms up their nature, but some foods that

are neutral or warm include apricots, blackberries, cherries, dates, figs, grapes (best to choose red for the Heart), guava, kumquat, longan, lychee/litchi, papaya, peach, pineapple, plum, pomegranate, quince, raspberry, and umeboshi plum.

- If you're used to waking up to a cold bowl of cereal, yogurt, a smoothie, or something else cold, consider starting your day with something warm and nourishing. Conversely, if you like a stick-to-the-ribs hearty, rich breakfast and you have heart issues, you are best to tone down the bacon and sausages, but, of course, you already knew that.
- Oats, rice, rye, and spelt are neutral and warming grains. Quinoa is a warming seed that you cook like a grain, and because it's rich in omega-3 fatty acids, protein, and fiber, it's a heart-healthy choice.
- Because legumes, nuts, and seeds are particularly nourishing to the TCM Kidneys, and since Kidney Yang deficiency contributes to Heart Yang deficiency, make sure to bump up these foods. If you're not used to legumes, increase them gradually in your diet so you don't get too gassy. Black beans, fava/broad beans (I can't think of these beans without thinking of their reference in the movie *The Silence of the Lambs*), garbanzo beans/chickpeas, kidney beans, lentils, and peas are great options. Pick a seed or nut, any seed or nut—they are pretty much all neutral or warm in nature. Walnuts are particularly good at tonifying Yang energy.
- If you dig seafood, anchovy, eel, mussel, salmon, shrimp/prawn, and trout are all warming in nature.
- Meats are generally warm in nature, but make sure you choose lean options, as too many saturated fats from animal sources can up your cardiovascular risks.
- Think heart-healthy food needs to be boring? Think again. Most culinary herbs and spices are warming and flavorful. Ones that can warm the Heart or Kidney Yang include aniseed, basil, cayenne, chili, cinnamon, clove, fennel, fenugreek, garlic, ginger, hawthorn, horseradish, juniper, oregano, pepper, rosemary, sage, savory, and thyme.

Heart Blood Deficiency

Once more, many of the symptoms are similar to Heart Qi deficiency—palpitations, fatigue, and pale complexion—but the palpitations here are often more noticeable in the evening. In addition, the mental and emotional symptoms can be more pronounced and show up as insomnia, dream-disturbed sleep, anxiety, being easily startled, and having a poor memory. Because of the Blood deficiency, dizziness and more pale signs (pale lips, pale nails, pale tongue) and possibly anemia will show up.

- Because an agitated nervous system is one of the common symptoms of Heart Blood deficiency, it is also a good plan to avoid caffeine and too much sugar, as they are overstimulating. If you love your coffee, try instead some coffee-like, caffeine-free beverage options like dandelion or chicory. Decaf coffee is another option, but remember that it does contain some caffeine.

- You could also choose green tea or non-caffeinated herbal tea options as mentioned in the Heart Qi Deficiency section above.

- According to TCM food cures, dark leafy greens help tonify the Blood, and a look into why shows that they contain several nutrients that nourish the blood and support a healthy heart. Folate and vitamin C have been shown to decrease the risk of heart attack and stroke. Calcium, magnesium, and potassium help with the balance of muscle contraction and relaxation (essential for the most important muscle in your body—your heart) and maintain a healthy blood pressure. Vitamin K is key to the proper blood clotting as well as helping prevent calcification of the arteries. Iron is the main mineral people usually think of when thinking about building the blood, as it is needed for the proper formation of red blood cells that carry oxygen to all your tissues. And indeed, you'll find that meat isn't the only option; dark leafy greens are a good source of iron too.

- Other vegetables that help nourish Blood include alfalfa sprouts, artichoke, beets/beetroot, sweet potato, kelp, and reishi and shiitake mushrooms.

- Hoping that there are also some Blood-building fruit options for you? No problem. Go for apricot, avocado, cherries, dates, grapes (especially red or dark ones), longan, lychee/litchi, blackberries, strawberries, and raspberries. Mulberries and lemons are listed as ones that calm the mind.

- Grain options are aplenty too, including barley, Job's tears (yi yi ren, coix, hato mugi), oats, rice, and wheat (especially wheat germ). In fact, complex carbohydrates help maximize the presence of L-tryptophan in the brain, which aids in the formation of the neurotransmitter serotonin. Serotonin is needed to calm the mind and promote sound sleep.

- Many of the previously mentioned legumes, nuts, and seeds also build Blood. Say yes to adzuki beans, black beans, kidney beans, soybeans, tempeh, tofu, coconut, hazelnuts, peanuts, and sesame seeds.

- Because they also contain blood, many animal-source foods are also nourishing for the Blood, including carp, salmon, tuna, eel, mussel, oyster, octopus, squid, beef, chicken, duck, lamb, pork, eggs, and milk products.

- While not many culinary herbs and spices are specific for tonifying Heart Blood, you could benefit from having some nettle tea (cooling Blood tonic) and adding and eating more parsley (warming Blood tonic) to your meals. Dill and basil are also said to have a calming effect.

Heart Yin Deficiency

Blood is part of Yin, so Heart Yin deficiency has some similar signs to Heart Blood deficiency, particularly when it comes to the insomnia and anxiety. Where it is most likely to differ is that Yin deficiency may create more Heat signs like night sweats, feeling flushed, and red face and tongue, instead of paleness. There will be dryness signs like dry eyes, mouth, lips, throat, and skin.

- Don't further deplete Yin by having foods that are too warming (meaning energetically, not temperature) or drying. This means avoiding hot, spicy foods or too many diuretics like caffeine. Also limit some of the pungent foods like onions and garlic.
- While you can read above to see which foods tonify Heart Blood, also include some Yin-nourishing vegetables (some of which overlap with the Blood tonics) like alfalfa sprouts, artichoke, asparagus, mung bean sprouts, potato, tomato, yam, kelp, nori, and wakame.
- Because they are juicy, fruits are generally nourishing to the Yin and they are often cooling, helping to reduce the Heat signs that build because of the lack of Yin cooling energy. Your best picks are apples, apricot, avocado, banana, mulberries, orange, pear, persimmon, plum, raspberries, and strawberries.
- Kamut and wheat are your best grain options for nourishing Heart Yin, but if you're going for gluten-free, try millet.
- Mung beans and peas are the most supportive legumes for Heart Yin, but you could also include Yin-boosting kidney beans, lima beans, peas, soybeans, and tofu.
- Coconut milk, flax seeds, hemp seeds, and sesame seeds are all Yin tonics.
- If you want to savor some seafood, consider abalone, clam, cuttlefish, mullet (I thought that was just hockey hair), octopus, sardine, and scallop.
- If you have Heat signs, you could choose small amounts of Yin-nourishing duck, goose, pork, rabbit, cheese, milk, yogurt, and egg, but otherwise, Yin tonic meats that are warm include beef and chicken.

- Nettle is your best bet for cooling and nourishing the Kidney Yin, which helps then nourish Heart Yin.
- Also follow the calming food recommendations listed in the Heart Blood deficiency category.

Heart Fire

While Heart Fire may sound a lot like heartburn, it's not that. Once again, palpitations are a key symptom of a Heart imbalance diagnosis. Just like the Heart Blood and Yin deficiency patterns, insomnia and dream-disturbed sleep is another symptom. But this is the first Heart pattern that is excess instead of deficiency, and symptoms like agitation and impulsiveness help to differentiate it.

Because of the Heat signs, this pattern can cause feeling hot, being thirsty, and having a bitter taste in the mouth. In addition, because Fire is a more extreme form of Heat, mouth and tongue ulcers (canker sores) are commonly seen. And because Heart Fire can move to its partner organ, the Small Intestine, which then releases the Heat into the Urinary Bladder, blood in the urine or dark urine can occur.

- What food and drink things would add fuel to the fire and are best avoided or limited? Hot spices like cayenne and chili, but also warming spices like ginger, clove, cinnamon, cardamom, mustard seeds, nutmeg, oregano, and horseradish. Many meats are also warming, so best limited. Sorry to report that alcohol, especially spirits (you know that burning feeling in your throat), and coffee are warming too.
- Now for the foods that can help put out the fire. Think cooling and moist.
- Endive/chicory and lotus root are vegetables that cool Heart Fire, but you can also include a slew of other cooling veggies like alfalfa sprouts, asparagus, bamboo shoots, bok choy, broccoli, burdock root (gobo), button mushrooms, cabbage, celery, Swiss chard, cucumber, dandelion greens, lettuce, seaweeds, spinach, tomato, water chestnut, and zucchini/courgette.
- Your best bets in the fruit category to clear Heart Fire are apples, persimmon, and watermelon, but they aren't the only cooling fruits. Additional options are avocado, banana, blueberry, bilberry, cantaloupe, cranberry (especially if you have signs of a urinary tract infection), grapefruit, kiwifruit, lemon, lime, mandarin, melon, mulberry, orange, pear, pomelo, rhubarb, strawberry, and tangerine.
- Just as kamut and wheat are your best options for tonifying Heart

Yin, they are also top choices for clearing Heart Fire. But you can also choose from barley, buckwheat, Job's tears, and millet.

- Mung beans and adzuki beans are at the top of the beans list, while other legumes to choose from include kidney beans, soybeans, and tofu.
- Nuts and seeds are generally nourishing to Yin, which can help tame the excess Yang of Fire, and neutral and cooler in nature are coconut milk, flax seeds, and hemp seeds.
- Many animal-source foods are richly nourishing, tonifying Qi and Blood, but they tend not to be as likely to help clear Heat, so it's better to limit them. Of the animal-source foods, your best choices are clam, crab, octopus, quail, and egg whites.
- You know that, on a hot day, a cup of mint tea, whether hot or cold, can help you feel cooler. This is part of Food Cures 101. Other culinary herbs and spices that can clear Heat include aloe, purslane, and sage.

Phlegm Misting the Heart/Mind

When most people think of phlegm (and, of course, everyone thinks about phlegm often, right?), they think of something they can physically clear from the throat or that they can feel rattle in their chest when they're sick. But TCM has another version of phlegm, called "hidden," "invisible," or "insubstantial" Phlegm. This type of Phlegm can block (or "mist") the meridians/channels that supply the Heart and Mind, causing mental confusion, dementia, unconsciousness, dizziness, stroke, sudden sensory loss, convulsions, and some types of mental illness (bipolar, schizophrenia, obsessive-compulsive disorder).

While I would be hard pressed to suggest that any of the dietary changes recommended here will cure someone of these serious health conditions, they may help and can be used preventatively if someone is displaying early warning signs.

- Because the creation of Phlegm involves Dampness, supporting Spleen Qi and drying or draining excess Dampness is one way to help prevent this imbalance. You can do this by checking out the food recommendations in the Spleen Qi Deficiency section under Earth—Late Summer/Seasonal Transitions, as well as the Dampness section shortly after that.
- Limit Damp-producing foods like dairy, excess sweet foods, refined or overly processed foods, and greasy fried foods.
- Choose more vegetables, especially cooked ones, to make them easier to digest.

- If you eat meat, limit the quantity, especially of the richer and heavier meats like duck, lamb, bacon, and beef.
- That doesn't mean avoiding fats. It means having high-quality fats rich in omega-3s, like flaxseed oil, hemp seeds, chia seeds, buckwheat, walnuts (looks like a brain and said to be good for the brain), wild salmon, herring, mackerel, and sardine.
- Whole grains (not in flour format) that can help remove excess Dampness include amaranth, Job's tears, and rye.
- Some of the legumes can also help drain excess Damp, including adzuki beans, black-eyed beans, fava/broad beans, garbanzo beans/chickpeas, kidney beans, and lentils.

Heart Blood Stagnation

Heart Blood stagnation can be a serious problem, causing the classic signs that result in you calling an ambulance: pain in the chest that may radiate down the left arm and/or a feeling of constriction, strong pressure, or discomfort in the chest. In other words, a heart attack.

It can also closely resemble the Western diagnosis of angina pectoris, translated as chest pain. This pain is caused when heart muscle doesn't get enough blood, usually due to narrowing or blockage of arteries to the heart. Those who've been diagnosed with this condition know that it occurs usually after physical exertion, after an emotional stressor, during exposure to very hot or cold temperatures, after heavy meals, or because of smoking. It usually lasts for less than five minutes and is better after resting or taking medication (nitroglycerin).

Blood stagnation can also be identified by poor circulation to the limbs and purplish color of the lips, tongue, or nails.

Heart Blood stagnation evolves from other conditions which should also be treated. Check the sections on Heart Yang Deficiency, Heart Blood Deficiency, Heart Fire, and Liver Blood Deficiency to see which pattern best fits, and address that.

In addition, choose foods that can help move Qi and Blood.

- Blood-moving foods include eggplant/aubergine, chili, chive, onion, scallions/spring onions, leek, kohlrabi, radish, turnip, mustard leaf, hawthorn berry, peach, chestnut, chicken, egg, pepper, saffron, rose, and turmeric.
- Qi-moving foods include carrot, fennel, squash, watercress, grapefruit, plum, orange or tangerine peel, basil, caraway, cardamom, cayenne, clove, cilantro/coriander, dill seed, garlic, marjoram, peppermint, and star anise.

Excess Heat in the Small Intestines

Because the Small Intestines are part of the digestive system, too much hot, spicy food can result in Heat in the Small Intestines, which is then often transmitted to the Urinary Bladder. The consequence of this is abdominal pain and urinary issues like urine that is small in amount and dark in color, painful and burning to pass, and sometimes bloody.

Urinary tract infections (UTIs), cystitis, and interstitial cystitis are common Western diagnoses of this pattern. SIBO (small intestinal bacterial overgrowth) may also be present, but to distinguish that this is the correct TCM pattern to link it to, you need to look for other symptoms.

Because of the pairing to the Heart, stress and anxiety can cause Heat in the Small Intestines, and it can be a vicious cycle, also causing more sleep issues and mental restlessness. As one of the tissues related to the Heart is the tongue, Heat in either the Heart or the Small Intestines can result in ulcers (canker sores) on the tongue. The Heat accumulation can also cause thirst, dry or hot throat, and a flushed face.

Since the Small Intestines channels end at the ear, sudden hearing loss is a possible symptom.

- The first food tip should be obvious (read the first sentence in this pattern section): avoid hot, spicy food.
- Include some cooling foods (but not only cooling foods, as you don't want to throw the imbalance in the other direction) like alfalfa sprouts, asparagus, broccoli, cabbage, celery, cucumber, eggplant/aubergine, kelp and other seaweeds, lettuce, watercress, apple, grapefruit, lemon, pear, watermelon, barley, millet, mung beans, tofu, egg white, mint, and peppermint.
- If you have UTI symptoms, cranberry is usually a good go-to food or drink, but even though it's very tart, don't add sugar. You can get it in capsules if the taste is too intense. Bamboo shoots and cornsilk are food/herbs used in TCM to work as diuretics and help clear the UTI.
- As a cooling food that is also rich in good bacteria, yogurt is another wonderful food option.

Small Intestines Deficiency and Cold

When too much raw and cold food is consumed or when Spleen Yang is deficient, this pattern can arise. It can cause abdominal pain that feels better with warmth and pressure, borborygmus (fancy word for stomach rumbling), diarrhea, undigested food in the stool, and frequent, copious urination. Other signs of Cold include feeling cold, a preference for warm food, drink, and environment, and a pale or slightly bluish color of the tongue, skin, or nails.

SIBO may also manifest from this pattern, provided enough of the other symptoms fit the category. Many disorders of malabsorption also fit this TCM diagnosis.

- Clearly a first step is to limit or avoid raw and cold foods to allow the body to regain some warmth.
- Although raw food can be healthy, it's not for everyone, especially not all the time. For those who insist on eating raw only, choose foods listed in this book as warming, including ginger, hot peppers, durian (if you can bear the smell), fennel, leek, mustard greens, onions, pumpkin, squash, date, oats, quinoa, black beans, pumpkin seeds, walnuts, lamb, trout, cardamom, cinnamon, clove, pepper, fennel seed, and rosemary.
- Check out Spleen Yang Deficiency in the Earth—Late Summer/Seasonal Transitions section to get more details about helpful foods.

Small Intestines Qi Stagnation

Liver Qi stagnation and poor dietary choices (including even too much raw, otherwise healthy food) are common causes of Qi stagnation of the Small Intestines.

Twisting, cramping pain in the lower abdomen that may radiate to the low back, colic, abdominal distension and pain that is worse with pressure, gas, and borborygmus are common symptoms of this imbalance. Testicular pain and inguinal (groin) hernia can also occur.

If anger, frustration, and irritability are common emotions for you, then it's important to check out Liver Qi Stagnation in the Wood—Spring section here for food tips. If you eat a lot of cold, raw foods and you often feel cold, then consider the recommendations under the Small Intestines Deficiency and Cold section above.

CHAPTER 7

Modern Food

I read a lot of books on nutrition, and I've yet to find one that has recommended eating a diet rich in processed foods. When it comes to good, healthy nutrition, the emphasis is on whole foods. Real foods. Now, of course, there are many "real foods" and a seemingly unlimited number of diets telling you how to choose and prepare those foods for your optimal wellness. But this chapter is about the problems and benefits of the modern diet, and the various ways to "keep it real."

The Olden Days

"In myyyyyy day," Grandpa Simpson says on the popular TV show *The Simpsons*. He starts with a rant on some silly way that things were better when he was younger, but then rambles off on something unrelated (just like this sentence). There's often a sense that things were better in the old days, particularly by those of us above the age of 40. And, yes, some things may have been better. But some things were worse.

While it sounds romantic and wonderful to be nostalgic about food grown on our own property and made fresh from scratch every single day, the reality is that most of us simply don't have the time or space to do that. There's a reason we created "convenience foods."

Unfortunately, we've gone too far. Hydrogenated fats, artificial dyes and flavors, butylated hydroxytoluene (BHA), sodium nitrite, high-fructose corn syrup, artificial sweeteners, and more have allowed us to store food for longer and enhance flavors, but they are also associated with many health conditions and diseases.

But not all food processing is bad, and we've actually been processing our foods for a long, long time. Cooking our food with fire began approximately 1.8 million years ago. Bread came somewhere around 30,000 years ago. And because of bread, beer making started maybe around 7000 BC, made from a by-product of bread making. Next came tortillas, wine, cheese, olive oil, pickles, noodles, chocolate, mustard, and so forth. Pickling, canning, cooking, freezing, drying, smoking, fermenting, and sprouting are all examples of processing.

The Good and the Bad of the Rise of Canning

I should mention that I've never canned anything other than jam. Once. With the help of my mom. That is, she did all the work, and I decorated the jars.

The Start of Canning

In 1795, the French government offered a 12,000 Franc prize to whoever could find a way to preserve a wide variety of foods. They wanted to be able to feed their soldiers around the globe. In 1810, Nicolas Appert won that prize with a canning process that involved cooking the food in glass jars and then sealing those jars with cork. British inventor Peter Durand "borrowed" this invention for a British patent using similar canning techniques with food sealed in either glass jars or tin containers.

It didn't always go well, unfortunately. Sometimes those canned goods resulted in botulism or other bacterial-caused illness. In the late 1800s and early 1900s, people, justifiably, were wary of canned foods. As a result, the Heinz Company required all its employees to shower regularly, change their underwear regularly, and have weekly manicures to avoid having bacteria from the workers contaminating the food they were canning. Doesn't sound unreasonable or objectionable to us these days!

It was hard to find a happy balance of enough heat to kill microbes without destroying the taste, texture, and appearance of canned foods. Someone figured out that adding salt worked. But, of course, that's one of the problems with canned food. Too much sodium results in high blood pressure.

Thankfully, it was discovered that sterilizing the cans or jars first helped immensely in reducing bacteria-laden, illness-causing canned foods.

I used to hate canned food. My dad, however, loved canned foods. It was an easy way to feed us kids if our mom was out. I remember having mushy canned "green" (they weren't that green anymore) beans, blandly flavored yellow beans, oddly textured creamed corn, and syrupy baked beans.

Canning Options Today

But canned foods are a viable healthy option now. Don't have time to soak some beans and cook them? Canned legumes are a quick and easy alternative. Canned tomatoes are higher in the antioxidant carotenoid called lycopene than raw tomatoes. Canned tuna, salmon, sardines, herring, or oysters provide you easy access to relatively inexpensive seafood even if you don't live close to any body of water. And I use canned pureed pumpkin or sweet potato blended with a nut to make my own sweet nut butter blend.

Just make sure to choose cans that have a BPA-free lining. And, if you have sodium restrictions, look for low-sodium options.

Or, perhaps, can your food yourself! A lot of people have joined the home canning revolution. It's a great way to preserve fruits or vegetables from your garden—though your neighbors may be sad that you are no longer dumping off your extra cucumbers, tomatoes, and berries to them.

Modern Food Chemistry

Modern food chemistry arrived around the late 1800s when trans fats were invented and then entered our food supply in the 1910s. We began the descent into processed convenient foods with hotdogs, Crisco, Oreo cookies, and Hellman's mayonnaise. Then it was MSG, Wonder Bread, pop, Kool Aid, Froot Loops (changed their name because they don't contain any fruit), Batchelors Super Noodles, Velveeta, Easy Cheese spray, Spam, Mr Kipling cakes, chicken nuggets, high-fructose corn syrup, candy bars, Ritz crackers, Cheetos, Cheezels, Tang, Pringles, Gatorade, Stove Top Stuffing, Hamburger Helper, Happy Meals, Lean Cuisine, and so forth.

Chemists playing with food has resulted in a long list of food flavorants, preservatives, colorants, and other additives. Some food chemicals are still in the GRAS (Generally Recognized As Safe) category, others have been firmly added to the "definitely do not eat" category, while a bunch of others sit somewhere in between. They might be categorized as "It's okay, but don't have too much," "We don't know much about it, so probably don't eat too much," or "It used to be considered safe, but now we're saying don't eat it."

To make matters even more confusing, some countries have banned some chemical food substances, while others still allow them. For example, Europe has banned azodicarbonamide (ADA), but Canada and the United States still allow its use in food. It's found in donuts, buns, and pizza, especially at your fast-food joints like Tim Horton's and McDonald's. This is the infamous "yoga mat" chemical that you may have heard about when Subway decided to get rid of it (Landau, 2014).

Red dye #40 (aka Allura Red or FD&C Red 40) is probably one you've heard about. About 20 years ago, when my cousin was just a little kid, even he knew to avoid that ingredient. He said it made him go "crazy off the wall" (i.e., hyperactive). It's also banned in Europe, but not Canada or the US. Ditto yellow dye #5 and 6 (Tatrazine and Sunset Yellow FCF). In fact, in Europe, M&Ms and Smarties use natural foods to dye their candies. But they still sell the chemical versions in North America (wbur, 2014). This is because the European Union follows what it calls the "Precautionary Principle," which "aims at ensuring a higher level of environmental protection through preventative decision-taking in the case of risk" (Eur Lex, n.d.).

Chemicals are used to grow the food faster, kill the bugs and pests that would otherwise eat it and contaminate it, slow or speed up ripening, alter the color, enhance the flavor, replace the flavor or color that was lost in growth or processing, extend the shelf life, keep things mixed (like oil and water staying together in a salad dressing or mayonnaise), substitute for sugar or fat, and are even used in the food packaging that can leach into the foods contained.

Your farmed salmon may have red dye in it to make it look pinker because otherwise it may have an "unappetizing grey colour" (Langer and Bio, 2003). That fat-free packaged food you bought may cause "anal leakage" if it contains olestra (Silverstein, 1997)! Not making that up.

Because the world of food chemicals is ever-changing and massive in number, I won't list them, but it's a good idea to read your labels, and try to follow the general rule of limiting your intake.

"Natural Flavors"

Okay, so we get it. Maybe it's a good idea to avoid or at least limit artificial colors and flavors. But what about "natural flavors"? They're all right, aren't they? Maybe, but they aren't necessarily natural. Natural flavor additives originally come from natural sources that are then extracted and concentrated.

So a single chemical naturally found in a strawberry could be taken, altered, and added into your food as a "natural flavor."

What distinguishes a "natural flavor" additive from an "artificial flavor" additive is whether the origin on the molecule was purified and altered in a lab or whether it was synthesized entirely. Not much difference (Woerner, 2015).

And to make things even more convoluted, though you might pay more for something with "natural flavor," thinking it'll be healthier, that might not be the case. In fact, because artificial flavorings are simpler to make and are also better regulated, they may actually be safer. Maybe. Either way, natural flavors like almond flavor doesn't necessarily mean crushed almonds were added to your food. Additionally, the natural flavorings might be more harmful to our environment. For example, natural coconut flavorings use a chemical called massoya lactone which comes from the massoya tree in Malaysia. Reaping this chemical kills the tree. So, for your coconut-flavored snack that has coconut flavor added to make it sufficiently coconutty to your liking, you are paying more and destroying forests (Scientific American, 2002). Eek!

Ultra-Processed Foods

Many of these foods are termed "ultra-processed," which is defined generally as any foods that cannot be made at home; more specifically, these have been described as "formulations mostly of cheap industrial sources of dietary energy and nutrients plus additives, using a series of processes" (Monteiro et al., 2017). For example, corn on the cob is unprocessed, canned corn is processed, and Doritos are ultra-processed. A growing number of studies have been done to investigate the impact of these foods on our health. And this quote makes me laugh because of its directness: "No study reported an association between UPF [ultra-processed foods] and beneficial health outcome" (Elizabeth et al., 2020).

In a population-based study of over 105,000 adults over a median of 5.2 years, researchers found that a 10 percent increase in the consumption of ultra-processed foods (UPF) resulted in a 12 percent increase in cardiovascular disease, a 13 percent increase in coronary heart disease, and an 11 percent increase in cerebrovascular disease (Srour et al., 2019). That's significant because all those diseases can be lethal.

A Spanish study of almost 20,000 adults over ten years showed a 62 percent increased risk of death ("all cause mortality") for those consuming more than four servings per day (e.g., a serving of processed meat, a pastry, a soft drink) of UPF versus less than two servings per day. And, for each additional serving of UPF, the mortality risk increased by 18 percent (Rico-Campà *et al.*, 2019).

Other studies have found an increased risk of cancer (Chang *et al.*, 2023), irritable bowel disease, depression, respiratory diseases, and type 2 diabetes (Marti, 2019). Furthermore, diets high in UPFs are linked with an increase in calorie consumption (about 500kcal/day more) and significant weight gain, further compounding health risks (Hall *et al.*, 2019).

So, who's eating these foods? Turns out a lot of people! While it's difficult to obtain specific numbers, residents of the United States and United Kingdom have been reported as having more than 50 percent (and as much as 70 percent in the United States) of their energy intake coming from UPFs, while Mediterranean countries like Italy came in as low as 10 percent. Children and adolescents show the worst numbers, ranging from 55 to 65 percent in the UK, US, and Canada (Marino *et al.*, 2021).

Why do these numbers matter? Because hopefully they shock you at least a little. It's important to recognize the problem that UPFs contribute to our health so that we can make changes.

Other Things We've Done to Food

It's a long list, each with its own book-worthy focus, so here's a short list of some of the things we've done. And, for better or worse, this is the legal stuff. Some of this sounds futuristic!

- Change the genetics of our foods to make genetically modified organism (GMO) foods.
- Irradiate our food to kill off microbes.
- Plump up our chicken meat with salt water to make it look juicier, but also making it high in sodium.
- Use methods to speed up our food processing, while resulting in foods, flavors, and health benefits entirely different from the original methods (e.g., fermentation, curing, and ripening). Have you ever tried a black olive in Greece? I really dislike the black olives I get in cans or bottles at home in Canada, but then I had a Greek salad in Crete, and it turns out I actually love black olives. Just not the standard processed version here.
- We've now developed artificial, lab-grown meat—meat grown from stem cells.
- Some are even trying to create "note-by-note" cuisine, the making of a food completely with chemicals to taste and feel and look exactly like the real deal (Science History Institute (SHI), 2014).

- And an inventor, Pablos Holman, is trying to make edible 3D-printed food (SHI, 2014).

Seasonally, Locally Available Foods

We once ate what was seasonally, locally available. Live far from the Equator? Well, then, you wouldn't have had coffee and a banana for breakfast this morning. However, we've now created ways to keep our foods seemingly fresh, even though they may have traveled thousands of miles to arrive on our grocery store shelves.

Planes, Trains and Automobiles is a funny movie from 1987 that you should watch if you haven't seen it already. But it's not ideal for your food to have arrived via that combination, having traveled long distances before landing on your plate. Food that collects Air Miles or does a cross-country road trip is picked before it's ready, leaving it potentially less flavorful and less nutritious.

Did you know your apples (and other produce) might have been sprayed with a chemical called methylcyclopropene? It sounds much nicer if you call it SmartFresh, but it's a gas that's pumped into crates of apples or bananas to help them last longer. I've bought conventionally grown grocery store apples that looked good on the outside—firm with no obvious bruising or discoloration—but on the inside were brown. It could be because of multiple sprays of this chemical.

And, of course, there's the issue of environmental impact. What happens when the average North American meal is transported 1500 miles (2414 km) before landing on your plate? It's estimated that it costs us 10 kcal of fossil fuel energy for every 1 kcal of food energy that we get. That's a lot of energy consumed and pollution created so we can have dinner (Foodwise, n.d.).

When I was in Hawaii visiting a local coffee plantation, I was surprised to hear that they send their coffee beans to Vancouver, BC (my home city) to have the beans decaffeinated before shipping them back to Hawaii for roasting and packaging. And then, of course, the beans would be shipped out to be sold in cities all around the world, including Vancouver.

Obviously, coffee beans don't grow everywhere in the world, but sometimes we import foods that can be—and are—grown or produced much closer to where we live. When possible, it's a good idea to focus on eating locally, seasonally available foods.

This is a principle of modern TCM because we understand that nature has the wisdom to deliver what we need. Where we need it. Of course, if you live in the Arctic, or something along that line, then yes, you will quite possibly benefit from stepping outside of the 100-mile diet and having some of your food delivered from far away. But many of us are buying lettuce that has come from across the country (or across the sea) instead of from a local farm or even growing it in our own yards.

Genetically Modified Organisms (GMO)

We've also engineered or selectively bred some of our foods so that they can withstand a more specific type of environmental condition, while producing more food for us.

We've done this for about 10,000 years, choosing to breed animals or collect the seeds of plants that had traits we desired. For example, we wanted wheat that was easy to harvest. Wild wheat dropped its ripe kernels to the ground so the plant could reseed itself. When a random mutation produced a wheat plant that didn't do that, we kept that plant and seeded that one specifically. We've even bred a sheep that can live on nothing but seaweed—the North Ronaldsay sheep of the Orkney Islands (Henton, n.d.). Yup, truth is often stranger than fiction.

Many of the fruits and vegetables you find in stores today were not available anywhere hundreds of years ago. Carrots were not orange. They were purple or yellow (The Economist, 2018).

Apples were small and very sour. As the famous writer Henry David Thoreau wrote, though he preferred the "spirited flavor" of the wild apple, he did say that some bites were "sour enough to set a squirrel's teeth on edge and make a jay scream" (Rupp, 2014).

Watermelon, peaches, bananas, eggplant/aubergine, and corn are all just some of the other fruits and vegetables that you would have trouble identifying if you were to be presented their wild ancestors (Liberatore, 2016).

We didn't like the way a plant looked or tasted, so we bred it to suit our desires. Sweeter, juicier, bigger, and more edible portions were common traits we selected.

But now we've gone much further...

It's hard to write about GMO with just pure information and no opinion of pro or con, and this book isn't necessarily the place to get into that debate. Read up on GMO for yourself to form your own educated thoughts. The basics of it is that it is an

> organism whose genome has been engineered in the laboratory in order to favor the expression of desired physiological traits or the products of desired biological products... Recombinant genetic technologies are employed to produce organisms whose genome have been precisely altered at the molecular level, usually by the inclusion of genes from unrelated species

of organisms that code for traits that would not be obtained easily through conventional selective breeding. (Diaz and Fridovich-Keil, 2018)

In other words, scientists can take the gene from a plant, animal, bacterium, or virus and place it into the genes of another plant or animal. This is why GMO foods are sometimes nicknamed Frankenfoods. Want a tomato that resists insects? Take a gene from a specific bacterium and splice it into the tomato's genetic makeup.

One of the concerns about GMO foods is that we still don't have a strong grasp on the effect of gene manipulation. We used to think that one gene coded for one protein. We've since learned that that's wrong. We're now educated enough to know that there's so much more we don't know. Genes are complex. How they interact with each other is complex. And the changes that can result from alterations in genes is, as a result, very complex.

Currently, the foods most likely to be GMO (unless labeled "non-GMO"—not required by companies—or certified organic) include canola, corn, soy, sugar beets, papaya (from Hawaii), squash (from the US), cottonseed oil, and milk products (from the US). There are, of course, other foods currently in development (or maybe they are already common by the time you read this), including salmon, potato, alfalfa, and a non-browning apple (Royal Society, n.d.).

A New Awareness

The good news about our food choices is that many of us have a wide variety of options, and we can easily become much more informed consumers. More and more of us are paying attention to food labels and are choosing to focus on shopping the grocery store perimeters (instead of the aisles where most of the processed foods fight for prime shelf space) or from the farmers themselves. And, while I kind of underplayed it at the start of this chapter, many are also finding ways to grow, prepare, and cook their own food from scratch—there's no better way to know about your food than that!

CHAPTER 8

Food Allergies, Sensitivities, and Intolerances

Is it a Food Allergy?

Allergies are reactions of the immune system to exposure to something that the body considers an enemy—an allergen. Allergies may be something we have from childhood or something we develop later in life. They can also disappear on their own or with treatment. Virtually anything can become an allergen, even temperature changes (some develop hives, while others sneeze and become congested immediately upon large temperature shifts from indoors to outdoors or vice versa), sunlight (some medications—like tetracycline antibiotics and sulfa-based drugs—increase this risk), and our own bodies (there is a long list of autoimmune disorders).

Some people who believe they have food allergies may instead have a food sensitivity or intolerance. A food allergy is an immune system response to a food protein that is mistakenly identified by the body as being harmful.

When Is a Food Allergy Not a Food Allergy?

Nearly 19 percent of 40,443 US adults surveyed for a 2019 study believe that they have a food allergy (Gupta *et al.*, 2019). However, only 4–8 percent of children and 4–11 percent of adults actually have food allergies, depending on the study (American College of Allergy, Asthma, and Immunology, 2022). One problem is that the term "allergy" is sometimes misused. Simply "feeling bad" when you eat a food doesn't constitute a food allergy.

Because an allergy requires an immune response, any reaction that does not involve the immune system is not an allergy. For example, what people might term a "dairy allergy" is more commonly actually a lactose intolerance (though dairy allergies are possible).

Some may also have pharmacological reactions to chemicals present in foods. An example of this is an adverse reaction (migraines are common) to theobromine in chocolate or tyramine in aged cheese.

When I did part of my TCM training in China, I tried to learn some Mandarin. I've since forgotten most of the very limited phrases I learned, except for one: "*Wo bu yao fang wei jing.*" There are specific tones with each of those syllables, so I was sometimes not understood, but what it means is "I don't want MSG." I learned this on behalf of two friends I did my training with. Upon eating MSG, one would get headaches and the other would break out with acne. They had a food intolerance to this chemical food additive.

There are two main groups of immune reactions:

1. IgE-mediated:
   a. Immediate IgE-mediated allergies occur almost immediately after allergen exposure.
   b. Immediate plus late-phase IgE-mediated allergies occur immediately and then are followed by prolonged symptoms.
2. Non-IgE-mediated. These are not yet well understood but are thought to be T-cell-mediated, and the allergic responses are usually delayed 4–28 hours after exposure to the allergen.

IgE is the short form for immunoglobulin E antibody. It is one of the five major types of antibodies the body makes to defend itself against foreign substances. IgE antibodies—found in the lungs, mucous membranes, and skin—defend against pollen, animal dander, fungus spores, parasites, and more. They are also often involved in allergic reactions to foods and medicines.

With an IgE-mediated food allergy, histamine is released, and symptoms occur within minutes or up to about an hour after eating, touching, or even just smelling a food allergen.

IgE-Mediated Food Allergy Symptoms
Skin Reactions
Acute Urticaria or Angioedema

These medical terms are more commonly recognized as hives (urticaria) and deep swelling often around the eyes or lips (angioedema). This response is common with a food allergy and may happen within minutes of consuming a trigger food. Chronic hives are rarely caused by a food allergy.

Eczema

Careful consideration for food allergies needs to be investigated for infants and young children with atopic eczema, as close to one-third of them have an IgE-mediated food allergy. The most common food allergens for children are eggs, milk, and peanuts.

Gastrointestinal
Oral Allergy Syndrome

This often happens to patients who also have hay fever or allergic rhinitis. A type of contact hives, symptoms include itchiness in the mouth and throat, and may also include swelling of the face and/or tingling sensation of the lips, tongue, palate, and throat.

Some people develop an itchy mouth or throat when eating an uncooked vegetable or fruit. It may not be a food allergy but could be an oral allergy from a reaction to pollen on the food. Heating the food destroys the pollen, allowing it to be consumed without problem.

Allergic Eosinophilic Esophagitis, Gastritis, or Gastroenteritis

All these conditions are inflammation of the corresponding tissues. You know this because of the "itis" at the end of the words relating to particular body tissues. Eosinophils are white blood cells that create an inflammatory response to destroy viruses, bacteria, and parasites that attack your body. They also are a main player in the inflammation that occurs with allergies and asthma.

Allergic eosinophilic esophagitis is inflammation from a buildup of eosinophils in the lining of the esophagus—the tube that delivers food and drink from your mouth to your stomach. Many with eosinophilic esophagitis have symptoms that are similar to gastroesophageal reflux (GERD), including acid reflux, heartburn, chest pain, upper abdominal pain, and problems swallowing. It can also cause food to get caught when you swallow, vomiting after eating, weight loss, or failure to thrive, and it does not improve with anti-reflux medication. In children, it is sometimes overlooked because it is thought that the child is fussy, simply eats too quickly, or doesn't chew enough (could be these things too, of course).

Allergic eosinophilic gastritis and allergic eosinophilic gastroenteritis are thought to be rare conditions caused by inflammation resulting from an accumulation of eosinophils in the lining of the stomach (gastritis) and stomach and small intestines (gastroenteritis). Abdominal pain is the most common symptom, but other symptoms include nausea and vomiting after eating, diarrhea, and weight loss. Malnutrition, anemia, and fatigue are common with these conditions.

Anaphylaxis
Anaphylaxis is a potentially life-threatening allergic response causing swelling, hives, itching, difficulty with breathing and swallowing, abdominal pain, vomiting, or diarrhea. The heart rate increases and blood pressure drops, and in severe cases, the person goes into shock and requires immediate medical attention. Many with severe allergies will carry an EpiPen—a shot of epinephrine—to help quickly reverse the symptoms of anaphylaxis by preventing the blood pressure from dropping too low, redirecting blood to vital organs, relaxing and opening the airways for breathing, and stimulating the heart to beat faster and stronger.

Non-IgE-Mediated Food Allergies
Gastrointestinal
Food Protein-Induced Enterocolitis Syndrome (FPIES)
This is a severe gastrointestinal reaction that mostly happens to infants being newly exposed to cow's milk, soy, eggs, rice, oats, and some other solid foods. Two to six hours after eating the problem food, symptoms include vomiting, bloody diarrhea, irritability, and abdominal distension.

In adults, symptoms include severe nausea, repetitive vomiting, and abdominal cramping, and the most likely food cause is crustaceans (e.g., shrimp/prawn, lobster, and crab).

FPIES can lead to dehydration and may resemble a viral illness or bacterial infection.

Respiratory
Heiner Syndrome (Food-Induced Pulmonary Hemosiderosis)
This is a rare allergy occurring mainly in infants hypersensitive to cow's milk, though reports of issues with pork and egg have also been reported. Symptoms include recurrent episodes of pneumonia, cough, wheezing, coughing up blood, problems breathing, fever, vomiting, diarrhea (sometimes with blood), and failure to thrive.

Common Food Allergens

Any food can be a food allergen, but there are some foods that are more likely to cause allergic reactions. These include:

- chicken egg
- fish
- milk (cow or goat)
- peanut
- shellfish (crab, lobster, oyster, scallops, shrimp/prawn)
- soy
- tree nuts (almond, Brazil nut, cashew, hazelnut/filbert, pine nut, pistachio, walnut)
- wheat
- seeds such as sesame and mustard seeds, which are categorized as major allergens in some countries.

Allergic Cross-Reactivity

Allergic reactions to some foods or inhaled substances can cause the development of allergies to other foods and inhaled substances with a similar protein structure (see Table 16). This means that someone can suffer from an allergic reaction even if they avoid all the foods they know they have an allergy to. For example, someone with a peanut allergy can develop a reaction to other legumes like soy, peas, beans, and lentils. Another example—the most researched cross-reactivity allergy—is the cross-reactivity between birch pollen and apples (but also with carrots, celery, hazelnuts, pit fruits, and raw potato).

Table 16: Allergen Cross-Reactivity

Allergen	Food allergens (not all inclusive)
Birch, alder, ash, elm, and hazel pollen	Apple, apricot, carrot, celery, cherry, chestnut, green pepper, kiwifruit, nectarine, peach, pear, peanut, plum, raw potato, tomato, anise, basil, caraway seeds, cilantro/coriander, dill, fennel, marjoram, oregano, paprika, pepper, tarragon, thyme, almond, Brazil nut, hazelnut, walnut
Mugwort pollen	Apple, carrot, celery, green pepper, melon, parsnip, anise, basil, caraway seeds, chamomile, cilantro/coriander, dill, fennel, marjoram, oregano, paprika, parsley, pepper, tarragon, thyme, sunflower seeds
Grass pollen	Melon, orange, tomato, pea, peanut
House dust mites	Shellfish
Latex rubber	Avocado, banana, chestnut, fig, kiwifruit, mango, melon, papaya, tomato

Note that these cross-reactions for allergies do not happen all the time. Many can have reactions to one item and not another, and reactions to spices and herbs are rare.

What About Gluten?

Gluten was once part of the vocabulary of relatively few people—health professionals, researchers, and celiacs. It now seems virtually impossible to go a day without hearing or seeing "gluten" something. "Gluten-free" is written on the packages of many grocery store products, just like "cholesterol-free," "fat-free," and "sugar-free" have had their rounds.

So, what is gluten? Gluten is a protein found in wheat, rye, and barley. Actually made up of two different proteins, gliadin and glutenin, gluten plays an important role in nourishing the plant embryo. It's also something that humans have come to alternately love and hate. We love it because gluten adds a soft chewiness to the baked goods we eat. We hate it when our bodies have a negative health reaction to it.

Celiac Disease

According to the Celiac Disease Foundation (2017), it is estimated that 1 in 100 people worldwide have celiac disease, with many of them undiagnosed. Because it is a hereditary disease, those with a first-degree relative (parent, child, or sibling) with celiac has a 1 in 10 chance of developing celiac disease.

The symptoms of celiac disease can be vague and include fatigue, weight loss (but can be overweight), anemia, irritability, depression, migraines, bone and joint pain, easy bruising, mouth ulcers, chronic diarrhea, constipation, cramps, gas, abdominal bloating, and more. Additional symptoms for children include vomiting, poor growth, dental enamel defects, delayed puberty, and behavourial changes. Some with gluten-intolerance can also suffer an intense itchy and burning rash called dermatitis herpetiformis.

So, how do you know if you are celiac? Blood screening may be the first step if celiac disease is suspected, but the only conclusive way to know is a small bowel biopsy. To get an accurate diagnosis, a person must *not* be eating gluten-free prior to the blood and biopsy tests, so some choose not to get tested if they find that eliminating gluten from their diet makes them feel better.

It's very important that those with celiac disease do not consume gluten. Continued consumption can lead to other health conditions including anemia, vitamin and mineral deficiencies, osteoporosis, nervous system disorders, neurological diseases, gastrointestinal cancers, and a slew of autoimmune diseases like multiple sclerosis and type 1 diabetes.

Gluten Sensitivity

Table 17: Gluten-Containing and Gluten-Free Grains

Gluten-containing grains	Gluten-free grains
Wheat (listed below in its many forms): • Wheat starch • Wheat bran • Wheat germ • Couscous • Cracked wheat • Durum • Einkorn • Emmer • Farina • Faro • Fu • Gliadin • Graham flour • Kamut • Matzo • Oats (not gluten-containing, but often contaminated by gluten-containing grains) • Semolina • Spelt Also: • Barley • Bulgur • Rye • Seitan • Triticale Beware as well of potential hidden sources of gluten: • Barley malt • Chicken broth • Malt vinegar • Salad dressings • Seasonings and spice mixes • Soy sauce • Veggie burgers	• Buckwheat (yup, this is a tricky one with a name containing "wheat," but it is not a wheat product) • Corn • Millet • Oats (when certified gluten-free) • Rice • Sorghum • Quinoa (technically a seed, but often cooked and consumed like a grain)

Non-celiac gluten sensitivity is a term for those who cannot tolerate gluten and have symptoms similar to those with celiac disease, but do not have the antibodies and intestinal damage found with celiac disease. Those with non-celiac gluten sensitivity may experience "foggy-headedness," headaches, joint pain, fatigue, depression, hyperactivity, numbness in the limbs, and a variety of digestive health symptoms.

There is no blood or biopsy test for gluten sensitivity. The only way it can be determined is via exclusion. Tests can rule out celiac disease, and if symptoms improve after removing gluten from the diet, followed by a return of symptoms when gluten foods are reintroduced to the diet, non-celiac gluten sensitivity can be suspected (see Table 17 for a list of gluten-containing and gluten-free grains). However, there is research that indicates that gluten sensitivity alone may not be the culprit (Beyond Celiac, 2012; Biesiekierski et al., 2013). A group of poorly absorbed short-chain carbohydrates called FODMAPs (fermentable oligosaccharides, disaccharides, monosaccharides, and polyols) may be the problem. What makes it confusing is that gluten-containing grains are high in FODMAPs. (See the FODMAPs section below for more information.)

FODMAPs

FODMAPs are a group of short-chain carbohydrates (sugars) and sugar alcohols (not the boozy kind) that are found naturally in foods or as food additives (see Table 18). While not unhealthy compounds in and of themselves, some people do not absorb FODMAPs well in the small intestine, so these carbohydrates move on to the large intestine where they can ferment and draw water into the colon, causing gastrointestinal distress. They are a suspected cause of irritable bowel syndrome (IBS), causing bloating, abdominal pain, cramping, gas, and constipation or diarrhea.

Many people are surprised to find that common foods that they thought were healthy for them may be creating their digestive symptoms. Note that not all those with IBS need to avoid all the following foods (see Tables 19, 20 and 21 for a list of high- and low-FODMAP foods). Many find that they are fine with some of these foods, that they can eat most of these foods in limited quantities, and/or that they can improve their digestion and begin to re-add these foods back into their diet.

The following defines what FODMAPs are and gives a couple of ways to look at foods in relation to their FODMAP levels. Some may find that foods high in lactose are particularly troubling and will need to limit or avoid foods in that category. Others may find that foods high in fructose or polyols are the troublemakers. For those people, the first two charts of food listings are suitable for use. Still others will be best to avoid all FODMAP foods. For those folk, the last FODMAP food chart is the easiest to use, as it lumps all high-FODMAP foods together by food type and provides low-FOD-MAP alternatives within the same chart. Note that FODMAP quantities in foods may vary between countries because of differences in the nature of the ingredients or food processing.

Table 18: FODMAP Definition

F	Fermentable: Fermentable carbohydrates and sugars that are broken down (fermented) by bacteria in the large intestine. • When these sugars and carbohydrates are not well digested and absorbed, bacteria in the intestines break them down and result in bloating, gas, pain, and diarrhea.
O	Oligosaccharides: Carbohydrates that have three to ten simple sugars linked together. "Oligo" means few and "saccharide" means sugar. • Fructans (chain of fructose molecules) and galacto-oligosaccharides (chain of galactose molecules) are not broken down by human digestive systems, so are poorly absorbed in the small intestine.
D	Disaccharides: Carbohydrates with two simple sugars joined. "Di" means two. • Lactose, the sugar in milk and dairy products, is a disaccharide made up of glucose and galactose. Much of the population does not make enough lactase enzymes to break down this sugar well.
M	Monosaccharides: Single carbohydrate molecules. "Mono" means one. • Fructose is the sugar found in some vegetables and many fruits. The problem arises when fructose molecules outnumber the glucose molecules, as glucose helps fructose be completely absorbed. Fructose absorption also relies on the activity of sugar transporters in the intestinal wall, and the ability to absorb excess fructose varies between individuals.
A	AND
P	Polyols: Carbohydrates that are not sugars. They are used as sugar replacements because they mimic the sweetness of sugar. They are found in low-calorie, sugar-free, and diet products. • Xylitol, mannitol, maltitol, sorbitol, and erythritol are examples of polyols. Their absorption is very slow, so they are only partially processed in the small intestine.

Table 19: High-FODMAP Foods

Fructans	Galacto-oligo-saccharides	Lactose	Excess fructose	Polyols
Vegetables: • artichokes • asparagus • beetroot • chicory • dandelion leaves • garlic • leek • onions • raddicchi lettuce • spring onions (white part)	Legumes: • baked beans • black-eyed peas • borlotti beans • garbanzo beans/chickpeas • kidney beans • lentils • miso • soybeans • soy flour • some soy milks	High-lactose dairy: • buttermilk • chocolate • cream • creamy or cheesy sauces • custard • dairy desserts • ice cream • milk (cow's, goat's, sheep's, condensed, evaporated, powdered) • soft and unripened cheese (cottage, cream, mascarpone, ricotta) • sour cream • yogurt	Fruits: • apples • boysenberries • canned fruit • dried fruit • cherries • figs • mangoes • pears • watermelon	Fruits: • apples • apricots • avocados • blackberries • cherries • longans • lychee/litchi • nectarines • peaches • pears • plums • prunes
Grains: • barley • rye • wheat (in large amounts) • chicory root • inulin			Sweeteners: • agave • corn syrup solids • high-fructose corn syrup (HFCS) • honey	Vegetables: • cauliflower • green peppers • mushrooms • pumpkin • snow peas
Nuts: • cashews • pistachios			Alcohol: • fortified wines (sherry, port) • rum	Sweeteners: • sorbitol • mannitol • isomalt • maltitol • xylitol

Sources: IBS Diets (n.d.); International Foundation for Gastrointestinal Disorders (2021)

Table 20: Low-FODMAP Foods

Fructans	Galacto-oligo-saccharides	Lactose	Excess fructose	Polyols
Vegetables: • bean sprouts • bok choy • butter lettuce • carrots • celery • chives • corn • eggplant/ aubergine • green beans • spinach • tomatoes	Legumes: • firm tofu • tempeh	High-lactose dairy: • natural, aged, hard cheese has less lactose (cheddar, colby, parmesan, Swiss) • ripened soft cheese (brie, camembert, feta) • Greek yogurt	Fruits: • bananas (unripe) • blueberries • grapefruit • grapes • honeydew • lemons • limes • passion fruit • raspberries • strawberries • tangelos	Fruits: • bananas • blueberries • grapefruit • grapes • honeydew • kiwifruit • lemons • limes • oranges • passion fruit • raspberries
Grains: • gluten-free breads • cereals • flours • pastas (provided also no honey or other high-FODMAP sweetener)		Non-dairy milk alternatives: • almond, cashew, coconut, flax, hemp, rice milks • sherbet	Sweeteners: • maple syrup • table sugar (sucrose)	Sweeteners: • glucose • table sugar (sucrose)

Source: Stanford Health Care (n.d.)

Table 21: High- and Low-FODMAP Foods by Type of Food

Food group	High FODMAPs	Low FODMAPs
Fruits	Apples, apricots, avocados, blackberries, boysenberries, canned fruits, cherries, dates, dried fruits, figs, guava, longans, lychee/litchi, mangoes, nectarines, papayas, peaches, pears, persimmons, plums, prunes, watermelon	Bananas (ripe), blueberries, cantaloupe, grapefruit, grapes, honeydew, kiwifruit, lemons, limes, mandarins, oranges, passion fruit, pineapple, raspberries, rhubarb, strawberries, tangelos, tangerines

cont.

Food group	High FODMAPs	Low FODMAPs
Vegetables	Artichokes, asparagus, beetroot, cauliflower, chicory, dandelion leaves, garlic, green peppers, leek, mushrooms, onions, pumpkin, radicchio lettuce, snow peas, spring onions (white part), sugar snap peas	Alfalfa, bamboo shoots, bok choy, carrots, cabbage, celery, chives, corn, cucumbers, eggplant/aubergine, green beans, kale, lettuce, parsnips, potatoes, radishes, rutabaga/swede, seaweed (e.g., nori, dulse, kombu), spinach, squash, tomatoes, turnips, water chestnuts, zucchini/courgette
Grains	Barley, rye, wheat; limit quantity of foods made with inulin or chicory root	Gluten-free grains
Dairy and dairy alternatives	High-lactose dairy: buttermilk, chocolate, creamy and cheesy sauces, custard, ice cream, milk (cow's, goat's, sheep's, condensed, evaporated, powdered), soft and unripened cheese (cottage, cream, mascarpone, ricotta), sour cream, yogurt	Low-lactose dairy: aged cheese (cheddar, colby, parmesan, Swiss), ripened soft cheese (brie, camembert, feta), Greek yogurt Lactose-free dairy Non-dairy alternatives: almond, cashew, coconut, flax, hemp, rice milk; sherbet
Legumes	Baked beans, black-eyed peas, borlotti beans, garbanzo beans/chickpeas, kidney beans, lentils, miso, soybeans, soy flour, some soy milk	Firm tofu, tempeh
Nuts and seeds	Cashews, pistachios	Any other
Meats, eggs, poultry, fish	Foods processed with high-fructose corn syrup (HFCS)	Any other
Sweeteners	Agave, corn syrup solids, high-fructose corn syrup (HFCS), honey, sorbitol, mannitol, isomalt, maltitol, xylitol	Glucose, syrup, table sugar (sucrose)
Other	Fortified wines (sherry, port), rum Read labels on processed foods to look for high-fructose corn syrup (HFCS), especially in jam, jelly, pickles, relish, salsa, salad dressings, sauces, tomato paste. Processed foods may also contain garlic salt or powder, onion salt or powder, honey, agave, or one of the non-sugar sweeteners (sorbitol, mannitol, isomalt, maltitol, xylitol). Canned fruit in syrup, dried fruit, and fruit juice are higher in concentration of FODMAPs.	Although garlic and onion are high in FODMAPs, FODMAPs are not soluble in oil, so garlic or onion oils are often okay to use. Or they can be sautéed in oil for 1–2 minutes so the oil can absorb the flavor. Then remove the whole peeled garlic or onion slices. Canned legumes (lentils and garbanzo beans/chickpeas) that are rinsed prior to consumption are lower in FODMAPs, as the water-soluble galacto-oligosaccharides leach out of the legume into the brine. Pickling (e.g., artichokes) may also reduce the FODMAP content.

How Do I Find Out if I Have Food Allergies or Intolerance?

Food Diary

One of the simplest things you can do is to keep a food diary (see the end of the book). Writing down what you eat, symptoms you experience, and how long after eating these symptoms occur and for how long will help you and your health professionals narrow down potential food concerns.

The more thorough you are in keeping the diary notes, the better chance you'll have at determining which foods could be problematic, so don't "forget" to include those foods that you would rather pretend you didn't eat, even though you did. You might also think you don't need to write everything down, as you believe that you'll remember later. Maybe you do have an excellent memory, but most of us will forget at least some important pieces.

Elimination Diet

This is one of the best ways to determine food allergies, intolerances, and sensitivities. It can be effective, you can do it on your own, and it's cheap. It just takes a bit of planning and commitment.

There are a couple of things to note before taking on an elimination diet, however. Do not try to test foods that you think you have an anaphylactic reaction to (your throat tightens, you break out in hives, you use an EpiPen). Also, if you suspect you might be celiac, do not take out gluten until you are tested, as removing gluten prior can cause a false negative result. You'll also want to make sure that you get enough nutrition out of your food for the time you are on the elimination diet. If you have a serious illness or health condition or have an eating disorder (or a history of one), speak with a qualified health professional first.

It's a good idea to do a food diary for a week or two prior to an elimination diet. That way you'll have a better appreciation of how your body feels, what symptoms you have, and perhaps some clues about troublesome foods.

The most basic elimination diet takes out gluten, dairy, soy, peanuts, shellfish, eggs, corn, alcohol, and processed foods for three to four weeks. If there are other foods that you believe your body may be reacting negatively to, take those out as well. Additional foods that are commonly suspect are nuts, citrus fruits, coffee, legumes, beef, pork, chicken, and nightshade vegetables—tomatoes, potatoes, eggplant/aubergine, and peppers (bell, chili, paprika, cayenne, hot, and sweet). (See Table 22.)

This may seem quite limiting, but there are still many foods available, even on the most rigorous elimination diet.

Table 22: Elimination Diet Foods to Exclude and Include

	Foods to exclude	Foods to include
Vegetables	Tomatoes, potatoes (sweet potatoes and yams are okay), eggplant/aubergine, peppers (bell, chili, paprika, cayenne, hot, and sweet)	Most other vegetables (see the FODMAPs list if you have IBS-like symptoms)
Fruits	Citrus fruits	Most other fruit (see the FODMAPs list if you have IBS-like symptoms)
Dairy and dairy alternatives	Butter, cheese, cream and non-dairy creamers, ice cream, milk, yogurt	Unsweetened coconut or rice milk; you can also make your own gluten-free oat milk
Grains	Barley, kamut, rye, spelt, wheat, and other gluten-containing grains; corn, oats (if not labeled gluten-free)	Buckwheat, millet, rice
Nuts and seeds	All nuts and seeds	
Legumes	All beans (black, navy, kidney, etc.), lentils, peas, soybeans and soy products, including miso, tempeh, and tofu	
Meat and fish	Bacon, beef, canned meat, chicken, cold cuts, eggs, hotdogs, sausage, shellfish	Fish, turkey, wild game
Fats	Butter, margarine, processed and hydrogenated oils, mayonnaise	Good-quality coconut oil, flaxseed oil, ground flax seeds, and olive oil
Condiments and spices	Mayonnaise, soy sauce, ketchup, mustard, relish, most packaged sauces	Fresh herbs and spices (e.g., dill, cumin, ginger, oregano, parsley, rosemary, thyme, turmeric), sea salt or Himalayan salt, black or white pepper
Sweets and sweeteners	Chocolate, corn syrup, honey, high-fructose corn syrup, white or brown sugar	Stevia, small amounts of maple syrup, if needed
Beverages	Alcohol, caffeine (coffee, green or black tea, soft drinks)	Drink lots of water, herbal tea

The better you are able to fully eliminate suspect foods, the more illuminative your results will be. If you occasionally slip and consume a food that is causing you problems, you won't get the full effect of eliminating them. When your immune system makes antibodies—proteins that cause an immune reaction—it takes around 21 days to clear them from your body. So, if you have a reaction to dairy and eat something with dairy in it on day 14, your body will still be circulating antibodies to dairy when you complete your elimination diet.

Many will feel generally better—possibly more energy, weight loss, feeling of clearer mind and better focus, fewer aches and pains, etc.—at the end of an elimination diet (though it might be challenging at times during the process).

Upon completion of your elimination diet, it's important that you don't go on a food binge; otherwise, you'll still never know which food(s) is (are) a problem. On day one, you can reintroduce *one* food category, like gluten *or* dairy *or* citrus for *one* day. For example, if you want to test out gluten, have rye bread, whole wheat pasta, and cooked barley. On day two, eliminate that food again. See how you feel on days two and three. Do you have any negative reactions?

- If you *do* have a negative reaction, continue to keep that food out of your diet, and take out the next category of food.
- If you *don't* have any negative reaction with the reintroduction of that food, you may keep it in your diet and move on to introducing the next category.
- Continue until you've tried reintroducing each food category and have a clearer picture of which foods your body does not respond well to.
- If you find that taking them all out at once is too much, you can try them in phases. It takes longer, but might be easier for you to do, as you'll feel less limited. Keep alcohol and intoxicants out through the whole process for the best results because the sugar helps yeast and bad bacteria thrive in the body. They also disrupt sleep, interfering with healing.

Allergy Tests

There are options for food allergy testing done by a health professional.

Skin Prick Tests

A liquid with a small amount of a potential food allergen is put on the skin of the patient's arm or back. One spot will be a control test using a liquid with no allergen to allow for comparison. Then the skin is pricked with a small, sterile needle to allow the liquid to enter the skin. One spot of liquid and one prick is done for each allergen being tested. The test is positive for an allergy if a weal (a bump that may or may not be red and/or itchy) develops at one of those spots.

The problem with a skin prick test is that though a weal less than 3 mm in diameter is good evidence that the food is safe to consume (in other words, it tests negative), a positive test producing a weal of 3 mm or more may not be clinically relevant. This is called a "false positive." It's possible that the reaction on the skin may not cause a reaction when the food is consumed. For example, infants usually lose food sensitivity as they grow up, but the skin prick test may still test positive even after a tolerance to the food has developed. Nonetheless, large weals, especially to foods like cow's milk, egg, or peanut, are likely to indicate an allergy, and this test is relatively inexpensive and easy to perform (Birch and Pearson-Shaver, 2020).

Blood Tests

Blood is drawn to measure the amount of IgE antibody to specific foods that are being tested. This is less accurate than a skin prick test, and, again, a negative test result is useful in ruling out an allergy, while a positive result doesn't necessarily indicate an allergy.

Oral Food Challenge

This is also called a double-blind, placebo-controlled food challenge (DBP-CFC). Although this is the most accurate way to diagnose a food allergy, this test is conducted under medical supervision because a dangerous anaphylactic reaction is possible. The patient is fed tiny amounts of a suspected allergy food. The amount of food is increased slowly over time, and the patient is watched for a few hours after to observe if a reaction occurs. This test may be chosen if the previous tests are not conclusive, if a patient's history is not clear, or to conclude if an allergy has been outgrown.

How Do I Live with Food Allergies/ Sensitivities/Intolerance?
Trigger Food Avoidance

It makes sense that avoiding the food that is of concern is a first step. Be aware of hidden sources of the trigger food, in premade foods, processed foods, and when eating out. Read labels and know alternate names for your trigger food. For example, MSG contains a chemical (processed free glutamic acid) that causes negative reactions for many. This chemical is found in more than 40 food ingredients (Truth in Labelling Campaign, 2021), some of which are vaguely labeled. This long list includes glutamate, hydrolyzed protein, yeast extract, umami, and gelatin. And did you know that marshmallows may contain egg? I thought that marshmallows were made by magical unicorns—though that's a bit redundant, I think, as all unicorns must be magical! But seriously, egg is found in a lot of foods, including salad dressings, many pastas, processed meats, and, of course, mayonnaise, baked goods, and custards. Those with an egg allergy should also talk to their physician before getting a flu vaccine.

The amount you should avoid the trigger food depends on how sensitive your body is to the ingredient and how severe your body's response. Obviously, if you have an anaphylactic response, you should avoid that food altogether.

A growing number of companies and restaurants are making it easier to identify foods that contain the more common allergens. You'll now find "gluten-free," "dairy-free," "egg-free," "nut-free," and "soy-free" written on food packages and in restaurant menus. Workers serving food are taught to ask you "Is that a preference or allergy?" when you ask for "[something]-free." No one wants to have a patron go into anaphylactic shock because the waiter mistakenly said the soup didn't have any shrimp in it, only to find out later that the pre-prepped stock had shrimp or that the chef used the same spoon to stir the creamed broccoli soup as the seafood chowder.

If you are having to avoid a number of nutritious foods, consider talking with a qualified health professional to talk about food alternatives and dietary supplementation to avoid nutritional deficiencies.

Allergy Treatments

There are several allergy treatment options, including medications and immunotherapy. Immunotherapy is commonly called "allergy shots," as it's a series of injections of purified allergen extracts given usually over years. It may also be given as sublingual (under the tongue) tablets.

Natural therapies, including Traditional Chinese Medicine, also offer a variety of allergy treatment options. Common approaches include modulating (balancing the response of) the immune system, strengthening the digestive system, calming the nervous system, and improving the microbiome.

Time may also be a treatment. Yes, time alone might change your allergies and sensitivities, so re-testing and careful (supervised if your reaction has been severe in the past!) reintroduction of problem foods can be done.

Young children are the most likely to outgrow their IgE-mediated food allergies, while older children and adults might lose their hypersensitivity if the allergen is completely removed from the diet for long enough. For those people, the skin prick test and blood test results might still show positive (indicating an allergy) even though there is no clinical reaction. Those with nut, peanut, fish, and shellfish allergies rarely lose their reactions to those foods, and celiac patients must forever keep away from gluten.

CHAPTER 9

Common Diets and Cleanses

This could have been the longest chapter of the book, including descriptions about fat-free, carb-free, vegetarian, vegan, paleo, calorie counting, zone, food combining, or even the Twinkie diet (yes, there's a Twinkie diet, a version of calorie counting), and so forth. But then I realized that the whole point of this book is anti-diet, against choosing a way of eating based on one ideal way.

Plus, there are always a growing number of diets that would make this book obsolete in a short period of time. I want this book to be relevant for years, decades to come.

So, here it is, my shortest chapter.

CHAPTER 10

Basic Healthy Eating Tips

Cravings May Be Telling You Something

Your craving may be signaling something important. Or not. But either way, it's a good idea to pay attention to the cues your body is giving you to see if there is action you can take.

Cravings are tricky. Do you want that cookie because you need an energy kick, you're bored, you're lonely, you want comfort, you're reminded of a pleasant memory, or something else? Is it the flavor, texture, smell, or something else that you are wanting? Could it be a nutrient deficiency or physical imbalance that you need to address? Or maybe you just saw a commercial that prompted you.

Some common cravings and their possible physical need are listed here. But know that just because you are craving chocolate (or something else), don't think of it as free rein to binge. Sometimes a small amount is enough. And sometimes there are healthier alternatives.

Chocolate

Chocolate is comfort food for many. It causes a release of endorphins (feel-good hormones) and is also associated with serotonin (another feel-good hormone). Depending on the amount of sugar added, it can also be quite sweet. But even the bitter 70 percent+ chocolate, which gets more bitter with higher percentages (the kind I love—yum!), still makes us feel good. It has been called the "food of the gods" and is considered an aphrodisiac by some.

If you are craving chocolate, you may also be deficient in the mineral magnesium. Beware that chocolate is a possible migraine trigger, that white chocolate is a misnomer (it doesn't contain chocolate liquor or cocoa solids that contribute to chocolate's health benefits), and that chocolate is a stimulant that can trigger nervous-type symptoms.

A little goes a long way, and it's best to choose high-quality chocolate products, low in added sugars and high in cocoa percentage (70% or more). Other magnesium-rich foods include legumes, leafy greens, nuts, and seeds. If it's the good feeling you're craving, other things that can elicit this are caring or affectionate touch, exercise, and acupuncture!

Sugar and Sweet Foods

If you're craving sweet foods, you could be experiencing blood sugar fluctuations, or you may have candida yeast issues. Are you eating a lot of sugar already? If so, you are best to watch your sugar intake, up your fiber, and include protein and healthy fats to help regulate your blood sugar levels. Healthier sweet foods include fruit (see the Sweet Foods section in Chapter 2 for more information).

Salty Foods

Cravings for salty foods could signify adrenal depletion from chronic stress or some medical issues like adrenal insufficiency, as in Addison's disease, or kidney disease. You may also have a mineral deficiency, particularly calcium.

In our modern world, many are eating way too much salt (and sodium) because of processed foods—even ones that you wouldn't think of as salty, like some cookies, frozen waffles, and cereals. Just as with sugar cravings, you may be craving salt because you are used to eating a lot of salt. If this is the case, start working on rebalancing your system by tuning into other flavors and eating healthier unprocessed salty foods (see the Salty Foods section in Chapter 2 for more information).

Meat

I've met many vegetarians and vegans who have sometimes craved meat. What their bodies were often telling them was that they needed more iron and/or protein.

There are many non-meat sources for this, including beans and legumes. Unsulfured prunes, figs, other dried fruits, spinach, and pumpkin seeds are also high in iron. Combine those with foods rich in vitamin C—like citrus fruits, broccoli, strawberries, bell peppers, kiwifruit, and dark leafy greens.

Spicy Foods

You may have trouble cooling down, and you're craving hot spicy foods that will make you sweat so that you can cool off. You may also be addicted to the rush you get when you eat these foods (see the Pungent Foods section in Chapter 2 for more information).

Sour Foods

Traditional Chinese Medicine would assert that craving sour foods means that your Liver is needing support. Some pregnant women also crave sour foods like lemons, as their taste buds are just one more of the things that change along with everything else (see the Sour Foods section in Chapter 2 for more information).

Fatty Foods

Feel like you really need something deep-fried, cheesy, or other rich fatty food? If you're craving fat, it may be the essential fatty acids (EFAs) that your body needs.

Choose raw nuts, ground flax seeds, hemp seeds, chia seeds, and fatty fish like sardines, herring, mackerel, salmon, cod, or halibut for those brain-boosting, heart-healthy EFAs. Other filling good-fat choices include olives and olive oil, avocados (one of my faves!), and coconut oil (see the Fats section in Chapter 3 for more information).

Carbohydrates

Carbs are not the evil they are sometimes portrayed to be. They are a major macronutrient, needed to supply easy energy to the body. The brain needs glucose, a basic sugar. It's just that we have overdone it because of easy access to too many carbs, especially the simple carbs.

As with the sugar and sweet cravings, you may have issues with your blood sugar and need to watch your carbs and balance them with protein and good fats. Or maybe you really do need more carbs because of a high level of physical activity (see the Carbohydrates section in Chapter 2 for more information).

Crunchy Foods

Is it the texture you crave instead? Crunchy foods can relieve tension, anger, and frustration, but can lead to overeating. If this makes sense to you, try some other physical activity, or go in the opposite direction and try meditation, breathing exercises, or relaxing music. Carrots and celery sticks are some examples of healthy crunchy food options.

Creamy Foods

Cravings for mashed potatoes, ice cream, or macaroni and cheese are common comfort foods, and perhaps you need to be soothed. It's no surprise that these foods are rich in carbohydrates and fat. Check out those categories above.

Caffeine

Ask yourself why you need it. Are you tired? Bored? Dissatisfied? Addicted? There is no nutritional caffeine deficiency. Or maybe it's simply a habit—a way to start your day, take a break, chat with friends—and you can try a decaf or non-caffeinated drink instead.

Pickles and Ice Cream

These are the foods most commonly associated with pregnancy cravings. Ice cream, okay, it's easy to understand why someone would crave that sugar and fat—it's evolution talking there. Plus, ice cream is cold, and many women find they feel like furnaces when they are pregnant. Is that part of the reason for the term "bun in the oven"? I looked it up; apparently, it's not, but it fits anyway.

How about pickles? Could be the salt that's needed, though there isn't evidence to support this. Having said this, my mom craved seaweed when she was pregnant with my sister and me. Back to the pickles, some women just like the crunchy texture, and, again, the taste buds change during pregnancy.

Weird Cravings?

Pica is the craving for dirt, paint, cigarette butts, laundry soap, matches, or other things that have no nutritional value. If someone is experiencing these cravings, they should be assessed for mental disorders like obsessive-compulsive disorder or intellectual or developmental disabilities. However, children and pregnant women have also been noted to experience pica cravings. Sometimes the craving may indicate nutritional deficiencies.

Dirt, Clay

Eating dirt may be something that we think of just for kids. Remember mud pies? I don't recall ever eating any of that. In some areas, however, eating dirt is not uncommon. It's called geophagy. Some have thought that eating dirt helps supplement minerals. However, more recent research shows that it may be helpful in staving off pathogens in the gut.

Kaolin clay is found in some nutrition stores, and it is recommended for cleansing. The problem is that while it can draw out impurities from the gut, it can also absorb important nutrients that you consume along with it, meaning the clay pulls that out too.

Chalk

Although you may never have actually tasted a stick of chalk, you may have tried a calcium pill and tasted it as chalky. Turns out we can taste calcium, it does taste chalky, and it's generally a taste we'd rather avoid. We perceive its flavor in the same realm as bitter.

A study on mice showed that though most mice agreed that calcium-enriched liquid was ick, preferring water instead, one mouse strain called PWK actually chose the calcium drink over water. Those mice were found to have a different set of genes responsible for the taste receptors on their tongues, and one of those genes was the same as part of the receptor that picks up on sweet and savory flavors. We don't yet know if we have that same version of genes, but it's possible. If you crave chalk, you probably could use more calcium in your diet (Wenner, n.d.).

Ice

Craving ice (called pagophagia—there really is a specific term for nearly everything) is often associated with iron-deficiency anemia, but it's not really clear. Since you're not going to get iron from ice, if you have low levels of iron, choose iron-rich foods like meat, legumes, spinach, dried fruit, and pumpkin seeds instead. If you chew ice as a way to de-stress, find alternative ways to manage that, especially as chewing ice can damage your teeth.

How to Eat

Just because we've been doing something for a long time doesn't mean we're doing it properly. The same way that most of us breathe poorly in some way—too fast, too shallow, through the mouth—many of us also have poor eating habits. It's not just *what* we eat but *how* we eat that affects our health.

Chew More

Digestion begins in the mouth. The process of chewing breaks down food and stimulates the release of saliva which moistens the food so it can be swallowed more easily. Saliva also contains an enzyme called amylase that helps break down starches. Saliva is also key in helping to protect the enamel on your teeth.

I wondered if chewing helps reduce stress and anxiety in humans because it does this for dogs. I checked the research on this, and it turns out that chewing does do this for humans too! It also may be associated with supporting healthy cognitive function (Kubo *et al.*, 2015). Your masseter muscles (the ones that pop out a bit at the corner of your jaw when you bite down) are the strongest muscles in your body for their weight, so don't put them to waste.

Avoid Drinking with Meals

Most people sitting for a meal will have a drink along with their food. But here's the problem. We often end up taking a bite of that food, chewing it a bit, and then swallowing it down with a drink. That means less chewing and more diluted saliva and digestive juices. In other words, worse digestion and absorption of nutrients.

Have your drinks between meals rather than with them. You'll still need to hydrate, of course, so don't deprive yourself of that, but by timing your beverages before or after meals, you'll improve your digestion.

Eat Mindfully

Mindful eating means slowing the process of eating, chewing more, savoring each bite, and paying attention to the aroma, taste, and texture of the food. It means focusing on eating when you're eating instead of multitasking during mealtimes. Doing so can increase your feeling of satisfaction and fullness, also known as satiety, giving you more time to digest your food and making it less likely that you'll overeat. Plus, eating with a calm mind is more likely to put your body into a parasympathetic state, recognized as "rest and digest" rather than the sympathetic state or "fight or flight."

Eat Until You're 80 Percent Full

"*Hara hachi bu.*" This is a Japanese expression that translates to eating until the stomach feels just 80 percent full, not more. While it can be tempting to fill your plate and eat it all, "get your money's worth" when you go to a buffet, or show your appreciation by going for seconds and thirds when you are invited for a home-cooked meal, having to loosen your belt isn't the healthiest way to eat.

How do you know that you're 80 percent full? Instead of stopping eating when you're full, stop eating when you're no longer hungry. That's a huge distinction to make, and it may take some practice and attention to notice the difference. Keep in mind that if you eat too quickly, you're unlikely to even notice when you're at that point.

Slow Down

Unless you're a competitive eater, you don't get a trophy for wolfing down your food. Except if you call indigestion, bloating, and gas a prize. I don't. Eating too quickly means you're missing many of the pieces I just covered.

If you're used to eating quickly, you might try some simple tricks to slow yourself down:

- Eat with your non-dominant hand.

- Put down your utensils between bites.
- Count your bites and aim for around 30 chews per mouthful.
- Take smaller bites of food.
- Eat with chopsticks, if you're not used to using them.
- Slow your breathing while you eat.

Final Word

This book is *not* about "good" and "bad" foods or one ideal way to eat. The goal is not making "perfect" choices around mealtimes.

This book *is* about offering nutritional information that you can use to make the best choices for yourself, based on your health condition, your health goals, the season, where you live, and what you enjoy. Don't let nutritional advice overwhelm you. Food can be and should be about more than nutrient-dense, superfood, clean eating. It is also about pleasure, memories, traditions, new experiences, creativity, connection, adventure, and so much more.

Food Diary

Table 23: Food Diary

	Foods	Notes on how I feel
Monday		
Tuesday		
Wednesday		

Thursday		
Friday		
Saturday		
Sunday		

Bibliography

af Geijerstam, P., Joelsson, A., Rådholm, K., and Nyström, F.H. (2024) `A low dose of daily licorice intake affects renin, aldosterone, and home blood pressure in a randomized crossover trial.' *The American Journal of Clinical Nutrition.* 119(3), 682 -691. https://doi.org/10.1016/j.ajcnut.2024.01.011

American College of Allergy, Asthma, and Immunology (2022) *Food allergy.* https://acaai.org/allergies/allergic-conditions/food

American Heart Association (2023, May 30) *Understanding blood pressure readings.* www.heart.org/en/health-topics/high-blood-pressure/understanding-blood-pressure-readings

American Thyroid Association (n.d.) *Hypothyroidism in pregnancy.* www.thyroid.org/hypothyroidism-in-pregnancy

Arthur (2023, July 26) *Historical consumption of sugar: A concise exploration of its evolution.* www.sugar-and-sweetener-guide.com/historical-consumption-of-sugar

Assunção, M.L., Ferreira, H.S., dos Santos, A.F., *et al.* (2009) 'Effects of dietary coconut oil on the biochemical and anthropometric profiles of women presenting abdominal obesity.' *Lipids, 44*(7), 593–601. https://doi.org/10.1007/s11745-009-3306-6

Aune, D., Navarro Rosenblatt, D.A., Chan, D.S.M., *et al.* (2015, January 1) 'Products, calcium, and prostate cancer risk: A systematic review and meta-analysis of cohort studies.' *American Journal of Clinical Nutrition, 101*(1), 87–117. https://pubmed.ncbi.nlm.nih.gov/25527754

Avena, N.M., Rada, P. and Hoebel, B.G. (2008) 'Evidence for sugar addiction: Behavioral and neurochemical effects of intermittent, excessive sugar intake.' *Neuroscience & Biobehavioral Reviews, 32*(1), 20–39. https://doi.org/10.1016/j.neubiorev.2007.04.019

Balch, P.A. and Balch, J.F. (2000) *Prescription for Nutritional Healing.* Avery Publishing Group.

Beinfield, H. and Korngold, E. (1992) *Between Heaven and Earth: A Guide to Chinese Medicine.* Ballantine.

Bell, P.G., Gaze, D.C., Davison, G.W., *et al.* (2014) 'Montmorency tart cherry (*Prunus cerasus L.*) concentrate lowers uric acid, independent of plasma cyanidin-3-O-glucosiderutinoside.' *Journal of Functional Foods, 11*, 82–90. https://doi.org/10.1016/j.jff.2014.09.004

Beyond Celiac (2012) *Non-celiac gluten sensitivity.* www.beyondceliac.org/celiac-disease/non-celiac-gluten-sensitivity

Biesiekierski, J.R., Peters, S.L., Newnham, E.D., *et al.* (2013) 'No effects of gluten in patients with self-reported non-celiac gluten sensitivity after dietary reduction of fermentable, poorly absorbed, short-chain carbohydrates.' *Gastroenterology, 145*(2), 320–328.e3. https://doi.org/10.1053/j.gastro.2013.04.051

Bilir, B., Sharma, N.V., Lee, J., *et al.* (2017) 'Effects of genistein supplementation on genome-wide DNA methylation and gene expression in patients with localized prostate cancer.' *International Journal of Oncology, 51*(1), 223–234. https://doi.org/10.3892/ijo.2017.4017

Birch, K. and Pearson-Shaver, A.L. (2020) 'Allergy Testing.' *PubMed.* StatPearls Publishing. https://www.ncbi.nlm.nih.gov/books/NBK537020

Breast Cancer Prevention Partners (BCPP) (2019) *Bovine Growth Hormone (rBGH) or Recombinant Bovine Somatotropin (rBST)*. Breast Cancer Prevention Partners (BCPP). https://www.bcpp.org/resource/rbgh-rbst

Canadian Sugar Institute (n.d.) *Consumption of sugars in Canada*. https://sugar.ca/sugars-consumption-guidelines/consumption-of-sugars-in-canada

Celiac Disease Foundation (2017, December 31) *What is celiac disease?* https://celiac.org/about-celiac-disease/what-is-celiac-disease

Chang, K., Gunter, M.J., Rauber, F., *et al.* (2023) 'Ultra-processed food consumption, cancer risk and cancer mortality: A large-scale prospective analysis within the UK Biobank.' *EClinicalMedicine, 56*, 101840. https://doi.org/10.1016/j.eclinm.2023.101840

Ciorba, M.A. (2012) 'A gastroenterologist's guide to probiotics.' *Clinical Gastroenterology and Hepatology, 10*(9), 960–968. https://doi.org/10.1016/j.cgh.2012.03.024

Clemente, J.C., Ursell, L.K., Parfrey, L. and Knight, R. (2012) 'The impact of the gut microbiota on human health: An integrative view.' *Cell, 148*(6), 1258–1270. https://doi.org/10.1016/j.cell.2012.01.035

Cogswell, M.E., Loria, C.M., Terry, A.L., *et al.* (2018) 'Estimated 24-hour urinary sodium and potassium excretion in US adults.' *JAMA, 319*(12), 1209. https://doi.org/10.1001/jama.2018.1156

Cronish, N. and Rosenbloom, C. (2015) *Nourish: Whole Food Recipes Featuring Seeds, Nuts and Beans*. Whitecap Books.

Curhan, G.C., Willett, W.C., Knight, E.L. and Stampfer, M.J. (2004) 'Dietary factors and the risk of incident kidney stones in younger women: Nurses' Health Study II.' *Archives of Internal Medicine, 164*(8), 885–891. https://doi.org/10.1001/archinte.164.8.885

Curhan, G.C., Willett, W.C., Rimm, E.B. and Stampfer, M.J. (1993) 'A prospective study of dietary calcium and other nutrients and the risk of symptomatic kidney stones.' *New England Journal of Medicine, 328*(12), 833–838. https://doi.org/10.1056/nejm199303253281203

Daures, M., Ngollo, M., Idrissou, M., *et al.* (2017) 'Soy phytoestrogens on DNA methylation in prostate cancer.' *Journal of Clinical Epigenetics, 3*(1). https://doi.org/10.21767/2472-1158.100046

Deans, E. (2011) *Magnesium and the brain: The original chill pill*. Psychology Today Canada. www.psychologytoday.com/ca/blog/evolutionary-psychiatry/201106/magnesium-and-the-brain-the-original-chill-pill

Deans, E. (2016) *Probiotics for depression*. Psychology Today Canada. www.psychologytoday.com/ca/blog/evolutionary-psychiatry/201602/probiotics-depression

De La Foret, R. (2017) *Alchemy of Herbs: Transform Everyday Ingredients into Foods and Remedies That Heal*. Hay House.

de Lemos, M.L. (2001) 'Effects of soy phytoestrogens genistein and daidzein on breast cancer growth.' *Annals of Pharmacotherapy, 35*(9), 1118–1121. https://doi.org/10.1345/aph.10257

Diaz, J.M. and Fridovich-Keil, J.L. (2018) 'Genetically modified organism.' In *Encyclopædia Britannica*. www.britannica.com/science/genetically-modified-organism

Drouin, G., Godin, J.-R. and Page, B. (2011) 'The genetics of vitamin C loss in vertebrates.' *Current Genomics, 12*(5), 371–378. https://doi.org/10.2174/138920211796429736

Elizabeth, L., Machado, P., Zinöcker, M., *et al.* (2020) 'Ultra-processed foods and health outcomes: A narrative review.' *Nutrients, 12*(7), 1955. https://doi.org/10.3390/nu12071955

Eur Lex (n.d.) *The precautionary principle*. https://eur-lex.europa.eu/legal-content/EN/TXT/?uri=LEGISSUM:l32042

Evans, S.S., Repasky, E.A. and Fisher, D.T. (2015) 'Fever and the thermal regulation of immunity: The immune system feels the heat.' *Nature Reviews Immunology, 15*(6), 335–349. https://doi.org/10.1038/nri3843

Fang, J.P. (1998) *Natural Remedies from the Chinese Cupboard*. Weatherhill.

Food and Agriculture Organization of the United Nations (n.d.) *The benefits of fermenting fruits and vegetables*. www.fao.org/3/x0560e/x0560e06.htm

Ferrières, J. (2004) 'The French paradox: Lessons for other countries.' *Heart, 90*(1), 107–111. www.ncbi.nlm.nih.gov/pmc/articles/PMC1768013

Foodwise (n.d.) *How far does your food travel to get to your plate?* https://foodwise.org/learn/how-far-does-your-food-travel-to-get-to-your-plate

Fraser, G.E., Jaceldo-Siegl, K., Orlich, M., *et al.* (2020) 'Dairy, soy, and risk of breast cancer: Those confounded milks.' *International Journal of Epidemiology, 49*(5). https://doi.org/10.1093/ije/dyaa007

Ganmaa, D., Cui, X., Feskanich, D., *et al.* (2012, June 1) 'Milk, dairy intake and risk of endometrial cancer: A 26-year follow-up.' *International Journal of Cancer, 130*(11), 2664–2671. https://pubmed.ncbi.nlm.nih.gov/21717454

Garg, M., Dalela, D., Dalela, D., *et al.* (2013) 'Selective estrogen receptor modulators for BPH: New factors on the ground.' *Prostate Cancer and Prostatic Diseases, 16*(3), 226–232. https://doi.org/10.1038/pcan.2013.17

Garg, R., Williams, G.H., Hurwitz, S., *et al.* (2011) 'Low-salt diet increases insulin resistance in healthy subjects.' *Metabolism, 60*(7), 965–968. https://doi.org/10.1016/j.metabol.2010.09.005

Geller, J., Sionit, L., Partido, C., *et al.* (1998) 'Genistein inhibits the growth of human-patient BPH and prostate cancer in histoculture.' *The Prostate, 34*(2), 75–79. https://doi.org/10.1002/(sici)1097-0045(19980201)34:2%3C75::aid-pros1%3E3.0.co;2-i

Golden, R.J., Noller, K.L., Titus-Ernstoff, L., *et al.* (1998) 'Environmental endocrine modulators and human health: An assessment of the biological evidence.' *Critical Reviews in Toxicology, 28*(2), 109–227. https://doi.org/10.1080/10408449891344191

Gupta, R.S., Warren, C.M., Smith, B.M., *et al.* (2019) 'Prevalence and severity of food allergies among US adults.' *JAMA Network Open, 2*(1), e185630. https://doi.org/10.1001/jamanetworkopen.2018.5630

Guthri, N., Morley, K.L., Hasegawa, S., *et al.* (2000) 'Inhibition of human breast cancer cells by citrus limonoids.' *Acs Symposium Series*, 164–174. https://doi.org/10.1021/bk-2000-0758.ch012

Haag, M. (2003) 'Essential fatty acids and the brain.' *The Canadian Journal of Psychiatry, 48*(3), 195–203. https://doi.org/10.1177/070674370304800308

Hall, K.D., Ayuketah, A., Brychta, R., *et al.* (2019) 'Ultra-processed diets cause excess calorie intake and weight gain: An inpatient randomized controlled trial of ad libitum food intake.' *Cell Metabolism, 30*(1), 67–77.e3. https://doi.org/10.1016/j.cmet.2019.05.008

He, F.J., Marrero, N.M. and MacGregor, G.A. (2008) 'Salt and blood pressure in children and adolescents.' *Journal of Human Hypertension, 22*(1), 4–11. https://doi.org/10.1038/sj.jhh.1002268

Henton, K. (n.d.) *Scotland's rare seaweed-eating sheep.* BBC. www.bbc.com/travel/article/20220712-the-orkney-sheep-reared-on-seaweed

Hoenselaar, R. (2011) 'The importance of reducing SFA intake to limit CHD risk.' *British Journal of Nutrition, 107*(3), 450–451. https://doi.org/10.1017/s0007114511006581

Hoenselaar, R. (2012) 'Further response from Hoenselaar.' *British Journal of Nutrition, 108*(5), 939–942. https://doi.org/10.1017/s0007114512000402

Hollmann, M., Runnebaum, B. and Gerhard, I. (1996) 'Infertility: Effects of weight loss on the hormonal profile in obese, infertile women.' *Human Reproduction, 11*(9), 1884–1891. https://doi.org/10.1093/oxfordjournals.humrep.a019512

IBS Diets (n.d.) *FODMAP food list.* www.ibsdiets.org/fodmap-diet/fodmap-food-list

International Foundation for Gastrointestinal Disorders (2021, March 8) *The low FODMAP diet approach—About IBS.* https://aboutibs.org/treatment/ibs-diet/low-fodmap-diet

Iorga, A., Cunningham, C.M., Moazeni, S., *et al.* (2017) 'The protective role of estrogen and estrogen receptors in cardiovascular disease and the controversial use of estrogen therapy.' *Biology of Sex Differences, 8*(1), 33. https://doi.org/10.1186/s13293-017-0152-8

Jandhyala, S.M. (2015) 'Role of the normal gut microbiota.' *World Journal of Gastroenterology, 21*(29), 8787. https://doi.org/10.3748/wjg.v21.i29.8787

Khalid, A.B. and Krum, S.A. (2016) 'Estrogen receptors alpha and beta in bone.' *Bone, 87*, 130–135. https://doi.org/10.1016/j.bone.2016.03.016

Kleanthous, B. (n.d.) *How much is a TRILLION?* www.thecalculatorsite.com/articles/finance/how-much-is-a-trillion.php

Korde, L.A., Wu, A.H., Fears, T., *et al.* (2009) 'Childhood soy intake and breast cancer risk in Asian American women.' *Cancer Epidemiology Biomarkers & Prevention, 18*(4), 1050–1059. https://doi.org/10.1158/1055-9965.epi-08-0405

Kubo, K., Chen, H., Zhou, X., *et al.* (2015) 'Chewing, stress-related diseases, and brain function.' *BioMed Research International, 2015*, 1–2. https://doi.org/10.1155/2015/412493

Kuehl, K.S., Elliot, D.L., Sleigh, A.E. and Smith, J.L. (2012) Efficacy of tart cherry juice to reduce inflammation biomarkers among women with inflammatory osteoarthritis (OA).' *Journal of Food Studies, 1*(1). https://doi.org/10.5296/jfs.v1i1.1927

Landau, E. (2014, February 6) *Subway to remove "dough conditioner" chemical from bread.* CNN. www.cnn.com/2014/02/06/health/subway-bread-chemical

Langer, O. and Bio, R. (2003) *Is there a bottom line in the wild salmon–farmed salmon debate? A technical opinion.* https://davidsuzuki.org/wp-content/uploads/2019/02/bottom-line-wild-salmon-farmed-salmon-debate-technical-opinion.pdf

Langlois, K. and Garriguet, D. (2011, September 21) *Sugar consumption among Canadians of all ages.* www150.statcan.gc.ca/n1/pub/82-003-x/2011003/article/11540-eng.htm

Lappé, F.M. (1971) *Diet for a Small Planet.* Random House.

Leggett, D. (1999) *Recipes for Self-Healing.* Meridian.

Leggett, D. (2005) *Helping Ourselves: A Guide to Traditional Chinese Food Energetics.* Meridian.

Lewis, R. and Robin, J.-L. (1985, August) 'Arachidonic acid derivatives as mediators of asthma [Review of arachidonic acid derivatives as mediators of asthma].' *The Journal of Allergy and Clinical Immunology.* www.jacionline.org/article/0091-6749(85)90639-6/fulltext

Liberatore, S. (2016, February 2) *Fruit and veg looked very different thousands of years ago.* Mail Online. www.dailymail.co.uk/sciencetech/article-3428689/What-fruit-vegetables-look-like-Researchers-banana-watermelon-changed-dramatically-ancestors-ate-them.html

Lu, H.C. (1989) *Chinese Systems of Food Cures: Prevention and Remedies.* Pelanduk Publications.

Lu, H.C. (1992) *Legendary Chinese Healing Herbs.* Sterling.

Lu, H.C. (1997) *The Chinese System of Using Foods to Stay Young.* Sterling.

Lu, H.C. (2005) *Chinese Natural Cures.* Black Dog & Leventhal.

Maciocia, G. (2005) *The Foundations of Chinese Medicine.* Churchill Livingstone.

Marino, M., Puppo, F., Del Bo', C., *et al.* (2021) 'A systematic review of worldwide consumption of ultra-processed foods: Findings and criticisms.' *Nutrients, 13*(8), 2778. https://doi.org/10.3390/nu13082778

Marques-Pinto, A. and Carvalho, D. (2013) 'Human infertility: Are endocrine disruptors to blame?' *Endocrine Connections, 2*(3), R15–29. https://doi.org/10.1530/EC-13-0036

Marti, A. (2019) 'Ultra-processed foods are not "real food" but really affect your health.' *Nutrients, 11*(8), 1902. https://doi.org/10.3390/nu11081902

McGill (n.d.) *Jerusalem artichokes.* Office for Science and Society. www.mcgill.ca/oss/article/food-health/jerusalem-artichokes

Mennella, J.A., Jagnow, C.P. and Beauchamp, G.K. (2001) 'Prenatal and postnatal flavor learning by human infants.' *Pediatrics, 107*(6), e88. https://doi.org/10.1542/peds.107.6.e88

Mergenthaler, P., Lindauer, U., Dienel, G.A. and Meisel, A. (2013) 'Sugar for the brain: The role of glucose in physiological and pathological brain function.' *Trends in Neurosciences, 36*(10), 587–597. https://doi.org/10.1016/j.tins.2013.07.001

Monteiro, C.A., Cannon, G., Moubarac, J.-C., *et al.* (2017) 'The UN Decade of Nutrition, the NOVA food classification and the trouble with ultra-processing.' *Public Health Nutrition, 21*(1), 5–17. https://doi.org/10.1017/S1368980017000234

Murray, M.T., Pizzorno, J.E. and Pizzorno, L. (2006) *The Encyclopedia of Healing Foods.* Time Warner International.

National Center for Health Statistics (2009) *Chartbook: Health, United States, 2008.* www.ncbi.nlm.nih.gov/books/NBK19623

National Institute on Alcohol Abuse and Alcoholism (NIAAA) (n.d.) *The basics: Defining how much alcohol is too much.* www.niaaa.nih.gov/health-professionals-communities/core-resource-on-alcohol/basics-defining-how-much-alcohol-too-much

National Institutes of Health (2017a) *Office of Dietary Supplements—Vitamin B6.* https://ods.od.nih.gov/factsheets/vitaminB6-healthprofessional

National Institutes of Health (2017b) *Office of Dietary Supplements—Chromium.* https://ods.od.nih.gov/factsheets/Chromium-HealthProfessional

Nevin, K.G. and Rajamohan, T. (2004) 'Beneficial effects of virgin coconut oil on lipid parameters and in vitro LDL oxidation.' *Clinical Biochemistry, 37*(9), 830–835. https://doi.org/10.1016/j.clinbiochem.2004.04.010

Ni, M. (2006) *Secrets of Longevity.* Ask Dr. Mao.

Ni, M. (2008) *Secrets of Self-Healing: Harness Nature's Power to Heal Common Ailments, Boost Your Vitality, and Achieve Optimum Wellness.* Avery.

Ni, M. and McNease, C. (2009) *The Tao of Nutrition.* Tao of Wellness Press.

O'Donnell, M., Mente, A. and Rangarajan, S. (2014) 'Urinary sodium and potassium excretion, mortality, and cardiovascular events.' *New England Journal of Medicine, 371*(7), 612–623. https://doi.org/10.1056/nejmoa1311889

O'Donnell, M.J., Yusuf, S., Mente, A., *et al.* (2011) 'Urinary sodium and potassium excretion and risk of cardiovascular events.' *JAMA, 306*(20). https://doi.org/10.1001/jama.2011.1729

Oregon State University (2014, April 22) *Calcium.* Linus Pauling Institute. https://lpi.oregonstate.edu/mic/minerals/calcium

Panahi, Y., Beiraghdar, F., Beiraghdar, N. *et al.* (2011) 'Comparison of piascledine (avocado and soybean oil) and hormone replacement therapy in menopausal-induced hot flashing.' *Iranian Journal of Pharmaceutical Research, 10*(4). www.ncbi.nlm.nih.gov/pmc/articles/PMC3813060

Parvez, S., Malik, K.A., Ah Kang, S. and Kim, H.-Y. (2006) 'Probiotics and their fermented food products are beneficial for health.' *Journal of Applied Microbiology, 100*(6), 1171–1185. https://doi.org/10.1111/j.1365-2672.2006.02963.x

Pasquali, R., Patton, L. and Gambineri, A. (2007) 'Obesity and infertility.' *Current Opinion in Endocrinology, Diabetes, and Obesity, 14*(6), 482–487. https://doi.org/10.1097/MED.0b013e3282f1d6cb

Pedersen, J.l., James, P.T., Brouwer, I.A., *et al.* (2011a) 'The importance of reducing SFA to limit CHD.' *British Journal of Nutrition, 106*(07), 961–963. https://doi.org/10.1017/s0007114511000506x

Pedersen, J.l., Norum, K.R., James, P.T., *et al.* (2011b) 'Response to Hoenselaar from Pedersen et al.' *British Journal of Nutrition, 107*(3), 452–454. https://doi.org/10.1017/s0007114511006593

Pflieger-Bruss, S., Schuppe, H.-C. and Schill, W.-B. (2004) 'The male reproductive system and its susceptibility to endocrine disrupting chemicals.' *Andrologia, 36*(6), 337–345. https://doi.org/10.1111/j.1439-0272.2004.00641.x

Ravnskov, U., Diamond, D., Karatay, M.C.E., *et al.* (2012) 'No scientific support for linking dietary saturated fat to CHD.' *British Journal of Nutrition, 107*(3), 455–457. https://doi.org/10.1017/S000711451100660X

Rich-Edwards, J.W., Spiegelman, D., Garland, M., *et al.* (2002) 'Physical activity, body mass index, and ovulatory disorder infertility.' *Epidemiology, 13*(2), 184–190. https://doi.org/10.1097/00001648-200203000-00013

Rico-Campà, A., Martínez-González, M.A., Alvarez-Alvarez, I., *et al.* (2019) 'Association between consumption of ultra-processed foods and all cause mortality: SUN prospective cohort study.' *BMJ, 365*, l1949. https://doi.org/10.1136/bmj.l1949

Round, J.L. and Mazmanian, S.K. (2009) 'The gut microbiota shapes intestinal immune responses during health and disease.' *Nature Reviews Immunology, 9*(5), 313–323. https://doi.org/10.1038/nri2515

Royal Society (n.d.) *What GM crops are being grown and where?* https://royalsociety.org/topics-policy/projects/gm-plants/what-gm-crops-are-currently-being-grown-and-where

Rozin, P. and Schiller, D. (1980) 'The nature and acquisition of a preference for chili pepper by humans.' *Motivation and Emotion, 4*(1), 77–101. https://doi.org/10.1007/bf00995932

Rozin, P., Gruss, L. and Berk, G. (1979) 'Reversal of innate aversions: Attempts to induce a preference for chili peppers in rats.' *Journal of Comparative and Physiological Psychology, 93*(6), 1001–1014. https://doi.org/10.1037/h0077632

Rupp, R. (2014, July 22) *The history of the "forbidden" fruit.* National Geographic. www.nationalgeographic.com/culture/article/history-of-apples

Saldeen, P. and Saldeen, T. (2004) 'Women and Omega-3 fatty acids.' *Obstetrical & Gynecological Survey, 59*(10), 722–730. https://doi.org/10.1097/01.ogx.0000140038.70473.96

Sanders, M.E. (2008) 'Use of probiotics and yogurts in maintenance of health.' *Journal of Clinical Gastroenterology, 42*(Supplement 2), S71–S74. https://doi.org/10.1097/mcg.0b013e3181621e87

Schnell, S., Friedman, S.M., Mendelson, D.A., *et al.* (2010) 'The 1-year mortality of patients treated in a hip fracture program for elders.' *Geriatric Orthopaedic Surgery & Rehabilitation, 1*(1), 6–14. https://doi.org/10.1177/2151458510378105

Science History Institute (SHI) (2014) *Processed: Food science and the modern meal.* Science History Institute. www.sciencehistory.org/stories/magazine/processed-food-science-and-the-modern-meal

Scientific American (2002) *What is the difference between artificial and natural flavors?* Scientific American. www.scientificamerican.com/article/what-is-the-difference-be-2002-07-29

Shu, X.O. (2009) 'Soy food intake and breast cancer survival.' *JAMA, 302*(22), 2437. https://doi.org/10.1001/jama.2009.1783

Silverstein, K. (1997, November) 'Procter & Gamble's academic "white hats."' *Multinational Monitor, 18*(11), 13.

Singh, M. and Das, R.R. (2013) 'Zinc for the common cold.' *The Cochrane Database of Systematic Reviews, 6*, CD001364. https://doi.org/10.1002/14651858.CD001364.pub4

Slattery, M.L., Benson, J., Ma, K.N., *et al.* (2001) 'Trans-fatty acids and colon cancer.' *Nutrition and Cancer, 39*(2), 170–175. https://doi.org/10.1207/S15327914nc392_2

Srour, B., Fezeu, L.K., Kesse-Guyot, E., *et al.* (2019) 'Ultra-processed food intake and risk of cardiovascular disease: Prospective cohort study (NutriNet-Santé).' *BMJ, 365*(8201), l1451. https://doi.org/10.1136/bmj.l1451

Stanford Health Care (n.d.) *Low FODMAP diet.* https://stanfordhealthcare.org/medical-treatments/l/low-fodmap-diet.html

Sterman, A. (2020) *Welcoming Food: Diet as Medicine for Home Cooks and Other Healers. Book 2, Recipes and Kitchen Practice.* Classical Wellness Press.

St Pete Urology (2022, March 15) *What dissolves kidney stones fast?* https://stpeteurology.com/what-dissolves-kidney-stones-fast

Taylor, E. and Curhan, G.C. (2013) 'Dietary calcium from dairy and nondairy sources, and risk of symptomatic kidney stones.' *Journal of Urology, 190*(4), 1255–1259. https://doi.org/10.1016/j.juro.2013.03.074

Taylor, E.N. (2004) 'Dietary factors and the risk of incident kidney stones in men: New insights after 14 years of follow-up.' *Journal of the American Society of Nephrology, 15*(12), 3225–3232. https://doi.org/10.1097/01.asn.0000146012.44570.20

The Economist (2018, September 26) *How did carrots become orange?* www.economist.com/the-economist-explains/2018/09/26/how-did-carrots-become-orange

Truth in Labelling Campaign (2021) *Names of ingredients that contain Manufactured free Glutamate (MfG).* www.truthinlabeling.org/hiddensources.html

Tucker, K.L., Morita, K., Qiao, N., *et al.* (2006) 'Colas, but not other carbonated beverages, are associated with low bone mineral density in older women: The Framingham Osteoporosis Study.' *The American Journal of Clinical Nutrition, 84*(4), 936–942. https://doi.org/10.1093/ajcn/84.4.936

United Nations (n.d.) *World Population Day.* www.un.org/en/observances/world-population-day

Ursell, L.K., Metcalf, J.L., Parfrey, L.W. and Knight, R. (2012) 'Defining the human microbiome.' *Nutrition Reviews, 70*(1), S38–S44.

Velasquez-Manoff, M. (n.d.) *Among trillions of microbes in the gut, a few are special.* Scientific American. www.scientificamerican.com/article/among-trillions-of-microbes-in-the-gut-a-few-are-special

Wang, J.X., Davies, M.J. and Norman, R.J. (2002) 'Obesity increases the risk of spontaneous abortion during infertility treatment.' *Obesity Research, 10*(6), 551–554. https://doi.org/10.1038/oby.2002.74

wbur (2014) *Why M&M's are made with natural coloring in the EU and not the U.S.* www.wbur.org/hereandnow/2014/03/28/artificial-dyes-candy

Wenner, M. (n.d.) *Like the taste of chalk? You're in luck—Humans may be able to taste calcium.* Scientific American. www.scientificamerican.com/article/osteoporosis-calcium-taste-chalk

Whelton, P.K. (2018) 'Sodium and potassium intake in US adults.' *Circulation, 137*(3), 247–249. https://doi.org/10.1161/circulationaha.117.031371

Willett, W.C. and Mozaffarian, D. (2007) 'Trans fats in cardiac and diabetes risk: An overview.' *Current Cardiovascular Risk Reports, 1*(1), 16–23. https://doi.org/10.1007/s12170-007-0004-x

Woerner, A. (2015, January 14) *What are natural flavors, really?* CNN. www.cnn.com/2015/01/14/health/feat-natural-flavors-explained

Wood, R. (2010) *The New Whole Foods Encyclopedia: A Comprehensive Resource for Healthy Eating.* Penguin Books.

World Health Organization (2023, 14 September) *Sodium reduction.* www.who.int/news-room/fact-sheets/detail/salt-reduction

Wu, A.H., Yu, M.C., Tseng, C-C. and Pike, M.C. (2008) 'Epidemiology of soy exposures and breast cancer risk.' *British Journal of Cancer, 98*(1), 9–14. https://doi.org/10.1038/sj.bjc.6604145

Wu, Y. and Fischer, W. (1997) *Practical Therapeutics of Traditional Chinese Medicine.* Paradigm Publications.

Yang, M., Kenfield, S.A., Van Blarigan, E.L., *et al.* (2015) 'Dairy intake after prostate cancer diagnosis in relation to disease-specific and total mortality.' *International Journal of Cancer, 137*(10), 2462–2469. https://doi.org/10.1002/ijc.29608

Yang, Q. (2011) 'Sodium and potassium intake and mortality among US adults.' *Archives of Internal Medicine, 171*(13), 1183. https://doi.org/10.1001/archinternmed.2011.257

Yehuda, S., Rabinovitz, S. and Mostofsky, D.I. (2005) 'Mixture of essential fatty acids lowers test anxiety.' *Nutritional Neuroscience, 8*(4), 265–267. https://doi.org/10.1080/10284150500445795

Appendix: Common and Relatively Accessible TCM Herbs

This is by no means a comprehensive list of foods that have health benefits or of Chinese herbs that are commonly used as foods (at least in China). However, these are foods that you might more easily find in a regular Western supermarket or in a local Asian food market. I've also listed just a few common uses for each, but that too is not a complete list because it would be an onerous effort to make and to read. The actions of the herbs are a mixture of TCM and Western. For more detailed information, you'll need to check herbal textbooks.

English name	Chinese herb name	Some common uses	Foods it might be good in	Notes
Aloe	Lu hui	Treats constipation, kills parasites	Add the gel to smoothies	Too much can cause cramping and diarrhea
Barley sprouts	Mai ya	Reduces food stagnation, inhibits lactation	Steam and add to salads, soups	Note that this contains gluten
Bitter melon	Ku gua	Lowers blood sugars, lowers cholesterol (if high)	Stir fries, smoothies, tea	Too much can cause diarrhea and abdominal pain
Cardamom	Sha ren	Treats diarrhea or vomiting, treats morning sickness	Tea, stews, curries, sauces, rice dishes, baking, smoothies	A little goes a long way

cont.

English name	Chinese herb name	Some common uses	Foods it might be good in	Notes
Chive/spring onion	Cong bai	Induces sweating to treat early-stage colds, treats abdominal pain or nasal congestion (due to Cold Yang Qi blockage)	Onions are the base of so many recipes, and chives are no exception	Chives are milder in flavor than other onions, so can be used as garnish or cooked lightly
Chrysanthemum flower	Ju hua	Helps treat early-stage common cold (Wind-Heat), calms irritated eyes	Tea, garnish on soups or in salads	
Cinnamon (twig)	Gui zhi	Helps treat common cold (Wind-Cold), relieves pain (Wind-Cold-Damp Bi syndrome), lowers blood sugar, good for heart health, improves circulation	An herb/spice that adds warmth and depth of flavor to soups, stews, oatmeal, roasted vegetables, tea, coffee, smoothies, baked goods	The cinnamon you buy in stores may be *Cassia* or *Ceylon*. The Chinese version is *Cassia*, which should not be consumed in larger than food quantities or as prescribed by a practitioner
Cinnamon (bark)	Rou gui	Warms the body, improves circulation, supports heart health, lowers blood sugar	Same as above	Warmer and deeper actions than *gui zhi*. Do not use more than 1 tsp daily unless guided by a practitioner
Clove	Ding xiang	Relieves stomach pain, diarrhea, vomiting (due to Stomach Cold), kills parasites, used topically for toothaches	Tea (e.g., chai), curries, baking, use to season meats	Only small amounts needed, as it's a strong herb/spice and can be harmful in larger quantities

Dandelion	Pu gong ying	Detoxifies, reduces abscesses and nodules, supports the liver, treats urinary tract infections, promotes lactation	Tea Roots: non-caffeinated coffee alternative Greens: salads, smoothies, soups Flowers: baking, stews	The greens are richer in iron than spinach and are high in vitamin K. This common "weed" has many medicinal benefits
Date	Da zao (black) Hong zao (red)	Supports digestion, nourishes Blood, supports good gut flora, provides energy	Snacks, sugar alternative, chutneys, baked goods, smoothies, tagines, salads	High iron content and rich in fiber and antioxidants. Even though high in sugar, they have a relatively low glycemic index
Garlic bulb	Da suan	Kills parasites, reduces abscesses, antibacterial, antiviral, supports heart health	Garlic tea to fight a cold, early stages; in stir fries, soups, stews— you name it; roasted	Those on blood thinner medications are often advised to limit or monitor
Ginger (dried)	Gan jiang	Warms (especially the Stomach), treats diarrhea, nausea, and vomiting (Cold syndromes), treats thin phlegm cough	Tea, stews, curries, soups, hot pots, casseroles, baked goods, sauces, dressings	Warmer and better at treating internal issues than fresh ginger
Ginger (fresh)	Sheng jiang	Induces perspiration for common cold (Wind-Cold), treats nausea, vomiting, and cough (Cold syndromes)	Tea, smoothies, curries, soups, hot pots, casseroles, baked goods, sauces, dressing	Fresh ginger slices are better at treating "exterior" conditions (e.g., colds) than dried

cont.

English name	Chinese herb name	Some common uses	Foods it might be good in	Notes
Ginkgo nut	Bai guo	Helps expel phlegm from the lungs, reduces wheezing	Soups, stews, in chawanmushi (a Japanese steamed egg custard)	This is not the ginkgo supplement for brain health (that's the leaf). Limit consumption, as it is slightly toxic
Goji berry	Gou qi zi	Nourishes the eyes, addresses fatigue and weakness (nourish the Blood and Yin), antioxidant	Use them in place of raisins; soups, stews, pilafs, chilis, casseroles, smoothies, baked goods	Simplest way to use them is add to water and drink as a tea
Green tea leaves	Cha ye/lu cha	Treats nausea, vomiting, diarrhea, indigestion, headaches; provides energy (contains caffeine)	Tea (clearly!), used instead of water for many recipes	I mention ochazuke (green tea over rice) in the section on irritable bowel syndrome
Hawthorn berry	Shan zha	Supports digestion (especially of proteins and fats), supports heart health	Fresh berries can make jam, sauces, even used in baking; dried can be used in soups and tea	You can often find *shan zha* candy in Chinese food shops, but remember they are high in sugar
Hemp seeds	Huo ma ren	Treat constipation (gently moistens intestines); supports brain, cardiovascular, skin, joint health	Hemp milk, smoothies, seeds can be sprinkled on salads, soups, cooked vegetables, yogurt, oatmeal; can be baked, but will destroy essential fats	Rich source of protein, essential fatty acids, and fiber

Honey	Feng mi	Treats constipation, cough, used topically as antibacterial for wound care	What doesn't taste better with honey?	Because it is high in sugar, enjoy in moderation
Job's tears (coix seed, Chinese pearl barley, hato mugi)	Yi yi ren	Treats diarrhea and soft stools, reduces joint pain with stiffness (Wind-Damp Bi syndrome)	Add to congee or porridge, tea or drink, soup, stew	Even though it's called a type of barley, it is gluten-free
Kelp (kombu)	Kun bu	Treats goiter, improves hypothyroidism, softens nodules	Soups, stews, salads, soaking beans with kelp helps enhance the flavor and texture	Rich source of iodine. Be mindful that seaweeds can also be high in heavy metals and sodium. Those on levothyroxine need to be careful of too much iodine
Longan fruit	Long yan rou	Nourishes the blood, calms the nervous system, benefits the skin and hair	Tea, puddings, soups, baked goods, porridges, congees	
Papaya	Mu gua	Supports digestion, relieves diarrhea, treats arthritis (Wind-Damp Bi), reduces edema	Tenderizes meat; can be eaten as is, roasted, or poached; salads, desserts	Unripe papaya should be cooked before eating; contains papain which is often put in digestive enzyme supplements
Peppermint	Bo he	Helps treat common cold (Wind-Heat), treats headache, sore throat, red eyes, early-stage measles; improves IBS, supports digestion	Tea, salads, pestos, sauces, marinades, baked goods	Peppermint essential oil can also be used as aromatherapy or topically to relieve headaches, open sinuses, relieve pain

cont.

English name	Chinese herb name	Some common uses	Foods it might be good in	Notes
Perilla leaf	Zi su ye	Helps treat early-stage common cold (Wind-Cold), stops vomiting, supports digestion, supports respiratory health	Slice thinly and add to rice, salads, or to top meats, soups, or vegetables; use as a wrap; tea, pickled	From the mint family
Pumpkin seed	Nan gua zi	Expels parasites, supports prostate, bladder, heart, and breast health	Eat raw or roasted; garnish salads or soups; pumpkin butter; pestos, crackers, baked goods	Rich source of magnesium, essential fatty acids, fiber
Rice (sprouted)	Gu ya	Promotes digestion, improves appetite, may help calm nervous system	Cook and use like regular rice	Lower glycemic index than regular rice; rich in GABA
Safflower	Hong hua	Treats menstrual cramping, improves blood circulation, relieves pain (due to Blood stasis)	Salads, soups, garnish, sauces	TCM uses the dried flower
Sargassum seaweed	Hai zao	Treats goiter, improves hypothyroidism, softens nodules	Soups, stews, salads	Same as for kelp
Sesame seed (black)	Hu ma ren	Treats constipation, reduces joint pain, lowers cholesterol and blood pressure (if high)	Topping for stir fries, cooked vegetables, salads, porridges, congees; baked goods, smoothies, dressings	Rich source of fiber, omega 3 fatty acids, magnesium

Soybean, black (fermented)	Dan dou chi	Treats early-stage common cold, especially fever and headache	Douchi is added to stir fries, soups, or braises; black bean sauces may also use douchi	*Dan dou chi* is different from natto, miso, and tempeh, though they are all fermented soybeans; high in sodium
Tangerine peel	Chen pi Ju hong/ju pi (aged)	Supports digestion, treats vomiting and hiccups, treats phlegmy cough	Can be eaten as is, tea, sauces, marinades, soups, baked goods	You can learn to make your own. The benefits are said to be better the longer the dried peels are aged
Turmeric	Jiang huang	Treats pain and inflammation, supports liver and heart health	Tea, smoothies, curries, soups, stews, baked goods	In TCM, it is combined with different herbs to target specific types of pain
Watermelon (flesh and rind)	Xi gua	Treats heat stroke, hydrates and cools	Eat as is; juice, drinks, smoothies, salads	
Winter melon	Dong gua	Treats edema, clears phlegm, cools the body, lowers blood sugar	Soups, stews, stir fries, tea	The seeds are also a TCM herb, *dong gua zi*

Subject Index

Sub-headings in *italics* indicate figures and tables. Sub-headings in **bold** indicate main sections.

Author Index